Recreational Water Illnesses

Recreational Water Illnesses

Special Issue Editor

Erica Leoni

MDPI • Basel • Beijing • Wuhan • Barcelona • Belgrade

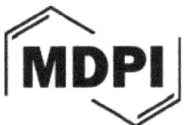

MDPI

Special Issue Editor
Erica Leoni
University of Bologna
Italy

Editorial Office
MDPI
St. Alban-Anlage 66
4052 Basel, Switzerland

This is a reprint of articles from the Special Issue published online in the open access journal *International Journal of Environmental Research and Public Health* (ISSN 1660-4601) from 2018 to 2019 (available at: https://www.mdpi.com/journal/ijerph/special_issues/Recreational_Water_Illnesses)

For citation purposes, cite each article independently as indicated on the article page online and as indicated below:

LastName, A.A.; LastName, B.B.; LastName, C.C. Article Title. *Journal Name* **Year**, *Article Number*, Page Range.

ISBN 978-3-03897-578-6 (Pbk)
ISBN 978-3-03897-579-3 (PDF)

Contents

About the Special Issue Editor vii

Preface to "Recreational Water Illnesses" ix

Athena Mavridou, Olga Pappa, Olga Papatzitze, Chrysa Dioli, Anastasia Maria Kefala,
Panagiotis Drossos and Apostolos Beloukas
Exotic Tourist Destinations and Transmission of Infections by Swimming Pools and Hot
Springs—A Literature Review
Reprinted from: *IJERPH* **2018**, *15*, 2730, doi:10.3390/ijerph15122730 1

Lucia Bonadonna and Giuseppina La Rosa
A Review and Update on Waterborne Viral Diseases Associated with Swimming Pools
Reprinted from: *IJERPH* **2019**, *16*, 166, doi:10.3390/ijerph16020166 21

Erica Leoni, Federica Catalani, Sofia Marini and Laura Dallolio
Legionellosis Associated with Recreational Waters: A Systematic Review of Cases and
Outbreaks in Swimming Pools, Spa Pools, and Similar Environments
Reprinted from: *IJERPH* **2018**, *15*, 1612, doi:10.3390/ijerph15081612 32

Franciska M. Schets, Harold H. J. L. van den Berg, Harry Vennema, Manon T. M. Pelgrim,
Cees Collé, Saskia A. Rutjes and Willemijn J. Lodder
Norovirus Outbreak Associated with Swimming in a Recreational Lake Not Influenced by
External Human Fecal Sources in The Netherlands, August 2012
Reprinted from: *IJERPH* **2018**, *15*, 2550, doi:10.3390/ijerph15112550 51

Xiaohong Wei, Juntao Li, Shuiping Hou, Conghui Xu, Hao Zhang, Edward Robert Atwill,
Xunde Li, Zhicong Yang and Shouyi Chen
Assessment of Microbiological Safety of Water in Public Swimming Pools in Guangzhou, China
Reprinted from: *IJERPH* **2018**, *15*, 1416, doi:10.3390/ijerph15071416 60

Antonios Papadakis, Dimosthenis Chochlakis, Vassilios Sandalakis, Maria Keramarou,
Yannis Tselentis and Anna Psaroulaki
Legionella spp. Risk Assessment in Recreational and Garden Areas of Hotels
Reprinted from: *IJERPH* **2018**, *15*, 598, doi:10.3390/ijerph15040598 72

Anthony C. Otigbu, Anna M. Clarke, Justine Fri, Emmanuel O. Akanbi and Henry A. Njom
Antibiotic Sensitivity Profiling and Virulence Potential of *Campylobacter jejuni* Isolates from
Estuarine Water in the Eastern Cape Province, South Africa
Reprinted from: *IJERPH* **2018**, *15*, 925, doi:10.3390/ijerph15050925 87

Daniela E. Koeck, Stefanie Huber, Nadera Hanifi, Manfred Köster, Martina B. Schierling and
Christiane Höller
Occurrence of Antibiotic-Resistant Bacteria in Therapy Pools and Surrounding Surfaces
Reprinted from: *IJERPH* **2018**, *15*, 2666, doi:10.3390/ijerph15122666 102

Mahbubul H. Siddiqee, Rebekah Henry, Rebecca Coulthard, Christelle Schang,
Richard Williamson, Rhys Coleman, Graham Rooney, Ana Deletic and David McCarthy
Salmonella enterica Serovar Typhimurium and *Escherichia coli* Survival in Estuarine Bank
Sediments
Reprinted from: *IJERPH* **2018**, *15*, 2597, doi:10.3390/ijerph15112597 120

Asja Korajkic, Brian R. McMinn and Valerie J. Harwood
Relationships between Microbial Indicators and Pathogens in Recreational Water Settings
Reprinted from: *IJERPH* **2018**, *15*, 2842, doi:10.3390/ijerph15122842 . . . . **133**

Laura M. Suppes, Kacey C. Ernst, Leif Abrell and Kelly A. Reynolds
Validation of Questionnaire Methods to Quantify Recreational Water Ingestion
Reprinted from: *IJERPH* **2018**, *15*, 2435, doi:10.3390/ijerph15112435 . . . . **172**

Federica Valeriani, Lory Marika Margarucci and Vincenzo Romano Spica
Recreational Use of Spa Thermal Waters: Criticisms and Perspectives for Innovative Treatments
Reprinted from: *IJERPH* **2018**, *15*, 2675, doi:10.3390/ijerph15122675 . . . . **178**

About the Special Issue Editor

Erica Leoni is Full Professor of Hygiene and Public Health at the Alma Mater Studiorum, University of Bologna (Italy). She is the academic referent of the Unit of Hygiene, Public Health, and Medical Statistics of the Department of Biomedical and Neuromotor Sciences of Bologna University. She obtained her degree in Biological Sciences and her degree in Medicine and Surgery from the University of Bologna, and her PhD in Microbiology at the University of Parma (Italy). She participated in continuative didactic activity in the fields of general and applied hygiene in different Bachelor, Master, and PhD courses at the University of Bologna. She was President and Coordinator of the Degree Course on Movement Sciences 2007–08 and 2012–13, and a member of the College of Professors of the Doctorate in "Health, Safety, and Urban Greening". She has supervised numerous PhD and post-doctoral students.

Her research work focuses on public health, epidemiology, environmental health, and the promotion of healthy lifestyles. She is a member of the scientific board of the work group in "Motor Sciences for Health" of the National Scientific Society of Hygiene and Preventive Medicine. As part of this role, she is actively involved in the development of Italian multi-centre studies concerning the safety of recreational environments and the promotion of healthy lifestyles, in particular, concerning the promotion of physical activity for primary and tertiary prevention. With reference to the last, she participates in a European multi-centre study funded by the European Community concerning Adapted Physical Activity (APA) administered for the tertiary prevention of osteoporosis. In the 2016–2018 biennium, she has been part of the National Committee for the assignment of the National Scientific Qualification of the Full/Associate University Professors for the subjects of Public Health, Nursing, and Medical Statistics.

Preface to "Recreational Water Illnesses"

Swimming and other water-based exercises are excellent ways to practice physical activity and to gain health and social benefits. However, recreational water use may expose people to different health risks due to exposure to chemicals or pathogens. The safety of recreational aquatic environments is affected by numerous variables such as water quality, the health conditions of users, and the correct functioning of the technological systems used for water treatment. This Special Issue aims to provide new knowledge on health risks related to recreational waters, together with the need to update prevention strategies. Such an approach will be essential for addressing the challenges posed by the increasing use of recreational waters by people with different age and health conditions. The editor wishes to thank all the contributors and the support of the *IJERPH* editorial staff, whose professionalism and dedication have made this Issue possible.

Erica Leoni
Special Issue Editor

International Journal of
*Environmental Research
and Public Health*

MDPI

Review

Exotic Tourist Destinations and Transmission of Infections by Swimming Pools and Hot Springs—A Literature Review

Athena Mavridou [1,*], Olga Pappa [1,2], Olga Papatzitze [1,3], Chrysa Dioli [1], Anastasia Maria Kefala [1], Panagiotis Drossos [1] and Apostolos Beloukas [1,4]

1   Department of Biomedical Sciences, University of West Attica, 12243 Egaleo, Greece;
    olpap79@gmail.com (O.P.); olgapapat@hotmail.com (O.P.); chrysrose57@gmail.com (C.D.);
    anastasia.m.kefala@gmail.com (A.M.K.); pdrossos2006@yahoo.gr (P.D.); abeloukas@uniwa.gr (A.B.)
2   Central Public Health Laboratory, Hellenic Centre of Disease Control and Prevention,
    15123 Maroussi, Greece
3   West Attica General Hospital, "Santa Barbara", 12351 Santa Barbara, Greece
4   Institute of Infection and Global Health, University of Liverpool, Liverpool L69 3BX, UK
*   Correspondence: amavridou@teiath.gr

Received: 5 October 2018; Accepted: 29 November 2018; Published: 3 December 2018

Abstract: A growing number of people undertake international travel, and yet faster growth of such travel is expected in the tropics. Information on the hazards presented by pool and hot spring waters in tropical countries is very limited. This review aims to collate available information on pool water quality, alongside data on cases and outbreaks associated with swimming in pools in tropical regions affecting both local populations and travellers. Bacteria species commonly causing cases and outbreaks in the tropics as well as elsewhere in the world were excluded, and the review focuses on studies related to pathogens that, with the exception of *Cryptosporidium*, are unusual in more temperate climates. Studies concerning subtropical countries were included in the light of climate change. Diseases transmitted by vectors breeding in poorly maintained, neglected or abandoned pools were also included. 83 studies dealing with Microsporidia, *Leptospira* spp., *Schistosomas* spp., *Cryptosporidium* spp., *Acanthamoeba* spp., *Naegleria* spp., *Clostridium trachomatis*, viruses, and vectors breeding in swimming pool and hot tub waters, and fulfilling predefined criteria, have been included in our survey of the literature. In conclusion, prevention strategies for pool safety in the tropics are imperative. Public health authorities need to provide guidance to westerners travelling to exotic destinations on how to protect their health in swimming pools.

Keywords: swimming pools; tropics; subtropics; pool assessment; infectious diseases

---

1. Introduction

An increasing number of people undertake international travel for professional, social, recreational and humanitarian purposes. Nowadays, more people travel greater distances and at greater speed than ever before, and this upward trend looks set to continue. Internationally, tourist arrivals have increased from 25 million globally in 1950 to 1235 million in 2016 [1] with travel for leisure and pleasure accounting for more than half of international tourism arrivals [2].

According to the research project "Tourism Towards 2030", the number of international tourist arrivals worldwide will increase by an average of 3.3% per year through to 2030. Greater growth is expected to occur in the tropical Asian and the Pacific regions, where arrivals are forecast to reach 535 million in 2030 (+4.9% per year). Countries of the tropical zone, such as those located in the Middle East and Africa regions are expected to double their arrival numbers during the same period, from 61 and 50 million to 149 and 134 million, respectively [1]. According to World Tourism highlights, 2001 the fastest developing region continues to be East Asia and the Pacific [3].

From a public health perspective, travellers are exposed to a variety of health risks in unfamiliar environments [2]. International travel can pose severe risks to health, depending both on travellers' health needs and on the type of travel undertaken. Accidents continue to be the primary cause of morbidity and mortality for international travellers, but infections also present an important health risk. Moreover, travellers interact dynamically with microbes and places. Travellers can carry these microbes and their genetic material, and, as Baker stated," can play multiple roles with regard to microbes, as victims, sentinels, couriers, processors, and transmitters of microbial pathogens" [4].

There is abundant information and guidance to travellers regarding precautions that need to be taken in respect of food, drinking water and air quality in tropical destinations. Nevertheless, information on the hazards presented by recreational and especially pool, spa and hot spring waters as a mode of transmission of pathogens is very limited, even though numerous infectious agents may threaten the health or comfort of pool and hot tub users [5]. As examples, the important World Health Organization (WHO) document [2] attributes only half, out of 244, pages to precautions related to the use of recreational waters [2]; the European Network on Imported Infectious Diseases Surveillance (TravelHealthPro) does not mention recreational waters on their webpage, which provides guidance to travellers on how to take care of their health [6]; the announced revision of the WHO Guidelines for recreational waters [3] has been suspended [3]; Page et al. do not refer to pool water in their outstanding review regarding attitudes of tourists towards water use in the developing world [7].

Climate changes are creating conditions in the subtropical zones similar to the tropics and these geographical regions were included in the review. For the purposes of our review, we considered both primary transmission from pool waters and secondary infections spread by the pool users. Tropical diseases encompass all diseases that occur solely, or principally, in the tropics. In practice, the term is often taken to refer to infectious diseases that thrive in hot, humid conditions, such as malaria, leishmaniasis, schistosomiasis, onchocerciasis, lymphatic filariasis, Chagas disease, African trypanosomiasis, and dengue [8]. Besides the "big three" diseases—malaria, tuberculosis, HIV/AIDS—which are well known causes of major global mortality, morbidity and burden, the term "neglected tropical diseases" has been introduced in the literature. They comprise a new field for travellers' health and the list includes 40 helminth, bacterial, protozoan, fungal, viral and ectoparasitic infections affecting local populations in the tropics, which are strongly associated with poverty and socio-ecological systems, but also presenting a serious health risk for travellers [9]. It is worth noting, however, that many of the so-called "tropical" diseases are not transmitted through recreational waters.

Objective

This review aims at collating information on pool water quality, and cases and outbreaks related to swimming in pools and hot springs in tropical and subtropical regions, and at carrying out a search and review of papers dealing with hazards deriving from the use of pools in the tropical and subtropical zones.

2. Materials and Methods

Search Strategy/Inclusion Criteria

Cochrane instructions for a systematic search that seeks to identify all studies dealing with incidences originating in tropical and subtropical countries were followed (https://ph.cochrane.org/sites/ph.cochrane.org/files/public/uploads/HPPH_systematic_review_handbook.pdf). The studies were required to meet pre-defined eligibility criteria, a major one being transmission via pool, spa or hot spring waters or the detection of the pathogens in such waters. Thus, studies reporting pathogens without confirmed transmission through recreational waters were excluded. For instance, the *Chikungunya* virus was the aetiological agent of an outbreak in Kenya in 2004, and major outbreaks followed in Indian Ocean island countries such as Reunion, Mauritius, Comoros, Seychelles and Madagascar in 2005 to 2006 [4,10]. *Burkholderia pseudomallei* has also caused melioidosis in the tropics [11]. Nevertheless, so far neither of these two pathogens' transmission has been confirmed to involve pool waters.

Diseases transmitted by vectors breeding in poorly maintained, neglected or abandoned pools were also included. As tourism presents seasonality a high number of pools stay inactive for several months, often still containing the water of the past season. This situation encourages the proliferation of pathogens and the extensive use of these waters by vectors in order to breed. Thousands of flooded swimming pools were abandoned in New Orleans following Hurricane Katrina and provided a natural experiment to examine colonization of a novel aquatic habitat by mosquito larvae and their aquatic predators [12–15].

A large number of cases and outbreaks described in the literature surely derive from unidentified sources, among which a number is likely to have been from swimming pools: reports of this kind or with a preconceived bias regarding the mode of transmission were excluded from this review.

Bacteria genera such as *Legionella*, *Salmonella* and *Pseudomonas*, commonly causing cases and outbreaks in the tropics, but also in the rest of the world [16,17] were excluded. The review endeavours to focus on infections transmitted by pool waters and caused by pathogens that, with the exception of *Cryptosporidium* spp. [18], are unusual in the moderate climates and common in the tropical and subtropical countries, including southern regions of Japan and North Australia, as shown in Figure 1.

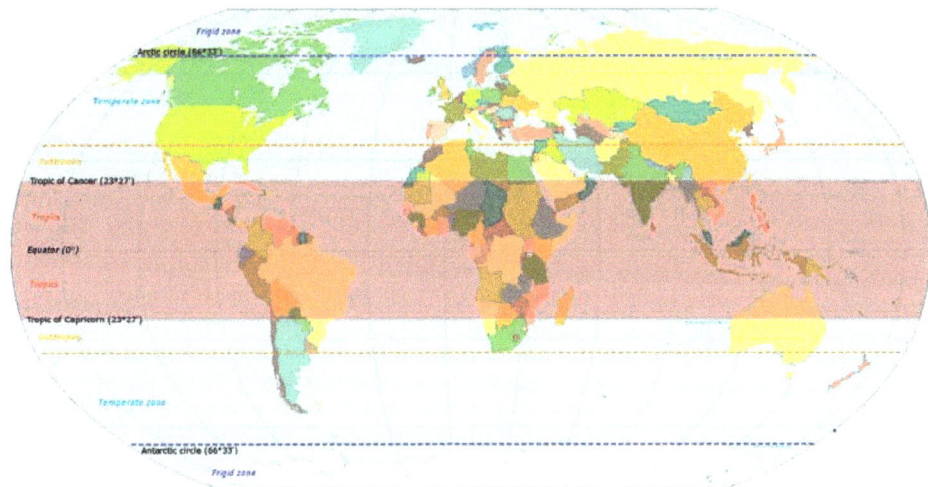

Figure 1. Map of the world indicating the tropical and subtropical zones.

Other eligibility criteria were: that the studies were published in English, though we did allow a few notable exceptions to this rule; and that the publications in question were scientific papers and reviews in scientific journals, national and international public health platforms, and journals and platforms related to tourism (for example UNWTO). PubMed, Google Scholar, Science Direct, CDC, ECDC and WHO platform and publications were systematically searched.

Further to the aforesaid eligibility criteria, we reviewed 83 studies on cases and outbreaks in tropical countries, 45 studies on modes and trends of pathogen transmission and selected outbreaks in western countries, and 3 studies on trends in the tourist industry. In addition, information was harvested from official national and international websites. They are presented in groups according to the pathogen involved. As mentioned above, viruses transmitted by vectors that breed in waters were also considered as waterborne pathogens.

3. Results

3.1. Assessments of Swimming Pools in Developing Tropical Countries

The repeated reference to health problems deriving from the use of swimming pools could be related to sub-optimal regulations, which do not address all factors contributing to the swimmers' well-being in a particular geographical area, or are poorly applied. For instance, countries around the Mediterranean basin are among the most popular tourist destinations. In a study, investigating pool and spa regulations in these countries, the conclusions were that the Africa and Middle East countries of this region possess satisfactory regulations comparable to the regulations of the European countries in the same area [19]. Similar conclusions were drawn from a report commissioned by Clúster de la Indústria Química de les Illes Balears in which a few countries worldwide were picked at random and their regulations presented and compared. Some tropical countries seem to adapt their regulations to specific issues. For instance, in the Mexican regulation, free living amoebae are included in the standard as water quality indicators along with bacterial parameters [20]. According to the authors of both reviews, the major question was whether regulations were applied, and if controls of the water quality and hygiene in the facilities were carried out by authorities.

Table 1. Assessments of swimming pools (SPs) located in tropical and subtropical countries.

Location/Country	Positive Results	Ref.
North Africa, Egypt	The authors suggest artificial plastic SPs as a prophylactic measure against infection with schistosomiasis in developing countries.	[21]
North Africa, Assiut Town, Egypt	In a survey of 2 SPs, which included 50 water samples *Dermatophytes*, *Aspergyllus* sp., *Penicillium*, *Altenaria*, *Syncephalastrium*, *Mucor* were detected.	[22]
North Africa, Alexandria, Egypt	Assessment of the environmental and health aspects of some SPs. Presence of pathogens indicated.	[23]
North Africa, Alexandria, Egypt	Assessment of 5 SPs, 30 water samples. Compliance of pool water with regulations regarding bacterial indicators was 56.7%. In 10% of the samples *Cryptosporidium* oocysts and *Giardia* cysts were detected.	[24]
Middle East, Ein Feshka, Dead Sea, Israel	Medical report of 10 cases of *Mycobacterium marinum* mimicking leismaniasis. Most of the infections were contracted in natural bathing pools.	[25]
Middle East, West Bank, Palestine	An assessment of 58 water samples, collected from 46 SPs. All unacceptable according to regulations. 21/23 water samples were positive for *Salmonella* spp.	[26]
Middle East, Amman, Jordan	Assessment of 85 SPs in Amman. Compliance of the pools' water with the microbial parameters was 56.5%.	[27]
Middle East, Nablus district, Palestine	In a survey of 3 SPs, 50 keratinophilic fungal species were recovered. The most frequently isolated species were *Acremonium strictum* & *Cladosporium cladiosporioides*. The most abundant species were *Acremonium strictum*, and *Aspergillus flavus*.	[28]
Sub Saharan Africa, Ghana	In a survey of 7 SPs, faecal coliforms, *E. coli*, total heterotrophic bacteria were recovered from all SPs; *E. coli* O157:H7 were recovered from 2 SPs. Antibiotic resistance tests revealed the highest resistance was in sulfamethoxazole (46%).	[29]
Asia, Guangzhou, China	A survey of 39 municipal SPs revealed protozoa (12.8%), *P. aeruginosa* (69.2%), total coliforms, *E. coli* (4%), *Cryptosporidium* & *Giardia* (12.8%), *E. coli* O157, *Shigella*, and *Salmonella*.	[30]
Asia, Ahwaz Iran	In a survey of 10 indoor SPs, 593 water and environmental samples (shower areas, dressing rooms, pool walls, slippers) revealed 372 saprophytic fungi species and 32 yeasts. The most common were *Aspergillus* & *Penicillium*.	[31]
Asia, Shahrekord City, Iran	In a seasonal assessment of 2 indoor SPs (459 pool water, shower & dressing room samples) faecal coliform *Pseudomonas aeruginosa*, *Legionella*, *Escherichia coli* and Heterotrophic Plate Count values exceeded regulations. The most prevalent fungi were in the showers, the most frequent being *Aspergillus* spp. (48.91%).	[32]

Information on the monitoring and the assessment of swimming pool waters in countries of the tropical and subtropical zones is limited (Table 1). It is possible that monitoring is carried out in some countries, but scarcely few data have been published. From the North Africa countries some studies have been published from Egypt [21–24] starting in the 1960s. In the Middle East, certain subtropical countries such as Israel, Palestine and Jordan provided some limited monitoring data [25–27] including a study from Palestine on the presence of fungi in pool water and facilities [28]. Setsoafia Saba et al. published a water quality assessment of swimming pools and the risk of spreading infections in Ghana, which is one of the very rare publications in Sub-Saharan Africa [29]. From the Asian countries, China [30], and most often Iran [31,32], have published assessments which include bacterial indicators, some tropical parasites and fungi related to the sanitary quality in the facilities [31,32]. In light of the above, the aim of the present review is to update our knowledge of waterborne outbreaks in the tropical and subtropical zones of the main tropical pathogens transmitted through the use of swimming pools, spas and hot tubs with a particular emphasis on tourist facilities.

3.2. Microsporidia

Microsporidia are newly emerging pathogens of humans and animals. They are tiny obligate intracellular parasitic fungi and as such are often still managed by diagnostic parasitology laboratories. Due to the small size of their spores and uncharacteristic staining properties they are difficult to detect. Accordingly, epidemiological studies to elucidate the sources of human-pathogenic Microsporidia and their routes of transmission are difficult to perform [33]. Faecal-oral transmission is the likely route of infection in humans with intestinal microsporidiosis [34]. The last two decades have seen several publications related to ocular microsporidiosis, in particular those forms affecting the cornea. Both immunocompetent, immunocompromised and AIDS patients are vulnerable to the acquisition of microsporidia and especially to keratoconjunctivitis, which is usually seen in immunocompromised individuals or in contact lens wearers. The organism is widespread in the environment and is considered a waterborne pathogen [34,35]. Exposure to soil, muddy water, and minor trauma are possible risk factors.

An analysis of risk factors for microsporidiosis showed that swimming in pools comprises an additional significant risk factor [36], even though conventional levels of chlorine (1–3 mg/L) used in swimming pools where water temperatures normally reach or exceed 22 °C should be adequate to greatly reduce or eliminate the infectivity *of* microsporidial species *E. intestinalis*, *E. hellem* and *E. cuniculi* spores after relatively short exposure times [37]. In Paris (France), in a survey of pools for microsporidia, *Cryptosporidium* spp. and *Giardia* spp., microsporidia were detected in only one out of 48 water samples [38].

The tropics seem to host most of the cases of microsporidial keratitis. A high prevalence has been documented in Singapore [39] and in India [40] and transmission through contact with water has been suggested. The present review identified 2 published studies (Table 2) clearly relating infection to the presence of microsporidia in pools in the tropics. In Paris, Curry et al. referred to a case of an HIV-negative patient from Bangladesh with bilateral keratitis who was found to be infected with a microsporidial parasite belonging to the genus *Nosema*. The patient had bathed in a rural pond 7 days prior to the development of ocular symptoms. *Nosema* parasites are common insect parasites and the source of this microsporidial infection was possibly from mosquito larvae developing in the pond in which the patient bathed [41]. In Taipei, Taiwan, a retrospective study included 10 eyes of 9 immunocompetent patients diagnosed with microsporidial keratitis. All of them were known to contract this disease after bathing in hot springs. The nine patients travelled and bathed in at least four different spa resorts located in two different areas [42].

3.3. Parasites

Waterborne parasitic protozoan diseases are distributed worldwide and comprise, in both developed and developing countries, reasons for epidemic and endemic human suffering. Looking at the trends of the prevalence of parasitic diseases in the developed world a significant decrease has been observed, which may be attributed to the substantial improvements in data reporting and the establishment of surveillance systems [43,44]. The highest prevalence of parasitic protozoan infections is known to occur in developing countries due to lower hygiene standards. In addition, developing countries that are more likely to be most affected by such waterborne disease outbreaks still lack reliable surveillance systems, and an international standardization of surveillance and reporting systems has yet to be established [45]. In 1999, the European Network on Imported Infectious Diseases Surveillance (TropNetEurop) was set up in order to collate reliable data on imported infectious diseases to Europe and assess trends over time [46].

A review by Lim et al. provided a comprehensive overview of the available data and studies on waterborne parasite occurrences among the Association of Southeast Asian Nations (ASEAN), which is comprised of ten member states (i.e., Brunei Darussalam, Cambodia, Indonesia, Lao People's Democratic Republic (PDR), Malaysia, Myanmar, the Philippines, Singapore, Thailand, and Vietnam) with the aims of identifying ways in which to progress. Many of these countries are booming tourist destinations. Swimming pools are included as a source of transmission. He points out the fact that there are massive gaps of knowledge in the occurrence, morbidity and mortality associated with parasitic diseases [47]. According to a review providing data related to neglected parasitic protozoa in the tropics reporting that only an estimated 1% of global outbreaks of waterborne parasitic protozoa outbreaks have occurred in Asia, it is evident that there is a paucity of information from this region where organized mechanisms of documentation of parasitic infections or waterborne outbreaks are lacking [48]. *Cryptosporidium*, *Amoebae* and *Schistosoma* spp. are the parasites with the highest public health significance when swimming pools are the route of transmission.

3.3.1. Schistosoma spp.

Schistosomiasis is caused by diagenetic blood trematodes. The three main species infecting humans are *Schistosoma haematobium*, *S. japonicum*, and *S. mansoni*. Two other species, more localized geographically, are *S. mekongi* and *S. intercalatum*. Other species of schistosomes, which parasitize birds and mammals, can cause cercarial dermatitis in humans [49]. Acute schistosomiasis was first described in 1847 in the prefecture of Katayama, Hiroshima district, Japan. A woman brought to the region to be married was found to become acutely unwell with a fever after she had been exposed to fresh water. Snails in fresh waters contribute to the life cycle of *Schistosoma* as, under optimal conditions, the eggs hatch and release miracidia, which swim and penetrate specific snail intermediate hosts [49].

Schistosomiasis has been rare in Europe and there is very limited published literature dealing with relevant outbreaks. In Corsica one outbreak involving 120 people infected after swimming in a fresh water swimming pool is one of the rare published cases [50]. Nevertheless, schistosomiasis is increasingly imported into temperate climates by immigrants and travellers to endemic areas [51–54]. Schistosomiasis in returning travellers is one of the most common imported tropical infections with potentially serious complications, which are preventable upon early diagnosis [55]. Human contact with water is required for infection by schistosomes.

Grobusch et al. studied imported schistosomiasis in Europe by seeking data from TropNetEurop. Three hundred and thirty-three reports of schistosomiasis have been analysed for their epidemiological and clinical features. The majority of patients were of European origin (53%), who travelled predominantly for tourism to endemic areas (52%). The majority of infections were acquired in Africa; 92 (%) infections were attributed to *Schistosoma haematobium* [56]. However, in a 15-year observational study at the Hospital for Tropical Diseases, London, the prevalence of schistosomiasis in presenting travellers is decreasing with predominant species *S. haematobium* [55].

Schistosomiasis is one of the endemic diseases that take advantage of environmental modifications due to water conveyance in the Saharan countries, for example Burgina Faso [57]. In Egypt, risk factors for *S. haematobium* infection were male gender, an age <21 years old, living in small communities, and exposure to canal water [58].

One of the first published reports on an epidemic of acute schistosomiasis concerned travellers returning from Mali. Imported schistosomiasis acquired in the Dogon country in Mali, West Africa, was first demonstrated in 1989 in three Spanish travellers [59]. More recently, 79 cases of acute schistosomiasis were reported by the Hospital of Tropical Diseases, London, between 1998 and 2012.

Most of these cases were young, male travellers who acquired their infection in Lake Malawi (53%). Most of the other cases were from West Africa, with only 13% acquiring their disease in East Africa, one in North Africa (Libya), and two in the Middle East (Saudi Arabia, Yemen). Most were on holiday (68%), while 16% had been working as volunteers. All of them reported contact fresh water in an area where schistosomiasis is endemic [60].

The present review identified five published studies clearly regarding schistosomiasis transmitted via swimming pools in the tropics, of which three were related to tourism (Table 2). In 1993, a 35-year-old Belgian woman was admitted to the University Hospital of Antwerp with schistosomiasis symptoms. She had swum with a group of travellers in a water pool in the Dongon valley in Mali. Sixty-two per cent (eight people) of the 13 travellers had acquired Schistosoma infection; seven of them had developed Katayama syndrome. All travellers, except one, who acquired a *Schistomoma* infection, had swum for at least 5 min in the pool [61]. In a study from the area of Belo Horizonte, Brazil, a group of 18 individuals was included. They had the impression that the water was clean and no snails were observed. *S. mansoni* was transmitted from non-symptomatic positive residents through infected intermediate hosts to visitors. The visitors came from an urban area who had never had contact with the disease before and who developed acute schistosomiasis [62]. Also in Brazil, transmission occurred in a non-endemic area of Brazil, which became a new point of transmission due to the immigration of infected workers [63]. In Upper Benue Valley in Cameroon, swimming in a pool for the local population was significantly associated with schistosomiasis infection [64]. The Department of Infectious Diseases, University Hospital of Leiden, The Netherlands, reported an outbreak of schistosomiasis among non-immunized travellers. Of 30 travellers in two consecutive groups, 29 who had swum in freshwater pools in the Dogon area of Mali, West Africa, were monitored for 12 months. Twenty-eight (97%) of those became infected; 10 (36%) of the 28 had cercarial dermatitis, and in 15 (54%), Katayama fever developed [65].

3.3.2. *Cryptosporidium spp.*

Transmission of *Cryptosporidium* has been on the increase over the last two decades. Currently, 31 valid *Cryptosporidium* species have been recognized and of these more than 17 have been found to infect humans. The most commonly reported species in humans worldwide are *C. parvum* and *C. hominis* [66]. This parasite has a low infectious dose, a small size that enables it to bypass water filtration systems, and resistance to chlorine disinfection at levels routinely used at swimming pools, water parks, and interactive fountains. It is the leading cause of outbreaks associated with disinfected recreational water and has also caused outbreaks in child care facilities. *Cryptosporidium* has the ability to cause community-wide outbreaks when transmitted in these venues [67] Swimming pool associated cases and outbreaks of cryptosporidiasis have been reported abundantly in the western world [68–72].

The burden of cryptosporidiosis is higher in tropical countries. In Australia, for instance, cryptosporidiosis seems to be an endemic problem in warm, remote areas and in Aboriginal and Torres Strait Islander population-dominated regions [73]. The most recent Global Burden of Disease Study listed *Cryptosporidium* as an important cause of disease and death of children under 5 years of age in Sub-Saharan Africa [74]. From 2004 to 2010, 199 outbreaks of human gastroenteritis due to the waterborne transmission of 59 enteric parasitic protozoa were reported worldwide and of these, *Cryptosporidium* spp. was the etiological agent in 60.3% of the outbreaks [60,61]. Bathing in contaminated swimming and therapeutic pools is a major mode of waterborne transmission of *Cryptosporidium* and other pathogens [75].

In a recently published review, Ryan et al. found that the necessary key barriers to limiting swimming-pool associated outbreaks of cryptosporidiosis (lack of uniform national and international standards, poor adherence and understanding of regulations governing staff and patron behaviour, and low levels of public knowledge and awareness) are not widely applied [76]. The present review identified three published studies clearly reporting cryptosporidiosis transmitted via swimming pools, or reporting detection of Cryptosporidium in pool waters, in tropical countries (Table 2).

A study of 35 pools in Beijing, including some hotel pools, showed that 16.7% and 15% were positive for *Cryptosoridium* oocysts and *Giardia* cysts, respectively [66]. Also, in the Philippines, in a total of 33 water samples taken from various environmental sources, including swimming pools, 45.5% were positive for *Cryptosporidium*. Two hundred seventy three children developed cryptosporidiosis after using a pool. Later on the same children used 10 swimming pools in a different prefecture and four of them were infected [77]. In Broom, Western Australia, another outbreak of cryptosporidiosis involving children who swam at the public pool was described [78].

3.3.3. *Acanthamoeba, Naegleria Species*

Free-living amoebae belonging to the genera *Acanthamoeba, Balamuthia, Naegleria* and *Sappinia* are important causes of disease in humans and animals. *Naegleria fowleri* produces an acute, and usually lethal, central nervous system (CNS) disease called primary Amoebic meningoencephalitis. *Acanthamoeba* spp. are opportunistic free-living amoebae capable of causing granulomatous amoebic encephalitis (GAE) in individuals with compromised immune systems [79]. *Acanthamoeba* spp., the Trojan horse of the microbial world, as it carries viruses, has two stages in its life cycle, an active trophozoite stage that exhibits vegetative growth and a dormant cyst stage with minimal metabolic activity. It is a causative agent of cutaneous lesions and sinus infections, vision-threatening keratitis and a rare but fatal encephalitis, known as granulomatous amoebic encephalitis [80]. *Acanthamoebae* and *Naegleria fowleri* are commonly found in warm freshwater environments such as hot springs, lakes, natural mineral water, and resort spas frequented by tourists. In an early survey of 13 swimming pools in Belgium, *Acanthamoeba* strains were detected in 43.6% of the samples [81]. Similarly, amoebae were detected in 27/30 swimming pools in New York State [82]. Previously thought to be a rare condition, the number of reported Primary Amoebic meningoencephalitis cases is increasing each year [83].

The present review identified 13 published studies reporting detection of free-living amoebae in pool waters in tropical countries [77,84–95] (Table 2). The earlier survey appeared in 1983 [84] and reported the presence of pathogenic and free-living amoebae in swimming pool waters of Mexico City. Among the organisms isolated, in their cystic or in their trophic stage, were *Naegleria fowleri Carter* and *Acanthamoeba castellanii Douglas* [84]. One study in Taiwan reported a fatality caused after swimming in hot springs [85]. The most recent one was carried out in two swimming pools in Alexandria (Egypt) [86].

3.4. *Leptospira spp.*

Leptospirosis also belongs to the spectrum of travel-related infections. Leptospirosis is a bacterial zoonosis caused by host-dependent spirochetes of the genus *Leptospira*, which is widespread throughout the world. Its main sources are rodents, particularly rats, which excrete the spirochete *Leptospira* spp. in urine. Humans are infected by direct contact with urine of infected animals or by contact with an infected environment such as surface water [96].

Leptospirosis is an important re-emerging tropical disease, especially in areas with a notable military presence. Several epidemics of leptospirosis have been reported worldwide during the past century, while leptospirosis is endemic in most of the urban areas in Southern and Western India, where outbreaks usually occur after flooding caused by heavy seasonal rainfall [97]. Almost every country in South and Southeast Asia, South and Central America and several island nations across the world are endemic to leptospirosis [98]. It is endemic in Sub-Saharan Africa; however, for most countries scarce epidemiological data, if any, exist.

The disease has been increasingly reported in travellers, particularly those travelling to tropical areas, due to the development of fresh-water sports and leisure activities [99,100], Leptospirosis is often reported in travellers to South Africa [96] and in travellers from Sub Saharan Africa. Returning from a water sports holiday in South Africa, a 49-year old man presented with acute leptospirosis [101]. In a recently published review from Rajarata University, Sri Lanka, the authors pointed out that a clear increase in the proportion of travel-associated leptospirosis over the time was observed.

According to their review, the countries with the highest number of cases detected in travellers returning from endemic regions are the US, Netherlands, Japan, France, Germany and Australia; among reports of systematically collected country level data, Israel reported the highest incidence of travel associated leptospirosis (41.7%) [102]. In a hospital study in Paris, France, fifteen cases of travel-related leptospirosis were reported. All travellers except one were returning from holidays in the tropics (seven from SE Asia, three from Sub-Saharan Africa, two from Reunion Island). The most frequent at-risk exposure was bathing in fresh water [103]. The clinical course of a leptospirosis outbreak at the Hash House Harriers Club on Guam, Micronesia, in the western Pacific Ocean, has been reported. Patients declared multiple exposures to wet river banks, mud, and swamps [104].

One case clearly connected a leptospirosis case to swimming in a pool (Table 2). A 25 year-old German woman visiting the Dominican Republic and staying for 3 weeks in a village became infected when swimming in the heavily chlorinated swimming pool during a trip to Samana [105].

3.5. Viruses

Viruses are considered a significant cause of recreationally associated waterborne diseases with a number of relevant outbreaks in western countries [106–109]. However, they have been difficult to document because of the wide variety of illnesses associated and limitations in detection methods. *Noroviruses* are the largest cause of outbreaks with just under half of the outbreaks occurring in swimming pools (49%) [110]. Some sporadic publications refer to transmission of *Hepatitis A virus (HAV)* [111,112] and *Echovirus* 30 [113].

The present review identified six published studies reporting the viruses' detection in swimming pool waters in tropical countries [114–119] (Table 2). The earliest was a study of a primary school outbreak of pharyngoconjunctival fever attributed to swimming in the swimming pool of a school camp [114]. Swimming pool water contaminated with *Human Adenovirus serotype 4 (HAdV-4)* was the most likely source of infection, although one instance of likely person-to-person transmission was noted [119].

3.6. Indirect Role of Swimming Pools in Water Related Diseases

Vector-borne diseases are human illnesses caused by parasites, viruses and bacteria that are transmitted by mosquitoes, sandflies, triatomine bugs, blackflies, ticks, tsetse flies, mites, snails and lice, causing more than 700,000 deaths globally. All the major vector-borne diseases, together, account for around 17% of all infectious diseases [8]. Swimming pools are considered major contributors to the disease burden, as proliferation sites for mosquitoes like *Anopheles*, transferring Malaria; *Aedes*, transferring *Dengue, yellow fever* and the *Zika viruses*; *Culex* transferring West Nile Fever. The latter became a major problem after the first cases and epidemics in western countries, starting in New York in 1999 [120]. Concerning the ecology of the *Culex* mosquitoes, Petersen et al., in their review of the spread of *West Nile Virus*, included density of poorly maintained swimming pools in the critical factors for *Arvoviral* proliferation [121]. Chen et al., in their review of the significance of the *Zika virus* as a new public health concern, emphasize the need to eliminate standing waters outside homes, including swimming pools [122].

Distribution of vector-borne diseases is determined by complex demographic, environmental and social factors. Global travel and trade, unplanned urbanization and making the transmission season longer or more intense or causing diseases to emerge in countries where they were previously unknown [8]. The world risk maps, demonstrated that for dengue fever Sub-Saharan areas and the central and northern countries of South America are the most dangerous zones [123]. Mackenzie et al., in his risk map, presents the spread and resurgence of Japanese encephalitis, West Nile and dengue encompassing all continents except Antarctica [124]. An important outbreak of dengue fever occurred recently in France [125], and of the *West Nile virus* in Greece [126].

Vectors are contributing to the dispersion of lethal diseases in the tropics, initially in agricultural and rural areas [127,128]. There are reports of westerners traveling in Southeast Asian countries who were infected by the *Zika virus*—an Australian traveller to Indonesia [129], a Canadian traveller to Thailand [130]—and the trends of the disease alter as time goes by with the symptoms getting more severe [131]. Nevertheless, in a review by De Sylva and Marshall dealing with the factors contributing to urban malaria transmission in Sub-Saharan Africa, the authors concluded that "artificial rather than natural vector breeding sites provide the most abundant sources of mosquito larvae in African urban centres. Africa's demography is rapidly changing with a fast increasing number of people moving to urban areas". According to the same review, urban malaria is considered an emerging problem in Africa because the populations of most large African cities have grown exponentially over the last 30 years. Ninety-five artificial vector breeding sites are referred to in this review, including swimming pools, in contrast with only 42 natural sites [132].

The present review identified five published studies reporting surveys of swimming pools in the tropics as environments encouraging vector's proliferation (Table 2). Impoinvil et al. conducted larval surveys in habitats located in urban Malindi, Kenya, and, out of the 250 habitats sampled, 66 were unused swimming pools. Of the 110 habitats found to be positive for mosquitoes, unused swimming pools represented 42.7% and 148 anopheline pupae were found in eight of the 66 unused swimming pools while none was found in the other habitats [133]. The same authors in an earlier study reported that, from a total of 889 *Anopheles* and 7217 culicine immatures found in diverse water body types, unused swimming pools comprised 61% of all water bodies found to serve as the main habitats for Anopheles immatures [134]. Studies have been carried out in Dakar [135] and in Brazil [136].

3.7. Chlamydia Trachomatis

Trachoma, caused by *Chlamydia trachomatis*, has been noted throughout history as a significant cause of blindness. *Chlamydia trachomatis* is one of four bacterial species in the genus and they are obligatory intracellular parasites. Trachoma is considered a neglected tropical disease. The causative organism is passed from person to person by flies, fomites and fingers, particularly among preschool-aged children [137]. In 1998, the World Health Assembly adopted the goal of Global Elimination of Trachoma as a cause of blindness; the year 2020 was set as the target date by a WHO Alliance set up to support the elimination agenda [138].

Interestingly, Warren et al. notes the suggestion that the construction of well-maintained and chlorinated public swimming pools could be a practical method to improve facial cleanliness and disinfection and consequently reduce trachoma rates among children in remote Indigenous communities in Australia [139]. Nevertheless, simultaneous use by travellers might enhance transmission of *Chlamydia trachomatis* through the use of the pool, even though such a case has not been reported to the present. As with all obligatory intracellular parasites, *C. trachomatis* is unlikely to be affected by chlorination and thus survives well in pool water. Ozone only, in a concentration of 4 ppm, was enough to inactivate *C. trachomatis* and *C. pneumonia* according to a study conducted mostly for medical purposes [140].

Table 2. List of surveillance studies of swimming pools (SPs), and respective cases and outbreaks of infections associated with swimming pools and hot springs in tropical and subtropical countries.

Microsporidia			
Location/Country	Type of Research	Positive Results	Reference
Rural areas, Bangladesh	Report of an incident of a traveller from Bangladesh returning to Paris, France	A man suffered from bilateral keratitis after bathing in a rural pond. The patient was found to be infected with a microsporidial parasite belonging to the genus *Nosema*.	[41]
Taipei, Taiwan	Retrospective study of patients diagnosed with microsporidial keratitis	All patients were known to have contracted microsporidial keratitis after bathing in hot springs.	[42]

Table 2. *Cont.*

Location/Country	Type of Research	Positive Results	Reference
Schistosoma spp.			
Dogon Valley, Mali	Study of an acute schistosomiasis in Belgian travellers returning from Dogon Valley, Mali	8/13 travellers infected with *Schistosoma*. 5/8 travellers had experienced swimmer's itch and developed Katayama syndrome.	[55]
Belo Horizonte, State of Minas Gerais, Brazil	Study of an outbreak of acute schistosomiasis in a holiday resort at an endemic area	17 cases infected with *S. mansoni*.	[56]
São João del Rei, Brazil	Study of an outbreak where an area became infected due to influx of infected workers from endemic areas, who infected water sources, including SPs	50 workers infected in the pool with *S. mansoni*.	[57]
Upper Benue Valley, North Cameroon	Study of the risk factors for human schistosomiasis in the local population	High prevalence of the disease depending on, among other factors, the intensity of contact with the water.	[58]
Dogon Valley, Mali	Study of an outbreak in two groups of 30 Dutch travellers returning from Dogon area of Mali where they swam in fresh water pools	29 infected with *S. intercalatum*, *S. haematobium*.	[59]

Location/Country	Type of Research	Positive Results	Reference
Cryptosporidium spp.			
Beijing, China	Survey of 35 randomly selected hotel SPs, 60 water samples	16.7% positive for *Cryptosporidium*, 15% positive for *Giardia*.	[66]
Various areas, Philippines	Survey of water sources including SPs	33% positive for *Cryptosporidium*.	[77]
Broome, Kimberley region, Western Australia	Investigation of outbreak of cryptosporidiasis	11/18 cases swam in the public pool. In faecal and pool water samples *Cryptosporidium ominis* was identified.	[78]

Location/Country	Type of Research	Positive Results	Reference
Acanthamoebae & Naegleria Species			
Mexico City, Mexico	Survey of six swimming pools	All SPs were positive for *Acanthamoebae*. The most commonly found were *Amoebae* of the species *Naegleria gruberi Schardinger*.	[84]
Taichung, Taiwan	Diagnosis of fatality	One fatal case of meningoencephalitis caused by *N. fowleri* and transmitted in hot springs was reported.	[85]
Alexandria, Egypt	Survey of two SPs	Both SPs were positive for *Acanthamoeba* spp. and *Naegleria* spp.	[86]
Kuala Lumpur, Malaysia	Survey of 14 pools. Four water samples and six samples using swabs were collected from each	*Acanthamoeba* species were detected in all sampling sites of all SPs, while *Naegleria* spp. was detected in 3 sampling sites of 8 SPs.	[87]
Mexico City, Mexico	Survey of three physiotherapy tubs and 11 SPs	All therapy tubs were positive for *Acanthamoeba* spp., while 7/11 SPs were positive for *Naegleria* spp.	[88]
Brazil, Porto Alegre	Survey of 65 water samples from SPs	Amoebae were detected in 20% of the SPs. 4/65 water samples were positive for *Acanthamoeba* spp. while 9/65 water samples were positive for free-living amoebae.	[89]
Egypt, various locations	Survey in various waters including two SPs	49.2% of pool water samples were positive for heat-tolerant *Acanthamoeba* spp.	[90]
Porto Alegre, Brazil	Survey in pools and spas	8/72 water samples were positive for *Acanthamoeba* spp. distributed in group genotypes T3, T5, T4, T15.	[91]
Brasilia District, Brazil	Study of the pathogenicity of strains from environmental sources	4/4 *Acanthamoeba* spp. isolates from pool waters were pathogenic.	[92]
Ahwaz, Iran	Survey of 110 water and soil samples including four SPs	In 71.6% of water samples *Acanthamoeba* spp. was detected SP isolates belong to T4 genotype.	[93]
Various areas, Philippines	Survey of rivers, ponds, dispensers, wells, taps, natural lakes and SPs	33.3% of SP water samples were positive for *Acanthamoeba* sp. While 9.1% of SP water samples were positive for *Naegleria* spp.	[77]
Adana, Afyon, Kutahya, Mersin and Nigde provinces, Turkey	Survey of hot springs and SPs	42% of water samples were positive for *Acanthamoeba* sp. belonging to T3, T4, T5 genotypes.	[94]
Malaysia Peninsular	A survey of recreational lakes, streams, SPs	*Naegleria sp* was detected in all samples.	[95]

Table 2. *Cont.*

Leptospira spp.			
Location/Country	**Type of Research**	**Positive Results**	**Reference**
Various places, Dominican Republic	Study of leptospirosis in travellers	A German woman developed leptospirosis after swimming in a chlorinated SP.	[105]

Viruses			
Location/Country	**Type of Research**	**Positive Results**	**Reference**
Queensland, Australia	Study of a primary school outbreak of pharyngo-conjunctival fever attributed to swimming in the SP of a school camp	40% of the students infected by *Adenovirus type 3*.	[114]
Pretoria, South Africa	A study of the risk of infection of *HAdVs* detected in a survey of 3 SPs, 92 water samples	*HAdVs* were detected in 15 samples.	[115]
Porto Alegre, Brazil	Survey of SPs for the detection of adenoviruses in *Acanthamoeba* strains	16 *Acanthamoeba* strains were detected, *HAdVs* were detected in 62.5% (10/16) of *Acanthamoeba* isolates.	[116]
South Africa	Investigation of an outbreak related to swimming in the school camp pool	90 children & the SP water were positive for *Echovirus 3*.	[117]
Taiwan, various areas	A study to determine the prevalence of *HAdVs* in hot springs. 57 hot springs and 14 public SPs were investigated, 57 water samples	*HAdVs* were detected in 28.1% of the samples from hot springs and 21.4% of SP water samples.	[118]
Beijing, China	A study of an outbreak of pharyngoconjunctival fever related to swimming in a University SP	50 patients used the same SP. *HAdV* type 4 was identified from the patients and SP water samples.	[119]

Vectors			
Location/Country	**Type of Research**	**Positive Results**	**Reference**
Malindi, Kenya	A systematic review of the factors contributing to urban transmission of malaria in Sub-Saharan Africa	*Anopheles gambiae* proliferating in SPs. Artificial rather than natural breeding sites provide most abundant sources for mosquito larvae.	[132]
Malindi, Kenya	A study on larvae surveys in urban environments and the productivity of unused SPs in relation to other habitats	Unused SPs accounted for 42.7% of all 110 positive habitats. *Anopheles gambiae s.l.* and *Culex quinquefasciatus* were detected.	[133]
Malindi, Kenya	A study on the abundance of immature *Anopheles* and culicines in various water body types in the urban environment	Unused SPs comprised 21.7% of water bodies serving as habitats for immature *Anopheles*.	[134]
Dakar, Senegal	An entomological survey on the determinants of malaria transmission in the city of Dakar	355 private properties were visited, including SPs. *Culicidae* larvae were found in 80 (23%) and *Anopheles* larvae in 11 (3%).	[135]
Sao Jose de Rio Preto, Brazil	A study on the evaluation of two sweeping methods for estimating the number of immature *Aedes aegypti*	*Aedes aegypti* was harvested in various types of containers including SPs.	[136]

4. Discussion

Global experience and research demonstrate that international travel can pose various risks to health, depending both on the health needs of the traveller and on the type of travel undertaken. Travellers may encounter sudden and significant changes in altitude, humidity, temperature and exposure to a variety of infectious diseases, which can result in illness. In addition, serious health risks may arise in areas where accommodation is of poor quality, hygiene and sanitation are inadequate, medical services are not well developed and clean water is unavailable [2]. Trends in the West towards novel, alternative "natural" ponds, deprived of disinfection with chemicals and using instead biological processes for cleaning the organic compounds in the water are expanding rapidly. Many European countries have adopted guidelines or regulations specific for natural ponds. These establishments require careful, scientifically sound management [141]. Some or all of these factors apply in numerous tropical and subtropical countries of the developing world. Also, the trend towards higher standard accommodation in tourist establishments and more water-intense activities—including the use of pools and hot springs—coincides with changes in the global climate system leading to declining water resources and poorer water quality in many regions [142]. Tourists' lack of awareness of their impact on the environment becomes an added factor aggravating sustainability in certain destinations [7].

A host of viral, bacterial, fungal, helminth and protozoal diseases that occur mainly in the tropics and subtropics remain neglected, and hence the phrase "neglected tropical diseases" is used to characterize them [9]. The growing number of people travelling to the tropics means that it is imperative that there be more effective management of various public health issues by local authorities in the countries concerned, as well as by international bodies, tourist agencies and social groups, to enhance prevention and protection. Travellers should be considered as an integral part of the global surveillance network for emerging infections. Research and the knowledge gained can be used to alert the global community to the presence or susceptibility patterns of pathogens in different regions; to inform strategies that can be used to control infections in developing countries; and to prepare travellers to those areas and guide the care for those returning [4].

Tropical diseases transmitted via swimming pools and hot spring waters are less well understood than the hazards deriving from the use of unsafe food or drinking water. Also, secondary transmission occurs when travellers return to their homeland. Today, transmission at home is frequently related to climate change. Any climate change may alter the disease burden resulting from exposure to pathogens transmitted through recreational waters. In a study examining the impact of temperature, humidity, and precipitation on the incidence of reported West Nile virus infections in the US, increasing weekly maximum temperature and weekly cumulative temperature were similarly and significantly associated with a higher incidence of reported WNV infections [143].

Eighty three studies dealing with *Microsporidia, Leptospira, Schistosoma, Cryptosporidium, Amoebae,* viruses, and vectors breeding in swimming pools and hot springs in the tropics, and fulfilling pre-set criteria, have been included in this survey of the literature. The survey indicated that papers dealing with the quality of pool waters in the tropics are scarce, and information about infected tourists using pools is even less. The published literature, at least in international languages, presenting assessments and surveys of swimming establishments in the developing world are also scarce. Reasons for this neglect seem to be manifold including, as noted above, lesser awareness on this issue, not only in the developing, but also in the developed world. On the other hand, it is true that cases and outbreaks have been difficult to document because by its very nature travelling makes it difficult to follow up the cases in question and to carry out an epidemiological investigation. An international collaboration on this issue, along the lines of the European Legionnaires' Disease Surveillance Network (ELDSNet), would certainly be an important step forward. As emphasized in a review published by RIVM, it is becoming imperative that recreational waterborne infectious diseases be prioritized and quantified [144].

Castor and Beach have made several recommendations for the prevention and control of disease transmission in swimming venues. They recommend the redesign of aquatic facilities, increased governmental oversight of swimming pool maintenance and training of staff, and education of the public regarding healthy swimming habits. In addition, they recommend that high-risk groups, such as the elderly and infirm and pregnant women, should be made aware of their increased risk of illness as a result of swimming, even in apparently adequately disinfected swimming waters [145]. Tourists in general, and in particular tourists travelling to the tropical and subtropical countries of the developing world, should be included in the list of vulnerable citizens and provided with specific advice, services and care.

5. Conclusions

There is abundant information and guidance to travellers regarding precautions that need to be taken in respect of food, drinking water and air quality in tropical destinations. Nevertheless, information on the hazards presented by recreational and especially pool, spa and hot spring waters as a mode of transmission of pathogens is limited. The survey indicated that papers dealing with the quality of pool waters in the tropics are scarce, and information about infected tourists using pools is even less. In addition, the ongoing climate change may alter the disease burden resulting from exposure to pathogens transmitted through recreational waters. Under the pressure of a growing number of people undertaking international travel, and yet faster growth of such travel in the tropical and subtropical zones, assessments of the swimming pool establishments, research and prevention strategies for pool safety in the tropics are imperative. Public health authorities need to provide guidance to westerners travelling to exotic destinations on how to protect their health in swimming pools. An international collaboration on this issue would certainly be an important step forward.

Funding: This research received no external funding

Acknowledgments: We would like to thank John C. Davis, DipTransIoL for editing the English text.

Conflicts of Interest: The authors declare no conflict of interest.

References

1. World Tourism Organization, Tourism Highlights. 2017. Available online: http://www2.unwto.org/publication/unwto-tourism-highlights-2017 (accessed on 20 July 2018).
2. World Health Organization, International Travel and Health, 2012. Available online: http://www.who.int/ith (accessed on 20 July 2018).
3. World Health Organization. *Water, Sanitation and Health Team. Guidelines for Safe Recreational Water Environments. Volume 2, Swimming Pools and Similar Environments*; World Health Organization: Geneva, Switzerland, 2006; Available online: http://www.who.int/iris/handle/10665/43336 (accessed on 20 July 2018).
4. Baker, D.M. Tourism and the health effects of infectious diseases: Are there potential risks for tourists? *Int. J. Saf. Secur. Tour./Hosp.* **2015**, *12*, 1–17.
5. Barna, Z.; Kádár, M. The risk of contracting infectious diseases in public swimming pools. A review. *Annali dell Istituto Superiore di Sanità* **2012**, *48*, 374–386. [CrossRef]
6. TravelHealthPro. Available online: https://travelhealthpro.org.uk/ (accessed on 24 July 2018).
7. Page, J.S.; Essex, S.; Causevic, S. Tourist Attitudes Towards Water Use in the Developing World: A Comparative Analysis. *Tour. Manag. Perspect.* **2014**, *10*, 57–67. [CrossRef]
8. World Health Organization: WHO. Available online: www.who.int (accessed on 24 July 2018).
9. Utzinger, J.; Becker, S.L.; Knopp, S.; Blum, J.; Neumayr, A.L.; Keiser, J.; Hatz, C.F. Neglected tropical diseases: Diagnosis, clinical management, treatment and control. *Swiss Med. Wkly.* **2012**, *142*, w13727. [CrossRef]
10. Charrel, R.N.; de Lamballerie, X.; Raoult, D. Chikungunya outbreaks—The globalization of vector borne diseases. *N. Engl. J. Med.* **2007**, *356*, 769–771. [CrossRef]
11. Rammaert, B.; Beauté, J.; Borand, L.; Hem, S.; Buchy, P.; Goyet, S.; Guillard, B. Pulmonary melioidosis in Cambodia: A prospective study. *BMC Infect. Dis.* **2011**, *11*, 126–174. [CrossRef]
12. Goodman, R.A.; Buehler, J.W. Delinquent Mortgages, Neglected Swimming Pools and West Nile Virus, California. *Emerg. Infect. Dis.* **2009**, *15*, 508–509. [CrossRef]
13. Marten, G.; Harrison, C.; Nguyen, M.; Sacket, S.; Thompson, G.; Carroll, M.; Riegel, C. The Use of Gambusia to Control Mosquito Larvae in Abandoned Swimming Pools: The New Orleans Experience. New Orleans Mosquito, Termite & Rodent Control Board. 2013, pp. 1–70. Available online: http://www.gerrymarten.com/publicatons/pdfs/GM_new-orleans-swimming-pools.pdf (accessed on 24 July 2018).
14. Horney, J.; Goldberg, D.; Hammond, T.; Stone, K.; Smitherman, S. Assessing the Prevalence of Risk Factors for Neglected Tropical Diseases in Brazos County, Texas. *PLoS Curr.* **2017**, *9*. [CrossRef]
15. Caillouët, K.A.; Carlson, J.C.; Wesson, D.; Jordan, F. Colonization of abandoned swimming pools by larval mosquitoes and their predators following Hurricane Katrina. *J. Vector Ecol.* **2008**, *33*, 166–172. [CrossRef]
16. Hlavsa, M.C.; Hill, R.V.; Beach, J.M. Immediate closures and violations identified during routine inspections of Public Aquatic Facilities—Network for Aquatic Facility Inspection Surveillance, United States, 2013. *MMWR Surveill. Summ.* **2016**, *65*, 1–26. [CrossRef]
17. Hlavsa, C.M.; Cikesh, L.B.; Roberts, A.V.; Kahler, M.A.; Marissa, M.; Hilborn, D.E.; Wade, J.T.; Roellig, M.D.; Murphy, L.J.; Xiao, L.; et al. Outbreaks Associated with Treated Recreational Water—United States, 2000–2014. *MMWR Surveill. Summ.* **2018**, *67*, 547–551.
18. Chalmers, R.M. Waterborne ourbreaks of cryptosporodiasis. *Ann. Ist Super Sanita.* **2012**, *48*, 429–446. [CrossRef]

19. Mavridou, A.; Pappa, O.; Papatzitze, O.; Blougoura, A.; Drossos, P. An overview of pool and spa regulations in Mediterranean countries with a focus on the tourist industry. *J. Water Health* **2014**, *12*, 359–371. [CrossRef]

20. CliQ: Towards a Clean Future. Swimming Pool Regulations and Pool Market Analysis in the Tourism Sector. Available online: https://cliqib.org (accessed on 26 July 2018).

21. Abd-Rabbo, H. A new suggestion. Artificial plastic swimming pools as prophylactic measures against infection with schistosomiasis in developing countries. *J. Trop. Med. Hyg.* **1968**, *71*, 18–19.

22. Maghazy, S.M.N.; Abdel-Mallek, A.Y.; Bagy, M.M.K. Fungi in Two Swimming Pools in Assiut Town, Egypt. *Zentralbl. Mikrobiol.* **1989**, *144*, 213–216. [CrossRef]

23. Abdou, M.H.; Akel, M.M.; El-Shal, W.I.; El-Naggar, A.S. Study of the environmental health aspects of swimming pools in Alexandria City. *J. Egypt. Public Health Assoc.* **2005**, *80*, 263–296.

24. Abd El-Salam, M.M. Assessment of water quality of some swimming pools: A case study in Alexandria, Egypt. *Environ. Monit. Assess.* **2012**, *12*, 7395–7406. [CrossRef]

25. Even-Paz, Z.; Haas, H.; Sacks, T.; Rosenmann, E. Mycobacterium marinum skin infections mimicking cutaneous leishmaniasis. *Br. J. Dermatol.* **1976**, *94*, 435–442. [CrossRef]

26. Al-Khatib, I.A.; Salah, S. Bacteriological and chemical quality of swimming pools water in developing countries: A case study in the West Bank of Palestine. *Int. J. Environ. Health Res.* **2003**, *13*, 17–22. [CrossRef]

27. Rabi, A.; Khader, Y.; Alkafajei, A.; Aqoulah, A.A. Sanitary conditions of public swimming pools in Amman, Jordan. *Int. J. Environ. Res. Public Health* **2008**, *5*, 152–157. [CrossRef]

28. Ali-Shtayeh, M.S.; Khaleel, T.K.; Jamous, R.M. Ecology of dermatophytes and other keratinophilic fungi in swimming pools and polluted and unpolluted streams. *Mycopathologia* **2003**, *156*, 193–205. [CrossRef]

29. Courage Kosi Setsoafia Saba; Saviour Kojo Tekpor. Water Quality Assessment of Swimming Pools and Risk of Spreading Infections in Ghana. *Res. J. Microbiol.* **2015**, *10*, 14–23. [CrossRef]

30. Wei, X.; Li, J.; Hou, S.; Xu, C.; Zhang, H.; Atwill, E.R.; Li, X.; Yang, Z.; Chen, S. Assessment of Microbiological Safety of Water in Public Swimming Pools in Guangzhou, China. *Int. J. Environ. Res. Public Health* **2018**, *15*, 1416–1428. [CrossRef]

31. Rafiei, A.; Amirrajab, N. Fungal Contamination of Indoor Public Swimming Pools, Ahwaz, South-west of Iran. *Iran. J. Public Health* **2010**, *39*, 124–128.

32. Fadaei, A.; Amiri, M. Comparison of Chemical, Biological and Physical Quality Assessment of Indoor Swimming Pools in Shahrekord City, Iran in 2013. *Glob. J. Health Sci.* **2014**, *7*, 240–248. [CrossRef]

33. Rinder, H. Transmission of microsporidia to humans: Water-borne, food-borne, air-borne, zoonotic, or anthroponotic? *Southeast Asian J. Trop. Med. Public Health* **2004**, *35*, 54–57.

34. Joseph, J.; Vemuganti, G.K.; Sharma, S. Microsporidia: Emerging ocular pathogens. *Indian J. Med. Microbiol.* **2005**, *23*, 80–91. [CrossRef]

35. Dowd, S.E.; Gerba, C.P.; Pepper, I.L. Confirmation of the human-pathogenic microsporidia Enterocytozoon bieneusi, Encephalitozoon intestinalis, and Vittaforma corneae in water. *Appl. Environ. Microbiol.* **1998**, *64*, 3332–3335.

36. Hutin, Y.J.; Sombardier, M.N.; Liguory, O.; Sarfati, C.; Derouin, F.; Modaï, J.; Molina, J.M. Risk factors for intestinal microsporidiosis in patients with human immunodeficiency virus infection: A case-control study. *J. Infect. Dis.* **1998**, *178*, 904–907. [CrossRef]

37. Li, X.; Fayer, R. Infectivity of microsporidian spores exposed to temperature extremes and chemical disinfectants. *J. Eukaryot. Microbiol.* **2006**, *53*, S77–S79. [CrossRef]

38. Fournier, S.; Dubrou, S.; Liguory, O.; Gaussin, F.; Santillana-Hayat, M.; Sarfati, C.; Molina, J.M.; Derouin, F. Detection of Microsporidia, cryptosporidia and Giardia in swimming pools: A one-year prospective study. *FEMS Immunol. Med. Microbiol.* **2002**, *33*, 209–213. [CrossRef]

39. Sharma, S.; Das, S.; Joseph, J.; Vemuganti, G.K.; Murthy, S. Microsporidial keratitis: Need for increased awareness. *Surv. Ophthalmol.* **2011**, *56*, 1–22. [CrossRef]

40. Vemuganti, G.K.; Garg, P.; Sharma, S.; Joseph, J.; Gopinathan, U.; Singh, S. Is microsporidial keratitis an emerging cause of stromal keratitis? A case series study. *BMC Ophthalmol.* **2005**, *17*, 19–33. [CrossRef]

41. Curry, A.; Mudhar, H.S.; Dewan, S.; Canning, E.U.; Wagner, B.E. A case of bilateral microsporidial keratitis from Bangladesh–infection by an insect parasite from the genus Nosema. *J. Med. Microbiol.* **2007**, *56*, 1250–1252. [CrossRef]

42. Fan, N.-W.; Wu, C.-C.; Chen, T.-L.; Yu, W.-K.; Chen, C.-P.; Lee, S.-M.; Lin, P.-Y. Microsporidial Keratitis in Patients with Hot Springs Exposure. *J. Clin. Microbiol.* **2012**, *50*, 414–418. [CrossRef]

43. Karanis, P.; Kourenti, C.; Smith, H. Waterborne transmission of protozoan parasites: A worldwide review of outbreaks and lessons learnt. *J. Water Health* **2007**, *5*, 1–38. [CrossRef]
44. Baldursson, S.; Karanis, P. Waterborne transmission of protozoan parasites: Review of worldwide outbreaks—An update 2004–2010. *Water Res.* **2011**, *45*, 6603–6614. [CrossRef]
45. Efstratiou, A.; Ongerth, E.J.; Karanis, P. Waterborne transmission of protozoan parasites: Review of worldwide outbreaks—An update 2011–2016. *Water Res.* **2017**, *114*, 14–22. [CrossRef]
46. TropNet: European Network for Tropical Medicine and Travel Health. Available online: http://www.tropnet.net/ (accessed on 26 July 2018).
47. Lim, A.L.Y.; Nissapatorn, V. Transmission of waterborne parasites in the Association of Southeast Asian Nations (ASEAN): Overview and direction forward. *Food Waterborne Parasitol.* **2017**, *8–9*, 75–83. [CrossRef]
48. Plutzer, J.; Karanis, P. Neglected waterborne parasitic protozoa and their detection in water. *Water Res.* **2016**, *101*, 318–332. [CrossRef]
49. Centers for Disease Control and Prevention (CDC). Available online: https://search.cdc.gov/search/?query=schistosomes&sitelimit=&utf8=√&affiliate=cdc-main (accessed on 26 July 2018).
50. Boissier, J.; Grech-Angelini, S.; Webster, B.L.; Allienne, J.F.; Huyse, T.; Mas-Coma, S.; Toulza, E.; Barré-Cardi, H.; Rollinson, D.; Kincaid-Smith, J.; et al. Outbreak of urogenital schistosomiasis in Corsica (France): An epidemiological case study. *Lancet Infect. Dis.* **2016**, *16*, 971–979. [CrossRef]
51. Meltzer, E.; Artom, G.; Marva, E.; Assous, M.V.; Rahav, G.; Schwartzt, E. Schistosomiasis among travelers: New aspects of an old disease. *Emerg. Infect. Dis.* **2006**, *12*, 1696–1700. [CrossRef]
52. Clerinx, J.; Bottieau, E.; Wichmann, D.; Tannich, E.; Van Esbroeck, M. Acute schistosomiasis in a cluster of travelers from Rwanda: Diagnostic contribution of schistosome DNA detection in serum compared to parasitology and serology. *J. Travel. Med.* **2011**, *18*, 367–372. [CrossRef]
53. Marchese, V.; Beltrame, A.; Angheben, A.; Monteiro, G.B.; Giorli, G.; Perandin, F.; Buonfrate, D.; Bisoffi, Z. Schistosomiasis in immigrants, refugees and travellers in an Italian referral centre for tropical diseases. *Infect. Dis. Poverty* **2018**, *7*, 55–65. [CrossRef]
54. Röser, D.; Bjerrum, S.; Helleberg, M.; Nielsen, H.V.; David, K.P.; Thybo, S.; Stensvold, C.R. Adventure tourism and schistosomiasis: Serology and clinical findings in a group of Danish students after white-water rafting in Uganda. *JMM Case Rep.* **2018**, *5*, e005141. [CrossRef]
55. Coltart, C.E.; Chew, A.; Storrar, N.; Armstrong, M.; Suff, N.; Morris, L.; Chiodini, P.L.; Whitty, C.J. Schistosomiasis presenting in travellers: A 15 year observational study at the Hospital for Tropical Diseases, London. *Trans. R. Soc. Trop. Med. Hyg.* **2015**, *109*, 214–220. [CrossRef]
56. Grobusch, M.P.; Mühlberger, N.; Jelinek, T.; Bisoffi, Z.; Corachán, M.; Harms, G.; Matteelli, A.; Fry, G.; Hatz, C.; Gjørup, I.; et al. Imported schistosomiasis in Europe: Sentinel surveillance data from TropNetEurop. *J. Travel Med.* **2003**, *10*, 164–169. [CrossRef]
57. Kpoda, N.W.; Sorgho, H.; Poda, J.N.; Ouédraogo, J.B.; Kabré, G.B. Schistosomiasis caused by Schistosoma mansoni in the Kou valley: Characterization of the transmission system and socioeconomic impact. *C. R. Biol.* **2013**, *336*, 284–288. [CrossRef]
58. El-Khoby, T.; Galal, N.; Fenwick, A.; Barakat, R.; El-Hawey, A.; Nooman, Z.; Habib, M.; Abdel-Wahab, F.; Gabr, N.S.; Hammam, H.M.; et al. The epidemiology of schistosomiasis in Egypt: Summary findings in nine governorates. *Am. J. Trop. Med. Hyg.* **2000**, *62*, 88–99. [CrossRef]
59. Corachan, M.; Ruiz, L.; Valls, M.E.; Gascon, J. Schistosomiasis and the Dogon country (Mali). *Am. J. Trop. Med. Hyg.* **1992**, *47*, 6–9. [CrossRef]
60. Logan, S.; Armstrong, M.; Moore, E.; Nebbia, G.; Jarvis, J.; Suvari, M.; Bligh, J.; Chiodini, P.L.; Brown, M.; Doherty, T. Acute Schistosomiasis in Travelers:14 Years' Experience at the Hospital for Tropical Diseases, London. *Am. J. Trop. Med. Hyg.* **2013**, *88*, 1032–1034. [CrossRef]
61. Colebunders, R.; Verstraeten, T.; Van Gompel, A.; Van den Ende, J.; De Roo, A.; Polderman, A.; Visser, L. Acute Schistosomiasis in Travelers Returning from Mali. *J. Travel Med.* **1995**, *2*, 235–238. [CrossRef]
62. Enk, J.M.; Amorim, A.; Schall, T.V. Acute schistosomiasis outbreak in the metropolitan area of Belo Horizonte, Minas Gerais: Alert about the risk of unnoticed transmission increased by growing rural tourism. *Mem. Inst. Oswaldo Cruz.* **2003**, *98*, 745–750. [CrossRef]

63. Lambertucci, J.R.; Drummond, S.C.; Voieta, I.; de Queiróz, L.C.; Pereira, P.P.; Chaves, B.A.; Botelho, P.P.; Prata, P.H.; Otoni, A.; Vilela, J.F.; et al. An outbreak of acute Schistosoma mansoni Schistosomiasis in a nonendemic area of Brazil: A report on 50 cases, including 5 with severe clinical manifestations. *Clin. Infect. Dis.* **2013**, *57*, e1–e6. [CrossRef]

64. Ndassa, A.; Mimpfoundi, R.; Gake, B.; Paul Martin, M.V.; Poste, B. Risk factors for human schistosomiasis in the Upper Benue valley, in northern Cameroon. *Ann. Trop. Med. Parasitol.* **2007**, *101*, 469–477. [CrossRef]

65. Visser, L.G.; Polderman, A.M.; Stuiver, P.C. Outbreak of schistosomiasis among travelers returning from Mali, West Africa. *Clin. Infect. Dis.* **1995**, *20*, 280–285. [CrossRef]

66. Xiao, S.; Yin, P.; Zhang, Y.; Hu, S. Occurrence of Cryptosporidium and Giardia and the Relationship between Protozoa and Water Quality Indicators in Swimming Pools. *Korean J. Parasitol.* **2017**, *55*, 129–135. [CrossRef]

67. Centers for Disease Control and Prevention: Parasites-Cryptosporodium (also known as 'Crypto'). Available online: https://www.cdc.gov/parasites/crypto/ (accessed on 26 July 2018).

68. Coetzee, N.; Edeghere, O.; Orendi, J.; Chalmers, R.; Morgan, L. A swimming pool-associated outbreak of cryptosporidiosis in Staffordshire, England, October to December 2007. *Euro Surveill.* **2008**, *13*, 19028.

69. Insulander, M.; Lebbad, M.; Stenström, T.A.; Svenungsson, B. An outbreak of cryptosporidiosis associated with exposure to swimming pool water. *Scand. J. Infect. Dis.* **2005**, *37*, 354–360. [CrossRef]

70. Shields, J.M.; Gleim, E.R.; Beach, M.J. Prevalence of Cryptosporidium spp. and Giardia intestinalis in Swimming Pools, Atlanta, Georgia. *Emerg. Infect. Dis.* **2008**, *14*, 948–950. [CrossRef]

71. Wheeler, C.; Vugia, D.J.; Thomas, G.; Beach, M.J.; Carnes, S.; Maier, T.; Gorman, J.; Xiao, L.; Arrowood, M.J.; Gilliss, D.; et al. Outbreak of cryptosporidiosis at a California waterpark: Employee and patron roles and the long road towards prevention. *Epidemiol. Infect.* **2007**, *135*, 302–310. [CrossRef]

72. Ichinohe, S.; Fukushima, T.; Kishida, K.; Sanbe, K.; Saika, S.; Ogura, M. Secondary Transmission of Cryptosporidiosis Associated with Swimming Pool Use. *Jpn. J. Infect. Dis.* **2005**, *58*, 400–401.

73. Lal, A.; Cornish, L.M.; Fearnley, E.; Glass, K.; Kirk, M. Cryptosporidiosis: A Disease of Tropical and Remote Areas in Australia. *PLoS Negl. Trop. Dis.* **2015**, *9*, e0004078. [CrossRef]

74. GBD Mortality Causes of Death Collaborators. Global, regional, and national age-sex specific all-cause and cause-specific mortality for 240 causes of death, 1990–2013: A systematic analysis for the Global Burden of Disease Study 2013. *Lancet* **2015**, *385*, 117–171. [CrossRef]

75. Dale, K.; Kirk, M.; Sinclair, M.; Hall, R.; Leder, K. Reported waterborne outbreaks of gastrointestinal disease in Australia are predominantly associated with recreational exposure. *Aust. N. Z. J. Public Health* **2010**, *34*, 527–530. [CrossRef]

76. Ryan, U.; Lawler, S.; Reid, S. Limiting swimming pool outbreaks of cryptosporidiosis—The roles of regulations, staff, patrons and research. *J. Water Health* **2017**, *15*, 1–16. [CrossRef]

77. Onichandran, S.; Kumar, T.; Salibay, C.C.; Dungca, Z.J.; Tabo, A.H.; Tabo, N.; Tan, T.C.; Lim, A.Y.; Sawangjaroen, N.; Phiriyasamith, S.; et al. Waterborne parasites: A current status from the Philippines. *Parasit. Vectors* **2014**, *7*, 244–252. [CrossRef]

78. Ng-Hublin, J.S.; Hargrave, D.; Combs, B.; Ryan, U. Investigation of a swimming pool-associated cryptosporidiosis outbreak in the Kimberley region of Western Australia. *Epidemiol. Infect.* **2015**, *143*, 1037–1041. [CrossRef]

79. Centers for Disease Control and Prevention: Parasites-Acantamobea. Available online: https://www.cdc.gov/parasites/acanthamoeba/ (accessed on 26 July 2018).

80. Visvesvara, G.S.; Moura, H.; Schuster, F.L. Pathogenic and opportunistic free-living amoebae: Acanthamoeba spp., Balamuthia mandrillaris, Naegleria fowleri, and Sappinia diploidea. *FEMS Immunol. Med. Microbiol.* **2007**, *50*, 1–26. [CrossRef]

81. De Jonckheere, J.F. Pathogenic free-living amoebae in swimming pools: Survey in Belgium. *Ann. Microbiol.* **1979**, *130B*, 205–212.

82. Lyons, T.B.; Kapur, R. Limax Amoebae in Public Swimming Pools of Albany, Schenectady, and Rensselaer Counties, New York: Their Concentration, Correlations, and Significance. *Appl. Environ. Microbiol.* **1977**, *33*, 551–555.

83. Heggie, T.W. Swimming with death: Naegleria fowleri infections in recreational waters. *Travel. Med. Infect. Dis.* **2010**, *8*, 201–206. [CrossRef]

84. Rivera, F.; Ramírez, P.; Vilaclara, G.; Robles, E.; Medina, F. A survey of pathogenic and free-living amoebae inhabiting swimming pool water in Mexico City. *Environ. Res.* **1983**, *32*, 205–211. [CrossRef]

85. Su, M.Y.; Lee, M.S.; Shyu, L.Y.; Lin, W.C.; Hsiao, P.C.; Wang, C.P.; Lai, S.C. A Fatal Case of Naegleria fowleri Meningoencephalitis in Taiwan. *Korean J. Parasitol.* **2013**, *51*, 203–206. [CrossRef]
86. Al-Herrawy, A.Z.; Khalil, M.I.; El-Sherif, S.S.; Omar, F.A.E.; Lotfy, W.M. Surveillance and Molecular Identification of Acanthamoeba and Naegleria Species in Two Swimming Pools in Alexandria University. Egypt. *Iran. J. Parasitol.* **2017**, *12*, 196–205.
87. Init, I.; Lau, Y.L.; Arin Fadzlun, A.; Foead, A.I.; Neilson, R.S.; Nissapatorn, V. Detection of free living amoebae, Acanthamoeba and Naegleria, in swimming pools, Malaysia. *Trop. Biomed.* **2010**, *27*, 566–577.
88. Rivera, F.; Ramírez, E.; Bonilla, P.; Calderón, A.; Gallegos, E.; Rodríguez, S.; Ortiz, R.; Zaldívar, B.; Ramírez, P.; Durán, A. Pathogenic and Free-living Amoebae Isolated from Swimming Pools and Physiotherapy Tubs in Mexico. *Environ. Res.* **1993**, *62*, 43–52. [CrossRef]
89. Caumo, K.; Frasson, A.P.; Pens, C.J.; Panatieri, L.F.; Frazzon, A.P.; Rott, M.B. Potentially pathogenic Acanthamoeba in swimming pools: A survey in the southern Brazilian city of Porto Alegre. *Ann. Trop. Med. Parasitol.* **2009**, *103*, 477–485. [CrossRef]
90. Al-Herrawy, A.; Bahgat, M.; Mohammed, A.; Ashour, A.; Hikal, W. Morpho-Physiological and Biochemical Criteria of Acanthamoeba spp. Isolated from the Egyptian Aquatic Environment. *Iran. J. Parasitol.* **2013**, *8*, 302–312.
91. Fabres, L.F.; Rosa Dos Santos, S.P.; Benitez, L.B.; Rott, M.B. Isolation and identification of Acanthamoeba spp. from thermal swimming pools and spas in Southern Brazil. *Acta Parasitol.* **2016**, *61*, 221–227. [CrossRef]
92. Alves Dde, S.; Moraes, A.S.; Nitz, N.; de Oliveira, M.G.; Hecht, M.M.; Gurgel-Gonçalves, R.; Cuba, C.A. Occurrence and characterization of Acanthamoeba similar to genotypes T4, T5, and T2/T6 isolated from environmental sources in Brasília, Federal District, Brazil. *Exp. Parasitol.* **2012**, *131*, 239–244. [CrossRef]
93. Rahdar, M.; Niyyati, M.; Salehi, M.; Feghhi, M.; Makvandi, M.; Pourmehdi, M.; Farnia, S. Isolation and genotyping of acanthamoeba strains from environmental sources in Ahvaz city, Khuzestan province, southern Iran. *Iran. J. Parasitol.* **2012**, *7*, 22–26.
94. Evyapan, G.; Koltas, I.S.; Eroglu, F. Genotyping of Acanthamoeba T15: The environmental strain in Turkey. *Trans. R. Soc. Trop. Med. Hyg.* **2015**, *109*, 221–224. [CrossRef]
95. Ithoi, I.; Ahmad, A.F.; Nissapatorn, V.; Lau, Y.L.; Mahmud, R.; Mak, J.W. Detection of Naegleria species in environmental samples from peninsular Malaysia. *PLoS ONE* **2011**, *6*, e24327. [CrossRef]
96. de Vries, S.G.; Visser, B.J.; Nagel, I.M.; Goris, M.G.; Hartskeerl, R.A.; Grobusch, M.P. Leptospirosis in Sub-Saharan Africa: A systematic review. *Int. J. Infect. Dis.* **2014**, *28*, 47–64. [CrossRef]
97. Patil, D.Y.; Dahake, R.V.; Chowdhary, A.S.; Deshmukh, R.A. Clinico-epidemiological observations of human leptospirosis from Mumbai, India. *J. Infect. Public Health* **2017**, *10*, 247–248. [CrossRef]
98. Sehgal, S.C. Epidemiological patterns of leptospirosis. *Indian J. Med. Microbiol.* **2006**, *24*, 310–311. [CrossRef]
99. Gelman, S.S.; Gundlapalli, A.V.; Hale, D.; Croft, A.; Hindiyeh, M.; Carroll, K.C. Spotting the spirochete: Rapid diagnosis of leptospirosis in two returned travelers. *J. Travel Med.* **2006**, *9*, 165–167. [CrossRef]
100. Leshem, E.; Segal, G.; Barnea, A.; Yitzhaki, S.; Ostfeld, I.; Pitlik, S.; Schwartz, E. Travel-Related Leptospirosis in Israel: A Nationwide Study. *Am. J. Trop. Med. Hyg.* **2010**, *82*, 459–463. [CrossRef]
101. Pimenta, D.; Democratis, J. Risky behavior: A rare complication of an uncommon disease in a returning traveler. *BMJ Case Rep.* **2013**. [CrossRef]
102. Bandara, M.; Ananda, M.; Wickramage, K.; Berger, E.; Agampodi, S. Globalization of leptospirosis through travel and migration. *Glob. Health* **2014**, *10*, 61–70. [CrossRef]
103. van de Werve, C.; Perignon, A.; Jauréguiberry, S.; Bricaire, F.; Bourhy, P.; Caumes, E. Travel-related leptospirosis: A series of 15 imported cases. *J. Travel Med.* **2013**, *20*, 228–231. [CrossRef]
104. Brinker, A.J.; Blazes, D.L. An outbreak of Leptospirosis among United States military personnel in Guam. *Trop. Dis. Travel Med. Vaccines* **2017**, *3*, 16. [CrossRef]
105. Grobusch, M.P.; Bollmann, R.; Schönberg, A.; Slevogt, H.; Garcia, V.; Teichmann, D.; Jelinek, T.; Flick, H.; Bergmann, F.; Rosseau, S.; et al. Leptospirosis in Travelers Returning from the Dominican Republic. *J. Travel Med.* **2003**, *10*, 55–58. [CrossRef]
106. Hauri, A.M.; Schimmelpfennig, M.; Walter-Domes, M.; Letz, A.; Diedrich, S.; Lopez-Pila, J.; Schreier, E. An outbreak of viral meningitis associated with a public swimming pond. *Epidemiol. Infect.* **2005**, *133*, 291–298. [CrossRef]

107. D'Angelo, L.J.; Hieholzer, J.C.; Keenlyside, R.A.; Anderson, L.J.; Martone, W.J. Pharyngoconjunctival fever caused by adenovirus type 4: Report of a swimming pool-related outbreak with recovery of virus from pool water. *J. Infect. Dis.* **1979**, *140*, 42–47. [CrossRef]

108. Maunula, L.; Kalso, S.; Von Bonsdorff, C.H.; Pönkä, A. Wading pool water contaminated with both noroviruses and astroviruses as the source of a gastroenteritis outbreak. *Epidemiol. Infect.* **2004**, *132*, 737–743. [CrossRef]

109. Morbidity and Mortality Weekly Report (MMWR). An Outbreak of Norovirus Gastroenteritis at a Swimming Club—Vermont. *Wkly Rep.* **2004**, *53*, 793–795. Available online: https://www.cdc.gov/mmwr/preview/mmwrhtml/mm5334a5.htm (accessed on 30 July 2018).

110. Sinclair, R.G.; Jones, E.L.; Gerba, C.P. Viruses in recreational water-borne disease outbreaks: A review. *J. Appl. Microbiol.* **2009**, *107*, 1769–1780. [CrossRef]

111. Mahoney, F.J.; Farley, T.A.; Kelso, K.Y.; Wilson, S.A.; Horan, J.M.; McFarland, L.M. An outbreak of hepatitis A associated with swimming in a public pool. *J. Infect. Dis.* **1992**, *165*, 613–618. [CrossRef]

112. Tallis, G.; Gregory, J. An outbreak of hepatitis A associated with a spa pool. *Commun. Dis. Intell.* **1997**, *21*, 353–354.

113. Faustini, A.; Fano, V.; Muscillo, M.; Zaniratti, S.; La Rosa, G.; Tribuzi, L.; Perucci, C.A. An outbreak of aseptic meningitis due to echovirus 30 associated with attending school and swimming in pools. *Int. J. Infect. Dis.* **2006**, *10*, 291–297. [CrossRef]

114. Harley, D.; Harrower, B.; Lyon, M.; Dick, A. A primary school outbreak of pharyngo-conjunctival fever caused by adenovirus type 3. *Commun. Dis. Intell.* **2001**, *25*, 9–12.

115. Van Heerden, J.; Ehlers, M.M.; Grabow, W.O. Detection and risk assessment of adenoviruses in swimming pool water. *J. Appl. Microbiol.* **2005**, *99*, 1256–1264. [CrossRef]

116. Staggemeier, R.; Arantes, T.; Caumo, K.S.; Rott, M.B.; Spilki, F.R. Detection and quantification of human adenovirus genomes in Acanthamoeba isolated from swimming pools. *An. Acad. Bras. Cienc.* **2016**, *88*, 635–641. [CrossRef]

117. Yeats, J.; Smuts, H.; Serfontein, C.J.; Kannemeyer, J. Investigation into a school enterovirus outbreak using PCR detection and serotype identification based on the 5′ non-coding region. *Epidemiol. Infect.* **2005**, *133*, 1123–1130. [CrossRef]

118. Shih, Y.J.; Tao, C.W.; Tsai, H.C.; Huang, W.C.; Huang, T.Y.; Chen, J.S.; Chiu, Y.C.; Hsu, T.K.; Hsu, B.M. First detection of enteric adenoviruses genotype 41 in recreation spring areas of Taiwan. *Environ. Sci. Pollut. Res. Int.* **2017**, *24*, 18392–18399. [CrossRef]

119. Li, J.; Lu, X.; Sun, Y.; Lin, C.; Li, F.; Yang, Y.; Liang, Z.; Jia, L.; Chen, L.; Jiang, B.; et al. A swimming pool-associated outbreak of pharyngoconjunctival fever caused by human adenovirus type 4 in Beijing, China. *Int. J. Infect. Dis.* **2018**, *75*, 89–91. [CrossRef]

120. Komar, N. West Nile virus: Epidemiology and ecology in North America. *Adv. Virus Res.* **2003**, *61*, 185–234.

121. Petersen, L.R.; Brault, A.C.; Nasci, R.S. West Nile Virus: Review of the Literature. *JAMA* **2013**, *310*, 308–315. [CrossRef]

122. Chen, H.L.; Tang, R.B. Why Zika virus infection has become a public health concern? *Chin. Med. Assoc.* **2016**, *79*, 174–178. [CrossRef]

123. Rogers, D.J.; Wilson, A.J.; Hay, S.I.; Graham, A.J. The Global Distribution of Yellow Fever and Dengue. *Adv. Parasitol.* **2006**, *62*, 181–220. [CrossRef]

124. Mackenzie, J.S.; Gubler, D.J.; Petersen, L.R. Emerging flaviviruses: The spread and resurgence of Japanese encephalitis, West Nile and dengue viruses. *Nat. Med.* **2004**, *10*, 98–109. [CrossRef]

125. Succo, T.; Noel, H.; Nikolay, B.; Maquart, M.; Cochet, A.; Leparc-Goffart, I.; Catelinois, O.; Salje, H.; Pelat, C.; de Crouy-Chanel, P.; et al. Dengue sero-survey after a 2-month long outbreak in Nîmes, France, 2015: Was there more than met the eye? *Euro Surveill.* **2018**, *23*. [CrossRef]

126. Patsoula, E.; Vakali, A.; Balatsos, G.; Pervanidou, D.; Beleri, S.; Tegos, N.; Baka, A.; Spanakos, G.; Georgakopoulou, T.; Tserkezou, P.; et al. West Nile Virus Circulation in Mosquitoes in Greece (2010–2013). *Biomed. Res. Int.* **2016**, *2016*, 2450682. [CrossRef]

127. Coulibaly, B.; Kone, R.; Barry, M.B.; Emerson, B.; Coulibaly, M.B.; Niare, O.; Beavogui, A.H.; Traore, S.F.; Vernick, K.D.; Riehle, M.M. Malaria vector populations across ecological zones in Guinea Conakry and Mali, West Africa. *Malar. J.* **2016**, *15*, 191–201. [CrossRef]

128. Matthys, B.; Koudou, B.G.; N'Goran, E.K.; Vounatsou, P.; Gosoniu, L.; Koné, M.; Gissé, G.; Utzinger, J. Spatial dispersion and characterization of mosquito breeding habitats in urban vegetable-production areas of Abidjan, Côte d'Ivoire. *Ann. Trop. Med. Parasitol.* **2010**, *104*, 649–666. [CrossRef]

129. Kwong, J.C.; Druce, J.D.; Leder, K. Zika virus infection acquired during brief travel to Indonesia. *Am. J. Trop. Med. Hyg.* **2013**, *89*, 516–517. [CrossRef]

130. Fonseca, K.; Meatherall, B.; Zarra, D.; Drebot, M.; MacDonald, J.; Pabbaraju, K.; Wong, S.; Webster, P.; Lindsay, R.; Tellier, R. First case of Zika virus infection in a returning Canadian traveler. *Am. J. Trop. Med. Hyg.* **2014**, *91*, 1035–1038. [CrossRef]

131. Salehuddin, A.R.; Haslan, H.; Mamikutty, N.; Zaidun, N.H.; Azmi, M.F.; Senin, M.M.; Syed Ahmad Fuad, S.B.; Thent, Z.C. Zika virus infection and its emerging trends in Southeast Asia. *Asian Pac. J. Trop. Med.* **2017**, *10*, 211–219. [CrossRef]

132. De Silva, M.P.; Marshall, J.M. Factors Contributing to Urban Malaria Transmission in Sub-Saharan Africa: A Systematic Review. *J. Trop. Med.* **2012**, *2012*, 819563. [CrossRef]

133. Impoinvil, D.E.; Mbogo, C.M.; Keating, J.; Beier, J.C. The role of unused swimming pools as a habitat for Anopheles immature stages in urban Malindi, Kenya. *J. Am. Mosq. Control Assoc.* **2009**, *24*, 457–459. [CrossRef]

134. Impoinvil, D.E.; Keating, J.; Mbogo, C.M.; Potts, M.D.; Chowdhury, R.R.; Beier, J.C. Abundance of immature Anopheles and culicines (Diptera: Culicidae) in different water body types in the urban environment of Malindi, Kenya. *J. Vector Ecol.* **2008**, *33*, 107–116. [CrossRef]

135. Gadiaga, L.; Machault, V.; Pagès, F.; Gaye, A.; Jarjaval, F.; Godefroy, L.; Cissé, B.; Lacaux, J.P.; Sokhna, C.; Trape, J.F.; et al. Conditions of malaria transmission in Dakar from 2007 to 2010. *Malar. J.* **2011**, *21*, 312–328. [CrossRef]

136. Dibo, M.R.; Fávaro, E.A.; Parra, M.C.; Santos, T.C.; Cassiano, J.H.; Deitz, K.V.; Pagliotto, A.M.; Zini, N.; Benetti, D.R.; Chiaravalloti-Neto, F. Evaluation of two sweeping methods for estimating the number of immature Aedes aegypti (Diptera: Culicidae) in large containers. *Rev. Soc. Bras. Med. Trop.* **2013**, *46*, 502–505. [CrossRef]

137. Courtright, P.; Rotondo, L.; MacArthur, C.; Jones, I.; Weaver, A.; Negash, B.K.; Olobio, N.; Binnawi, K.; Bush, S.; Abdala, M.; et al. Strengthening the links between mapping, planning and global engagement for disease elimination: Lessons learnt from trachoma. *Br. J. Ophthalmol.* **2018**, *102*, 1324–1327. [CrossRef]

138. 51st World Health Assembly, Geneva, Resolution WHA51.11, Global Elimination of Blinding Trachoma, 1988. Available online: http://www.who.int/blindness/causes/WHA51.11/en/ (accessed on 30 July 2018).

139. Warren, J.M.; Birrell, A.L. Trachoma in remote Indigenous Australia: A review and public health perspective. *Aust. N. Z. J. Public Health* **2016**, *40*, 48–52. [CrossRef]

140. Yamazaki, T.; Inoue, M.; Ogawa, M.; Shiga, S.; Kishimoto, T.; Hagiwara, T.; Matsumoto, T.; Hayashi, T. Inactivation of Chlamydia trachomatis and Chlamydia (Chlamydophila) pneumoniae by ozone. *Lett. Appl. Microbiol.* **2004**, *38*, 406–409. [CrossRef]

141. Giampaoli, S.; Garrec, N.; Donzi, G.; Valeriani, F.; Erdinger, L.; Romano Spica, V. Regulations concerning natural swimming ponds in Europe: Considerations on public health issues. *J. Water Health* **2004**, *12*, 564–572. [CrossRef]

142. Gössling, S.; Peeters, P.; Hall, M.C.; Ceron, J.-P.; Dubois, G.; Lehmann, V.; Scot, D. Progress in Tourism Management Tourism and water use: Supply, demand and security. An international review. *Tour. Manag.* **2012**, *33*, 1–15. [CrossRef]

143. Soverow, J.E.; Wellenius, G.A.; Fisman, D.N.; Mittleman, M.A. Infectious Disease in a Warming World: How Weather Influenced West Nile Virus in the United States (2001–2005). *Environ. Health Perspect.* **2009**, *117*, 1049–1052. [CrossRef]

144. de Roda Husman, A.M.; Schets, F.M. Climate Change and Recreational Water-Related Infectious Diseases, RIVM Publications, 2010. Available online: http://hdl.handle.net/10029/258107 (accessed on 30 July 2018).

145. Castor, M.L.; Beach, M.J. Reducing illness transmission from disinfected recreational water venues: Swimming, diarrhea and the emergence of a new public health concern. *Pediatr. Infect. Dis. J.* **2004**, *23*, 866–870. [CrossRef]

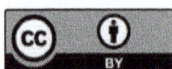

International Journal of
Environmental Research and Public Health

MDPI

Review

A Review and Update on Waterborne Viral Diseases Associated with Swimming Pools

Lucia Bonadonna * and Giuseppina La Rosa *

Italian National Institute of Health, Viale Regina Elena, 299-00161 Rome, Italy
* Correspondence: lucia.bonadonna@iss.it (L.B.); giuseppina.larosa@iss.it (G.L.R.); Tel.: +39-06-49902317 (L.B.); +39-06-49902718 (G.L.R.)

Received: 8 November 2018; Accepted: 5 January 2019; Published: 9 January 2019

Abstract: Infectious agents, including bacteria, viruses, protozoa, and molds, may threaten the health of swimming pool bathers. Viruses are a major cause of recreationally-associated waterborne diseases linked to pools, lakes, ponds, thermal pools/spas, rivers, and hot springs. They can make their way into waters through the accidental release of fecal matter, body fluids (saliva, mucus), or skin flakes by symptomatic or asymptomatic carriers. We present an updated overview of epidemiological data on viral outbreaks, a project motivated, among other things, by the availability of improved viral detection methodologies. Special attention is paid to outbreak investigations (source of the outbreak, pathways of transmission, chlorination/disinfection). Epidemiological studies on incidents of viral contamination of swimming pools under non-epidemic conditions are also reviewed.

Keywords: adenovirus; enterovirus; hepatitis A virus; norovirus; swimming pool; waterborne disease

1. Introduction

Swimming pools have been implicated in the transmission of infections. The risk of infection has mainly been linked to fecal contamination of the water, generally due to feces released by bathers or to contaminated source water. Failure in disinfection has been recorded as the main cause of many of the outbreaks associated with swimming pools.

The majority of reported swimming pool-related outbreaks have been caused by enteric viruses [1,2]. Sinclair and collaborators reported that 48% of viral outbreaks occur in swimming pools, 40% in lakes or ponds, and the remaining 12% in fountains, hot springs, and rivers (4% each) [1].

Viruses cannot replicate outside their host's tissues and cannot multiply in the environment. Therefore, the presence of viruses in a swimming pool is the result of direct contamination by bathers, who may shed viruses through unintentional fecal release, or through the release of body fluids such as saliva, mucus, or vomitus [3]. Evidence suggests that skin may also be a potential source of pathogenic viruses.

2. Materials and Methods

We carried out a comprehensive literature review aimed at investigating waterborne viral outbreaks linked to swimming pools, to explore the etiological agents implicated, pathways of transmission, associations between indicator organisms and disease, and key issues related to chlorination/disinfection procedures. Viral outbreaks are summarized in Table 1. The presence of enteric viruses in swimming pools under non-epidemic conditions was also reviewed. Different databases (Scopus, PubMed, and Google Scholar) were accessed using the terms norovirus, Norwalk virus, adenovirus, enterovirus, echovirus, coxsackievirus, and hepatitis A, in combination with terms recreation, swimming, pool, and water.

3. Viral Outbreaks Related to Swimming Pools

3.1. Adenovirus Outbreaks (N° = 15)

Adenoviruses are the enteric viruses most commonly associated with swimming pool-related outbreaks. Human adenoviruses (HAdVs) belong to the Adenoviridae family and are classified into seven species (A to G) and more than 90 types [4]. HAdVs are of major public health importance and can result in a variety of clinical manifestations, including gastroenteritis, respiratory, ocular and urinary tract infections [5]. Illnesses are common and ubiquitous with a worldwide distribution. HAdVs are highly stable in the environment and can survive for prolonged periods in water [6]. Transmission in swimming pools can occur by ingestion, direct contact with contaminated water, or through the inhalation of aerosol [7].

A Brazilian study recently detected HAdVs in *Acanthamoeba* isolated from water samples collected from swimming pools [8]. HAdVs were found in 62.5% (10/16) of amoebae with DNA copies up to 5.1×10^5 per milliliter, suggesting that *Acanthamoeba* may act as a reservoir and promote HAdV transmission through water.

The first swimming pool-related outbreak, published in 1953, described a 1951 outbreak in Greeley, Colorado, which thus came to be known as the "Greeley epidemic". The outbreak, involving 206 cases, caused a combination of symptoms, such as acute conjunctivitis, pharyngitis, muscle pain, and fever [9]. Between 25% and 50% of children swimming in the pool were affected. The transmission apparently occurred either by contact with contaminated objects, such as toys, or while swimming in a pool. The water was heavily chlorinated, with residual chlorine being close to 0.4 parts per million. No definite pathogen was identified at the time of publication. Serum samples from Greeley patients were later tested and showed a specific neutralizing antibody response to HAdV type 3 [10].

In 1954, an epidemic of pharyngeal-conjunctival fever occurred in Washington, D.C., with symptoms similar to those of the Greeley epidemic [10]. Over 300 cases were documented, with acute respiratory illness characterized by one or more of the following symptoms: fever, pharyngitis, and conjunctivitis. Cases occurred in all age groups, but predominantly in children. Adenovirus type 3 was isolated in 80 of 300 patients from eye, throat washings and stools. The disease occurred at different sites: in a children's summer day camp, in an orphanage, and in two residential neighborhoods. The suspected, but never confirmed, source of the epidemic was a swimming pool, even if cases due to direct contact were also recorded in houses and hospitals. The pool, chlorinated by hand, showed a low level of residual chlorine. Bell and collaborators were the first to suggest the term pharyngoconjunctival fever for this disease.

In August 1955, 112 cases of pharyngoconjunctival fever occurred in Toronto, linked to an indoor swimming pool. Seventy-four of the cases were children who had swum in the pool, while the others had swum in pools elsewhere, or had had direct contact with a case at home. Only one case had no history of either swimming or direct contact. Most of the children had pharyngitis, fever, malaise, and muscle pain. Conjunctivitis was absent or minimal in children, but was the main cause of discomfort in adults [11].

Another outbreak of pharyngoconjunctival fever was documented in August and September 1959 in Saitama Prefecture, Japan, among students of a primary and a middle school [12]. Epidemiological investigations suggested that the outbreak was mainly due to the contamination of a swimming pool used by the students of both schools. A total of 358 students were affected: 248 primary school students (attack rate, 20.6%) and 110 middle school students (attack rate, 19.2%). Laboratory findings suggested that the epidemic was due to HAdVs 3 and 7.

Foy and coworkers described an outbreak of pharyngoconjunctival fever (45 cases) in two swimming teams in Washington in 1966. Adenovirus type 3 was the etiological agent [13]. Most of the infected children had fever, pharyngitis, conjunctivitis, and diarrhea. In adults, symptoms were milder, with a high incidence of conjunctivitis. The attack rate was 65% and 67% for the two teams, respectively. Children had swum in the early morning, when the chlorinator of the pool was switched off, to avoid eye irritation with chlorine. Within one week, 25 of the 36 exposed swimmers became ill. Children swimming in the afternoon, when chlorination was still working, did not get sick. The infection was shown to spread in families having index cases (20 infected contacts). Analyses of water were done approximately 14 days after the presumed exposure. For this reason, attempts to isolate the virus from the water failed.

An outbreak of acute conjunctivitis due to HAdV type 7 occurred in Kansas, USA in 1973: 44 cases and one hospitalization were documented [14]. Eye symptoms predominated (red or pink eyes, swollen eyes), but a variety of other signs were also noted (mainly fever, headache, and nausea). A school swimming pool was identified as the source of infection. Chlorine concentration was low due to an equipment failure. The epidemic was easily controlled by raising the pool's chlorine level. Unfortunately, tests for viruses and bacterial indicators were carried out after super-chlorination and consequently results were negative.

In 1977, two outbreaks associated with swimming pools occurred in Georgia, USA. The first, due to HAdV type 3, involved at least 105 cases [15], with patients showing different symptoms, including sore throat, fever, headache, anorexia and conjunctivitis. In this case, a private swimming pool was the source of infection. A temporary malfunction in the water filtration system of the pool associated with inadequate chlorine levels was recorded. Both waterborne and person-to-person transmission occurred. In the second outbreak, HAdV type 4 was recognized as the etiological agent of pharyngoconjunctival fever in 72 persons [16]. An insufficient amount of chlorine was found in the water of the pool. To stop the spread of infection, the pool was closed during the summer and adequately chlorinated. Adenovirus was recovered from the water sampled from the pool.

In Oklahoma, USA, an outbreak of pharyngitis caused by HAdV type 7a was recorded in 1982 among 77 children attending a swimming pool [17]. Symptoms included conjunctivitis, fever, sore throat, headache, and abdominal pain. Two cases were hospitalized with dehydration from persistent vomiting. A malfunction of the automatic pool chlorinator was identified as the cause of the outbreak. In fact, during the two weeks preceding the epidemic, its failure forced the pool operator to manually add chlorine to the pool.

Another outbreak was recorded in 1995, in Greece, where 80 athletes under 18 years of age presented with fever, conjunctivitis, sore throat, weakness, and abdominal pain, after swimming in a pool [18]. Seven athletes were hospitalized. Virological analyses on clinical samples were not performed and the illness was attributed to HAdV on the basis of clinical symptoms alone. Water samples from both the pool and the distribution system were tested for HAdV, enterovirus, and hepatitis A virus by molecular methods. The water of the pool tested positive for HAdV and negative for the other viruses, demonstrating its role as the source of infection. Samples from the water system were negative for all viruses tested. Chlorine levels were found to be low, probably due to a malfunctioning of the pool chlorination system.

Five HAdV outbreaks associated with swimming were recorded in the 2000s.

In the year 2000, an outbreak of pharyngoconjunctival fever occurred in North Queensland, Australia, where, after a school camp, 34 children aged 4–12, got sick [19]. In addition to primary cases acquired at the camp (N° = 25), nine other cases were acquired within the households. The school camp had a large saltwater swimming pool. Adenovirus 3 was isolated from eye and throat swabs. A PCR analysis of water samples for HAdV did not yield positive results. It was, however, demonstrated that the pool was not properly maintained, and that the level of residual chlorine was inadequate.

An outbreak of pharyngoconjunctival fever affecting 59 children under 15 was recorded in a municipality of Northern Spain in July 2008 [20]. Forty-three cases were recognized as primary cases, all of whom attended a municipal swimming pool. The remaining 15 children were secondary cases, which had been in close contact with a primary case. Adenovirus type 4 was detected in pharyngeal swabs. Electrical system failures causing the intermittent breakdown of the pool's bromine dosing pumps and the slowing down of water circulation were assumed to have been the cause of the outbreak. Swimming was only allowed after the disinfection system was restored and appropriate concentrations of bromine were reached. Due to logistic problems, no water samples were taken from the swimming pool for virological analysis.

In 2011, children (4–9 years old) who had attended a swimming training center in Eastern China showed symptoms of pharyngoconjunctival fever. Adenovirus type 3 was recognized as the etiological agent [21]. A total of 134 cases were confirmed from among 900 amateur swimmers, with an incidence of 14.9%. Fourteen hospital admissions were documented. Fever, tonsillitis, sore throat, headache, sneezing, cough, conjunctivitis, fatigue, and diarrhea occurred among the bathers. The low level of residual chlorine in the water, along with excessive crowding in the pool were suggested as having caused the epidemic.

In the same year, in a primary school in Taiwan, an outbreak of HAdV infection occurred among 373 students, with four hospitalizations [22]. Most of the students attended a swimming course in two swimming facilities outside the school and presented with fever and symptoms of upper respiratory tract infection. Other symptoms included diarrhea, vomiting, skin eruptions and conjunctivitis. Throat swabs of affected students were tested for influenza virus, adenovirus, respiratory syncytial virus, coronavirus, metapneumovirus, parainfluenza types 1–4, and herpes simplex virus. Samples were found positive only for HAdV type 7. Water samples were not obtained from any of the facilities for virological analysis.

In 2013, an outbreak of pharyngoconjunctival fever involved 55 people (49 students and six staff) at a university in Beijing, China [23]. Fifty patients (91%) attending the same swimming pool two weeks before the onset of symptoms were considered primary cases. The other five subjects (9%) who had not swum in the pool were defined as secondary cases (person-to-person transmission). Human AdV type 4 was identified from both eye and throat swabs of the patients and from concentrated swimming pool water samples. Gene sequences obtained from the water samples exhibited a 100% match with the sequences obtained from swab samples. Control measures included the emptying and closing of the pool, and the disinfection with a high dose of sodium hypochlorite (500 mg/L).

3.2. Enterovirus Outbreaks (N° = 6)

Enterovirus is a genus in the family Picornaviridae, consisting of four human enterovirus species. Enteroviruses can cause many illnesses, including paralysis, meningitis, and cardiomyopathy, although most infections are asymptomatic or cause less severe conditions, such as colds and fever. A number of reports have described enterovirus infections linked to swimming pools.

The first enterovirus swimming pool-related outbreak occurred in 1987, at a municipal pool in Colorado, USA. Twenty-six children presented with fever along with at least one additional symptom such as malaise, headache, stomachache, nausea, or diarrhea [24]. It was found that the pool chlorination system was operating improperly, with chlorine levels close to zero. Stool specimens collected from the children affected were tested for common enteric bacterial pathogens (*Salmonella*, *Shigella*, *Aeromonas*, and *Campylobacter*), but not for viruses. Enterovirus was suggested as a likely etiological agent based on clinical manifestations, course of disease, incubation time, and the exclusion of likely bacterial pathogens.

An enterovirus outbreak occurred in Ireland in 1992, with 46 cases experiencing vomiting, diarrhea, and headache after attending an outdoor swimming pool in a small seaside village. One subject had vomited into the pool, and echovirus 30 was isolated from this case and from six other cases. Chlorine levels were found to comply with health standards, but were inadequate to contain the risk of infection from vomitus [25].

Another echovirus 30 outbreak occurred in Rome, Italy, in late 1997 [26]. Children from two schools showed clinical manifestations after swimming in a pool. Twenty children had meningitis-like symptoms (fever, headache, and vomiting), and six of them were hospitalized. Other 48 children had respiratory symptoms consistent with enterovirus infection. Echovirus 30 was isolated from the cerebrospinal fluid and stools of the hospitalized children. Based on the epidemiological characteristics, it was hypothesized that person-to-person transmission occurred both at the swimming pool and in a number of classrooms.

Data on chlorination at the time of the outbreak were not available. Virological analysis of pool water was performed one month after the outbreak, but yielded no positive results.

In South Africa, an outbreak involving 90 children occurred following a summer camp in 2001 [27]. Camp activities included swimming and other aquatic sports. Symptoms included mainly headaches, sore eyes, and/or abdominal discomfort, with one case of vomiting. Four children were hospitalized for meningitis. Echovirus 3 was detected in cerebrospinal fluid and stool samples from symptomatic and asymptomatic children. The presence of viruses in the pool was not investigated. Water contamination was confirmed through a total coliform count.

In Germany, 215 cases of aseptic meningitis were recorded from July to October 2001 [28]. Swimming in a public, nature-like pond was identified as a risk factor for disease. Up to 1500 people visited the pond each day during the summer holidays. Echovirus 3 and 30 were detected in cerebrospinal fluid samples taken from some of the patients. An echovirus 30 sequence obtained from one water sample collected from the pond showed a high level of genetic similarity (99% nucleotide homology) with sequences obtained from patient isolates.

In August 2003, an outbreak of meningitis occurred among campers staying at a campground in Connecticut, USA [29]. A total of 12 cases of aseptic meningitis, four hospitalized patients and 24 cases of enterovirus-like illness with symptoms such as headache, neck stiffness, photophobia, sore throat, chills, or exanthema were identified. Echovirus serotype 9 was detected in cerebrospinal fluid samples from three of the patients. The spread of the virus was associated with swimming in a crowded pool, which had low chlorine levels. As a result, the pool water was intermittently contaminated with enterovirus.

3.3. Hepatitis a Virus Outbreaks (N° = 3)

Hepatitis A is a virus causing mild to severe liver disease. Globally, there are an estimated 1.4 million cases of hepatitis A every year. The virus is transmitted mainly via the fecal/oral route through the ingestion of contaminated food and water, or through direct contact with an infected subject. There is evidence to suggest that hepatitis A can be acquired by swimming in contaminated water.

In September 1979, an outbreak of hepatitis A affecting 56 children (5–17 years old) and causing 31 hospitalizations was recorded in Hungary [30]. All of the children swam in a pool at a summer camp. The pool was a non-chlorinated thermal pool/spa, which was overcrowded during the month of August. It was concluded that crowding and poor hygienic conditions, with a suspected accidental fecal release, contributed to the outbreak.

Another outbreak of hepatitis A was described in the USA during 1989. It involved 20 cases, probably associated with a public swimming pool [31]. It was hypothesized that a cross-connection between a sewage line and the pool water intake line may have been the cause of the outbreak. According to another hypothesis, it was a swimmer who contaminated the water in the pool. However, disinfectant levels in the pools met local standards.

Seven hepatitis A cases among children from six families were documented in Australia in 1997 [32]. The children had attended an outdoor spa pool treated with hydrogen peroxide solution. It was hypothesized that hepatitis A virus was shed by the index case in the spa pool, and subsequently ingested by the others, who became secondary cases. Virological analyses of water samples were not performed.

3.4. Norovirus Outbreaks (N° = 7)

Noroviruses (NoVs), formerly known as Norwalk-like viruses, are small viruses within the family *Caliciviridae*, subdivided into at least seven genogroups (GI–VII), with GI, GII, and GIV infecting humans. They are recognized as a major cause of sporadic and epidemic gastroenteritis in both industrialized and non-industrialized countries.

Outbreaks have been associated with a variety of settings including childcare centers, hospitals, nursing homes, cruise ships and restaurants. Noroviruses are mainly transmitted via the fecal-oral route through contaminated food or water. Norovirus-contaminated water—both recreational and drinking water—can thus lead to waterborne infections. A number of NoV swimming-pool related outbreaks have been described.

In 1977, an outbreak of acute gastroenteritis with the typical symptoms of vomiting, cramping, nausea and diarrhea was documented among 103 students and teachers at a primary school in Ohio, USA [33]. Serologic studies suggested infection by Norwalk virus to be the cause of the outbreak. The first cases recorded were caused by swimming in a contaminated pool, and a person-to-person transmission followed. The water of the pool tested negative for both bacterial and viral pathogens. Water contamination was linked to both the pool chlorinator, which was accidentally turned off at the time of the school visits, and a leak in the water supply pipes.

A large outbreak of gastroenteritis due to NoVs was recorded in July 2001 in Helsinki. It involved 242 people (children and adults) after bathing in an outdoor wading pool [34]. Norovirus and astrovirus were detected in both patient stool samples and pool water, with identical nucleotide sequences. The pool was found to be heavily contaminated with human fecal material carried from public toilets. The pool water had been manually chlorinated three times per week, thus not continuously. To control the outbreak, the pool was emptied, refilled, and the water was heavily chlorinated (up to 10 mg/L of free chlorine). For the subsequent swimming season, the pool was equipped with both a continuous chlorination system and a water filtration system.

In 2002, a NoV outbreak associated with a swimming pool was reported in Minnesota, USA. Thirty-six persons of three different youth sports teams became ill after swimming in a hotel pool and spa [29]. Unfortunately, there is no other information available on this epidemic.

In 2004, an acute gastroenteritis epidemic affected 53 people who had swum in a pool in Vermont, USA. Vomiting and/or diarrhea occurred within 72 h of attending a private indoor pool. Specimens tested positive for NoV. At the time of the inspection, no equipment failures or irregularities were identified. Nevertheless, deficiencies in pool operation and maintenance, including poorly trained operators, inadequate maintenance checks, failure to alert management, and insufficient record keeping were reported [35].

Finally, Yoder and coworkers documented a NoV outbreak linked to a hotel pool in Wisconsin, USA in 2006, with 18 persons exhibiting symptoms of gastroenteritis, related to inadequate disinfection and continued use by ill swimmers [36].

Table 1. List of viral swimming pool-related outbreaks.

Caption	N° People Affected	Etiological Agent	Location	Virus Identified in Pool Waters	Year	Reference
Adenovirus	206	HAdV	Colorado, USA	Not tested	1951	[9]
	>300	HAdV 3	Washington	Not detected	1954	[10]
	112	HAdV 3	Canada	Not tested	1955	[11]
	358	HadV 3 and 7	Japan	Not tested	1959	[12]
	45	HAdV 3	Washington	No. Water analyses two weeks after the exposure	1966	[13]
	44	HAdV 7	Kansas	No. Samples were taken after hyperchlorination of the pool	1973	[14]
	105	HAdV 3	Georgia	Not tested	1977	[15]
	72	HAdV 4	Georgia	Yes. First swimming-pool related outbreak in which AdV was recovered from water samples	1977	[16]
	77	HAdV 7a	Oklahoma	Not tested	1982	[17]
	80	Unknow	Greece	Yes. Pool water samples tested found positive for AdVs, and negative for enteroviruses and hepatitis A virus	1995	[18]
	34	HAdV 3	Australia	No	2000	[19]
	59	HAdV 4	Spain	Not tested	2008	[20]
	134	HAdV 3	China	Not tested	2011	[21]
	373	HAdV 7	Taiwan	Not tested	2011	[22]
	55	HAdV 4	China	Yes. Gene sequences obtained from the water samples were 100% identical to the sequences obtained from the swab samples.	2013	[23]

Table 1. *Cont.*

Caption	N° People Affected	Etiological Agent	Location	Virus Identified in Pool Waters	Year	Reference
Enterovirus	26	Enterovirus-like	Colorado	Not tested	1987	[24]
	46	Echovirus 30	Ireland	Not tested	1979	[25]
	68	Echovirus 30	Italy	No. Virological analysis of pool waters was performed one month after the outbreak	1997	[26]
	90	Echovirus 3	South Africa	Not tested. Unclean swimming-pool water was confirmed by total coliform count	2001	[27]
	215	Echovirus 13 and 30	Germany	Yes. An echovirus 30 sequence obtained from pond water showed 100% amino-acid homology with sequence obtained from patient isolates	2001	[28]
	36	Echovirus 9	Connecticut	Not tested	2003	[29]
Hepatitis A virus	56	-	Hungary	Not tested	1987	[30]
	20	-	Louisiana, USA	Not tested	1989	[31]
	7	-	Australia	Not tested	1997	[32]
Norovirus	103	-	Ohio	No. Pool water were found negative for both bacterial and viral pathogens.	1977	[33]
	242	-	Finland	Yes. Identical sequence was detected in both patient stool and pool water	2001	[34]
	36	-	Minnesota	Not known	2001–2002	[24]
	53	-	Vermont	Not tested	2004	[35]
	18	-	Wisconsin	Not known	2006	[36]

4. Occurrence of Enteric Viruses in Swimming Pools under Non-Epidemic Conditions

To date, a limited number of studies examined the extent of viral contamination in swimming pools under non-epidemic conditions.

The first isolation of viruses from urban wading pools was documented in Albany, NY, USA in 1959 [37]. Two enteroviruses (echovirus 3 and echovirus 11) were identified from two chlorinated pools, both filled with water from the municipal supply. The same echovirus strains were found to be present in raw sewage sampled at the Albany treatment plant, reflecting widespread infection in the community.

In Toronto, Canada, Coxsackievirus B1 was isolated from children with pleurodynia, myalgia, and primary peritonitis during 1964. Examination for the virus content of a gauze swab, which was placed daily in a wading pool with high bather load located in a congested city area, revealed the presence of the same Coxsackievirus type [38].

In 1979 in Israel, swimming pool samples were found positive for enterovirus: three for Echovirus 7, two for Coxsackievirus B6, and one for Echovirus 6 [39]. Viruses were isolated from water samples with no detectable fecal or total coliform bacteria.

Different enteroviruses were detected in swimming pools and wading pools equipped with gas chlorine and sand/gravel filters in Texas, USA, in 1980 [40]. After virus concentration from water, samples were assayed on cell culture and plaque assays. Enteroviruses were found in 10/14 (71%) of the examined samples. Coxsackieviruses B3 and B4, poliovirus 1, and echovirus 7 were isolated in pool waters. No correlation was found with total coliform bacteria, as six among the positive virus samples were negative for coliforms. In three samples, viruses were detected in the presence of free chlorine exceeding 0.4 ppm and in the absence of coliforms, indicating that viruses can survive low levels of biocides in actively used pools. Cell cultures used in the study were suited for the isolation of enteroviruses, but it is likely that other viruses, not capable of growing on those cell lines, could also have been present in the water.

Three years later, in 1983, enteroviruses were detected in 28.4% of 116 water samples [41] collected from three outdoor swimming pools. A direct correlation was established between viral and microbial contamination, and the low exchange of water in the pools.

In 2004, van Heerden and coworkers detected HAdV in 12 of 64 samples (18.7%) from an indoor swimming pool and in three of 28 samples (10.7%) from an outdoor swimming pool [7]. Quantitative data were also obtained by Real-time PCR. Application of these results in an exponential risk assessment model, assuming a daily ingestion of 30 mL of water during swimming, indicated a daily risk of infection ranging from 1.92×10^{-3} to 3.69×10^{-3}. No acceptable microbial risk has thus far been established for swimming pool water. However, pool water quality is generally considered comparable to drinking water quality (absence of fecal indicators and pathogens). For this reason, a maximum of one infection per 10,000 consumers per year has been recommended as an acceptable level of microbial risk for swimming pools. The risk of HAdV infections calculated for the swimming pool water in the study exceeded this acceptable risk.

More recently, in 2007 in Cyprus, HAdVs and enteroviruses were detected in public swimming pools complying with bacteriological standards (such as fecal coliforms and enterococci) [42]. The investigation was performed over a period of 21 months, from April 2007 to December 2008. A total of 126 samples were obtained from swimming pools located in five major cities. Bacteriological marker analysis showed that 98% of pools complied with the national regulations. Enteroviruses were identified in four swimming pools, one containing echovirus 18, two containing echovirus 30 and one containing poliovirus Sabin 1. In four swimming pools, HAdVs were detected, all characterized as type 41.

In 2013–2014, a study investigated the presence of human enteric viruses (adenovirus, norovirus, and enterovirus) in indoor and outdoor swimming pool waters in Rome. Bacteriological parameters (fecal indicator bacteria, heterotrophic plate count, *Pseudomonas aeruginosa*, and *Staphylococcus aureus*) were also investigated [43]. Moreover, the study was the first to examine the occurrence of non-enteric viruses in swimming pool waters: human papillomavirus (HPV) and human polyomavirus (HPyV). Interestingly, enteric viruses were not detected, while both HPVs and HPyVs were identified in 9/14 swimming pool water samples, by means of molecular methods. Neither of these viruses had previously been recognized as potential recreational waterborne pathogens, although the WHO Guidelines for safe recreational water environments do include HPVs among non-fecally-derived viruses as viruses associated with plantar warts [3]. A variety of HPVs and HPyVs were found in another study investigating spa/pool waters in Rome [44].

Recently, disinfected water from sixteen pools and spa collected in Rome between 2015 and 2018 were examined for the presence of human enteric viruses (adenovirus, norovirus and enterovirus. Viruses were detected in 25% of the analyzed samples by molecular methods: two samples were positive for adenovirus (type 41) and three samples for norovirus GII (type GII.4) (Bonadonna et al., unpublished data).

5. Concluding Remarks

Starting with the first HAdV outbreak recorded in 1951, we reviewed all of the reports concerning swimming-pool related viral illness. The data collected here confirm the involvement of viruses in cases and outbreaks associated with swimming pool attendance.

A number of considerations emerge:

- The paper reviews 29 viral outbreaks due to adenovirus, enterovirus, hepatitis A virus, and norovirus, accounting for more than 3000 cases. Nevertheless, there are likely to have been many other undetected cases and outbreaks. In fact, waterborne diseases are difficult to record because of their wide variety, the difficulty associating symptoms with water use/contact, and the limitations of pathogen detection methods. In the studies described, viruses responsible for reported cases were detected in pool waters only in 21% of the outbreaks, and were found to match with viruses of clinical origin. Currently, better and more rapid methods for the detection of viruses in water samples are available than in the past, resulting in better studies and improved reporting of viral recreational outbreaks worldwide. This allows researchers to identify the causes of outbreaks and possible contributing factors for them. An excellent model to follow is the US-Waterborne Disease and Outbreak Surveillance System (WBDOSS) that has been collecting and reporting data related to occurrences and causes of waterborne disease outbreaks associated with drinking and recreational waters since 1971.

- Some of the studies found that waters meeting state or local water quality requirements contained enteric viruses and were the source of disease outbreaks, confirming that bacterial indicators are unreliable indicators of the presence of viruses and that enteric viruses are important hazardous waterborne pathogens. Indeed, despite the relatively low concentration of viruses in water, they may nevertheless pose health risks due to their low infectious doses (10–100 virions).
- The human illnesses associated with enteric viruses in the reviewed studies were diverse: the most commonly reported symptoms were gastroenteritis, respiratory symptoms, and conjunctivitis. More severe symptoms were also documented, however, including hepatitis and central nervous system infections (aseptic meningitis).
- The majority of the outbreaks described involved mainly children and young people less than 18 years of age. This may be attributable to differences in behaviors, susceptibility and/or immune defenses between children and adults. Children are known to experience more severe symptoms than adults.
- Low concentrations of disinfectant/disinfection malfunction in swimming pools were reported in the vast majority of the outbreaks. Only in one case the concentration of biocide was considered high.

In light of the health hazards posed by swimming pools, it is essential to constantly monitor water quality in swimming pools and to assess the effectiveness of treatment and disinfection processes and compliance with standards. Specifically, appropriate chemical and microbial evaluation of water quality should be carried out, especially when large numbers of bathers are expected to use the pools. Overcrowding should in any case be prevented. Since the behavior of swimmers may affect water quality, strict rules of behavior in the pool should be followed and enforced, including shower before entering the water, wash hands after using the toilet, take children to bathroom before swimming, and, importantly, avoid swimming while sick.

Author Contributions: L.B. and G.L.R. conceived and wrote the paper, and approved the submitted version.

Funding: This research received no external funding.

Conflicts of Interest: The authors declare no conflict of interest.

References

1. Sinclair, R.G.; Jones, E.L.; Gerba, C.P. Viruses in recreational water-borne disease outbreaks: A review. *J. Appl. Microbiol.* **2009**, *107*, 1769–1780. [CrossRef] [PubMed]
2. Barna, Z.; Kadar, M. The risk of contracting infectious diseases in public swimming pools. A review. *Ann. Ist. Super. Sanità* **2012**, *48*, 374–386. [CrossRef] [PubMed]
3. WHO: Guidelines for Safe Recreational Water Environments—Swimming Pools and Similar Environments. Available online: http://wwwwho.int/iris/handle/10665/43336 (accessed on 8 November 2018).
4. Human Adenovirus Working Group. Available online: http://hadvwg.gmu.edu/ (accessed on 14 December 2018).
5. La Rosa, G.; Suffredini, E. Adenovirus. In *Handbook of Foodborne Diseases*, 1st ed.; Liu, D., Ed.; CRC Press: Boca Raton, FL, USA, 2018.
6. Mena, K.D.; Gerba, C.P. Waterborne adenovirus. *Rev. Environ. Contam Toxicol.* **2009**, *198*, 133–167. [CrossRef] [PubMed]
7. Van Heerden, J.; Ehlers, M.M.; Grabow, W.O.K. Detection and risk assessment of adenoviruses in swimming pool water. *J. Appl. Microbiol.* **2005**, *99*, 1256–1264. [CrossRef] [PubMed]
8. Staggemeier, R.; Arantes, T.; Caumo, K.S.; Rott, M.B.; Spilki, F.R. Detection and quantification of human adenovirus genomes in Acanthamoeba isolated from swimming pools. *An. Acad. Bras. Cienc.* **2016**, *88* (Suppl. 1), 635–641. [CrossRef] [PubMed]
9. Cockburn, T.A. An epidemic of conjunctivitis in Colorado associated with pharyngitis, muscle pain, and pyrexia. *Am. J. Ophthalmol.* **1953**, *36*, 1534–1539. [CrossRef]
10. Bell, J.A.; Rowe, W.P.; Engler, J.I.; Parrot, R.H.; Huebner, R.J. Pharyngoconjunctival fever; epidemiological studies of a recently recognized disease entity. *J. Am. Med. Assoc.* **1955**, *157*, 1083–1092. [CrossRef]

11. Ormsby, H.L.; Aitchison, W.S. The role of the swimming pool in the transmission of pharyngeal-conjunctival fever. *Can. Med. Assoc. J.* **1955**, *73*, 864–866.

12. Fukumi, H.; Nishikawa, M.; Takemura, M.; Odaka, Y. isolation of adenovirus possessing both the antigens of types 3 and 7. *Jpn. J. Med. Sci. Biol.* **1961**, *14*, 173–181. [CrossRef]

13. Foy, H.M.; Cooney, M.K.; Hatlen, J.B. Adenovirus type 3 epidemic associated with intermittent chlorination of a swimming pool. *Arch. Environ. Health* **1968**, *17*, 795–802. [CrossRef]

14. Caldwell, G.G.; Lindsey, N.J.; Wulff, H.; Donnelly, D.D.; Bohl, F.N. Epidemic of adenovirus type 7 acute conjunctivitis in swimmers. *Am. J. Epidemiol.* **1974**, *99*, 230–234. [CrossRef] [PubMed]

15. Martone, W.J.; Hierholzer, J.C.; Keenlyside, R.A.; Fraser, D.W.; D'Angelo, L.J.; Winkler, W.G. An outbreak of adenovirus type 3 disease at a private recreation center swimming pool. *Am. J. Epidemiol.* **1980**, *111*, 229–237. [CrossRef] [PubMed]

16. D'Angelo, L.J.; Hierholzer, J.C.; Keenlyside, R.A.; Anderson, L.J.; Martone, W.J. Pharyngoconjunctival fever caused by adenovirus type 4: Report of a swimming pool-related outbreak with recovery of virus from pool water. *J. Infect. Dis.* **1979**, *140*, 42–47. [CrossRef] [PubMed]

17. Turner, M.; Istre, G.R.; Beauchamp, H.; Baum, M.; Arnold, S. Community outbreak of adenovirus type 7a infections associated with a swimming pool. *South. Med. J.* **1987**, *80*, 712–715. [CrossRef] [PubMed]

18. Papapetropoulou, M.; Vantarakis, A.C. Detection of adenovirus outbreak at a municipal swimming pool by nested PCR amplification. *J. Infect.* **1998**, *36*, 101–103. [CrossRef]

19. Harley, D.; Harrower, B.; Lyon, M.; Dick, A. A primary school outbreak of pharyngoconjunctival fever caused by adenovirus type 3. *Commun. Dis. Intell.* **2001**, *25*, 9–12. [PubMed]

20. Artieda, J.; Pineiro, L.; Gonzalez, M.; Munoz, M.; Basterrechea, M.; Iturzaeta, A.; Cilla, G. A swimming pool-related outbreak of pharyngoconjunctival fever in children due to adenovirus type 4, Gipuzkoa, Spain, 2008. *Eurosurveillance* **2009**, *14*, 19125.

21. Xie, L.; Yu, X.F.; Sun, Z.; Yang, X.H.; Huang, R.J.; Wang, J.; Yu, A.; Zheng, L.; Yu, M.C.; Hu, X.W.; et al. Two adenovirus serotype 3 outbreaks associated with febrile respiratory disease and pharyngoconjunctival fever in children under 15 years of age in Hangzhou, China, during 2011. *J. Clin. Microbiol.* **2012**, *50*, 1879–1888. [CrossRef]

22. Wei, S.H. An Adenovirus Outbreak Associated with a Swimming Facility. *SM Trop. Med. J.* **2016**, *1*, 1007.

23. Li, J.; Lu, X.; Sun, Y.; Lin, C.; Li, F.; Yang, Y.; Liang, Z.; Jia, L.; Chen, L.; Jiang, B.; et al. A swimming pool-associated outbreak of pharyngoconjunctival fever caused by human adenovirus type 4 in Beijing, China. *Int. J. Infect. Dis.* **2018**, *75*, 89–91. [CrossRef]

24. Lenaway, D.D.; Brockmann, R.; Dola, G.J.; Cruz-Uribe, F. An outbreak of an enterovirus-like illness at a community wading pool: Implications for public health inspection programs. *Am. J. Public Health* **1989**, *79*, 889–890. [CrossRef] [PubMed]

25. Kee, F.; McElroy, G.; Stewart, D.; Coyle, P.; Watson, J. A community outbreak of echovirus infection associated with an outdoor swimming pool. *J. Public Health Med.* **1994**, *16*, 145–148. [CrossRef] [PubMed]

26. Faustini, A.; Fano, V.; Muscillo, M.; Zaniratti, S.; La Rosa, G.; Tribuzi, L.; Perucci, C.A. An outbreak of aseptic meningitis due to Echovirus 30 associated with attending school and swimming in pools. *Int. J. Infect. Dis.* **2006**, *10*, 291–297. [CrossRef] [PubMed]

27. Yeats, J.; Smuts, H.; Serfontein, C.J.; Kannemeyer, J. Investigation into a school enterovirus outbreak using PCR detection and serotype identification based on the 5' non-coding region. *Epidemiol. Infect.* **2005**, *133*, 1123–1130. [CrossRef] [PubMed]

28. Hauri, A.M.; Schimmelpfennig, M.; Walter-Domes, M.; Letz, A.; Diedrich, S.; Lopez-Pila, J.; Schreier, E. An outbreak of viral meningitis associated with a public swimming pond. *Epidemiol. Infect.* **2005**, *133*, 291–298. [CrossRef] [PubMed]

29. Yoder, J.S.; Blackburn, B.G.; Craun, G.F.; Hill, V.; Levy, D.A.; Chen, N.; Lee, S.H.; Calderon, R.L.; Beach, M.J. Surveillance for waterborne-disease outbreaks associated with recreational water—United States, 2001–2002. *MMWR Surveill. Summ.* **2004**, *53*, 23–45.

30. Solt, K.; Nagy, T.; Csohan, A.; Csanady, M.; Hollos, I. An outbreak of hepatitis A due to a thermal spa. *Bp. Kozeu.* **1994**, *26*, 8–12.

31. Mahoney, F.J.; Farley, T.A.; Kelso, K.Y.; Wilson, S.A.; Horan, J.M.; McFarland, L.M. An outbreak of hepatitis A associated with swimming in a public pool. *J. Infect. Dis.* **1992**, *165*, 613–618. [CrossRef]

32. Tallis, G.; Gregory, J. An outbreak of hepatitis A associated with a spa pool. *Commun. Dis. Intell.* **1997**, *21*, 353–354.

33. Kappus, K.D.; Marks, J.S.; Holman, R.C.; Bryant, J.K.; Baker, C.; Gary, G.W.; Greenberg, H.B. An outbreak of Norwalk gastroenteritis associated with swimming in a pool and secondary person-to-person transmission. *Am. J. Epidemiol.* **1982**, *116*, 834–839. [CrossRef]

34. Maunula, L.; Kalso, S.; von Bonsdorff, C.H.; Ponka, A. Wading pool water contaminated with both noroviruses and astroviruses as the source of a gastroenteritis outbreak. *Epidemiol. Infect.* **2004**, *132*, 737–743. [CrossRef] [PubMed]

35. Podewils, L.J.; Zanardi, B.L.; Hagenbuch, M.; Itani, D.; Burns, A.; Otto, C.; Blanton, L.; Adams, S.; Monroe, S.S.; Beach, M.J.; et al. Outbreak of norovirus illness associated with a swimming pool. *Epidemiol. Infect.* **2007**, *135*, 827–833. [CrossRef] [PubMed]

36. Yoder, J.S.; Hlavsa, M.C.; Craun, G.F.; Hill, V.; Roberts, V.; Yu, P.A.; Hicks, L.A.; Alexander, N.T.; Calderon, R.L.; Roy, S.L.; et al. Surveillance for waterborne disease and outbreaks associated with recreational water use and other aquatic facility-associated health events—United States, 2005–2006. *MMWR Surveill. Summ.* **2008**, *57*, 1–29. [PubMed]

37. Kelly, S.; Sanderson, W.W. Enteric Viruses in Wading Pools. *Public Health Rep.* **1961**, *76*, 199–200. [CrossRef] [PubMed]

38. McLean, D.M.; Larke, R.P.B.; McNaughton, G.A.; Best, J.M.; Smith, P. Enteroviral Syndromes in Toronto, 1964. *Can. Med. Assoc. J.* **1965**, *92*, 658–661. [PubMed]

39. Marzouk, Y.M.; Goyal, S.M.; Gerba, C. Relationship of viruses and indicator bacteria in water and wastewater of Israel. *Water Res.* **1980**, *14*, 1585–1590. [CrossRef]

40. Keswick, B.H.; Gerba, C.P.; Goyal, S.M. Occurrence of enteroviruses in community swimming pools. *Am. J. Public Health* **1981**, *71*, 1026–1030. [CrossRef]

41. Cotor, F.; Zavate, O.; Finichiu, M.; Avram, G.; Ivan, A. Enterovirus contamination of swimming pool water; correlation with bacteriological indicators. *Virologie* **1983**, *34*, 251–256. [PubMed]

42. Bashiardes, S.; Koptides, D.; Pavlidou, S.; Richter, J.; Stavrou, N.; Kourtis, C.; Papageorgiou, G.T.; Christodoulou, C.G. Analysis of enterovirus and adenovirus presence in swimming pools in Cyprus from 2007–2008. *Water Sci. Technol.* **2011**, *63*, 2674–2684. [CrossRef] [PubMed]

43. La Rosa, G.; Della Libera, S.; Petricca, S.; Iaconelli, M.; Briancesco, R.; Paradiso, R.; Semproni, M.; Di Bonito, P.; Bonadonna, L. First detection of papillomaviruses and polyomaviruses in swimming pool waters: Unrecognized recreational water-related pathogens? *J. Appl. Microbiol.* **2015**, *119*, 1683–1691. [CrossRef]

44. Di Bonito, P.; Iaconelli, M.; Gheit, T.; Tommasino, M.; Della Libera, S.; Bonadonna, L.; La Rosa, G. Detection of oncogenic viruses in water environments by a Luminex-based multiplex platform for high throughput screening of infectious agents. *Water Res.* **2017**, *123*, 549–555. [CrossRef] [PubMed]

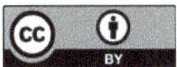

International Journal of
*Environmental Research
and Public Health*

MDPI

Article

Legionellosis Associated with Recreational Waters: A Systematic Review of Cases and Outbreaks in Swimming Pools, Spa Pools, and Similar Environments

Erica Leoni [1,*] , Federica Catalani [2] , Sofia Marini [3] and Laura Dallolio [1]

1   Unit of Hygiene, Public Health and Medical Statistics, Department of Biomedical and Neuromotor Sciences, University of Bologna, via S. Giacomo 12, 40126 Bologna, Italy; laura.dallolio@unibo.it
2   School of Hygiene and Preventive Medicine, Department of Biomedical and Neuromotor Sciences, University of Bologna, via S. Giacomo 12, 40126 Bologna, Italy; federica.catalani@studio.unibo.it
3   Department of Life Quality Studies, University of Bologna, Campus of Rimini; Corso d'Augusto 237, 47921 Rimini, Italy; sofia.marini2@unibo.it
*   Correspondence: erica.leoni@unibo.it; Tel.: +39-051-20948-07

Received: 12 July 2018; Accepted: 25 July 2018; Published: 30 July 2018

Abstract: *Legionella* spp. is widespread in many natural and artificial water systems, such as hot water distribution networks, cooling towers, and spas. A particular risk factor has been identified in the use of whirlpools and hot tubs in spa facilities and public baths. However, there has been no systematic synthesis of the published literature reporting legionellosis cases or outbreaks related to swimming/spa pools or similar environments used for recreational purposes (hot springs, hot tubs, whirlpools, natural spas). This study presents the results of a systematic review of the literature on cases and outbreaks associated with these environments. Data were extracted from 47 articles, including 42 events (17 sporadic cases and 25 outbreaks) and 1079 cases, 57.5% of which were diagnosed as Pontiac fever, without any deaths, and 42.5% were of Legionnaires' disease, with a fatality rate of 6.3%. The results are presented in relation to the distribution of *Legionella* species involved in the events, clinical manifestations and diagnosis, predisposing conditions in the patients, favourable environmental factors, and quality of the epidemiological investigation, as well as in relation to the different types of recreational water sources involved. Based on the epidemiological and microbiological criteria, the strength of evidence linking a case/outbreak of legionellosis with a recreational water system was classified as strong, probable, and possible; in more than half of the events the resulting association was strong.

Keywords: *Legionella* spp.; Legionnaires' disease; Pontiac fever; recreational water; hot tubs; whirlpools; spa pools; swimming pools

---

1. Introduction

Legionellosis is a disease transmitted through the inhalation of particles of aerosolized water contaminated by the opportunistic waterborne pathogen, *Legionella* spp. [1]. After the first recognition of legionellosis in 1976, when 221 participants of the annual convention of the American Legion contracted pneumonia and 34 of them died, surveillance systems were developed and implemented in several countries [2]. Legionellosis surveillance is a current public objective: In 2015, according to the European Centre for Disease Prevention and Control surveillance, 7034 cases were reported in Europe, concerning 1.4 cases per 100,000 inhabitants [3].

The majority of outbreaks described in the literature are correlated to *Legionella pneumophila*, in particular serogroup 1, but other serogroups and species were also associated to human disease, such as *L. micdadei* (now classified as *Tatlockia micdadei*), *L. dumoffii*, and *L. longbeachae* [4]. The two fundamental clinical pictures determined by these infective agents are Legionnaires' disease (LD) and Pontiac fever (PF): The former is generally characterized by an acute pneumonia and, rarely, by an extrapulmonary disease; Pontiac fever is a mild, self-limiting, flu-like illness, which resolves in a few days.

Legionella spp. are widely distributed in both natural (i.e., lakes, rivers, groundwater, thermal water) and man-made aquatic environments, such as the water systems of hospitals, hotels, private houses [5,6], cooling towers [7], dental units [8,9], and recreational [10,11] or therapeutic [12,13] facilities. Any system or equipment which contains, stores, or re-circulates non-sterile water that can be aerosolized is a source of legionellosis [14,15]. Considering these elements, the recreational use of water is an important potential way of exposure to *Legionella* spp., especially in hot water pools equipped with hydromassage systems. A recent review on outbreaks of LD and PF highlights that 14% of the reported outbreaks from 2006 to 2017 recognized pools or spas as an attributed or suspected source [16]. The role of these recreational facilities appears even more significant if one considers the growing popularity of private hot tubs and the increasing number of people frequenting public spa pools and similar environments.

Generally, the outbreak analysis and control measures, specific for each exposure setting, are essential tasks of Public Health Authorities, including outbreak surveillance and analysis specifically dedicated to the recreational water context. Epidemiological knowledge about these themes must be constantly updated. To our knowledge, no systematic synthesis or critical appraisal exists of the published literature reporting sporadic cases or outbreaks of LD and/or PF associated with recreational water. In the present study, we performed a systematic review and analysis of investigations on legionellosis cases or outbreaks related to treated and untreated recreational water, including natural waters, swimming pools, spa pools, and similar environments (hot tubs, whirlpools, hot spring baths, etc.), in accordance with the definitions given for these environments by World Health Organization (WHO) guidelines [17].

2. Materials and Methods

In line with the objective of the study, we set out to perform a systematic review of cases and outbreaks of LD and PF associated with recreational aquatic environments, such as swimming and spa pools or natural spas. The literature search was conducted in Medline, including publications from 1 January 1977 (since the disease was first described in 1976) to 31 May 2018, using the following search terms: (Legionella OR legionellosis OR "Pontiac fever" OR "Legionnaires' disease") AND (case* OR cluster* OR outbreak* OR infection* OR investigation OR surveillance) AND ("recreational water" OR spa OR pool OR "swimming pool" OR "hot tub" OR whirlpool OR bath OR "swim spa" OR "turkish bath" OR sauna OR Jacuzzi OR "natural spa" OR "hot spring" OR "thermal spring" OR "warm spring" OR spring OR thermal). The literature search was conducted without language restrictions, on the condition that the articles had an exhaustive abstract in English reporting the information of interest. A further selection of relevant publications was performed using the inclusion and exclusion criteria listed below.

Inclusion criteria:

- Primary studies describing cases/outbreaks of LD or PF originating from recreational water.

Exclusion criteria:

- Not recreational water (hot water system, cooling tower, fountain, network water, therapeutic water, water births);
- environmental studies without cases;
- not primary studies;

- articles focused only on clinical and laboratory aspects;
- abstract not available/ not complete or not exhaustive;
- articles focused on pools used for display only (retail premises, fairs, exhibitions, shows);
- articles evaluating only microbiological risk assessment; and
- hot tubs or pools on cruise ships (due to a recently published systematic review) [18].

Two researchers independently screened titles and abstracts to identify potentially relevant articles and to exclude articles incompatible with the first five exclusion criteria; any disagreements were resolved by discussion with a third author. After the application of the first five exclusion criteria, the full texts of the remaining articles were examined, and any publications exclusively focused on display spas were then excluded, since this type of exposure in environments used for retail premises, fairs, exhibitions, and shows is not directly linked to recreational use. The remaining articles were assigned to three categories related to three different recreational facilities or sources of infection:

(a) Private hot tub and similar facilities;
(b) public pools and spas and similar facilities, generally supplied by municipal network water; and
(c) spa facilities supplied by natural water, or hot spring/thermal water. Subsequently, we applied the last two exclusion criteria to each category.

Data extracted from these publications included: Year, country, case definition, clinical form, type of event (sporadic case or outbreak), number of cases, attack rate, number of hospitalizations and/or deaths, risk factors, laboratory diagnosis, *Legionella* spp. involved, environmental isolates and concentrations (cfu/L), type of recreational water, water supply, and the type of epidemiological study carried out (descriptive, analytical, presence/absence of environmental investigation). An event with multiple cases (at least two) linked in space and time, with a suspected common source, was defined as an outbreak. For each event (both sporadic cases and outbreaks), epidemiological and microbiological criteria were adopted to characterize the strength of evidence linking the legionellosis event with the suspected recreational water system. Table 1 summarizes these criteria.

Table 1. Strength of evidence linking a case/outbreak of legionellosis with a recreational water system.

Strength of Evidence	Epidemiological and Microbiological Criteria
Strong	• An analytical epidemiological study demonstrates a significant association between case/outbreak of legionellosis and exposure to the recreational water; and • the same species and serogroups of *Legionella* spp. are isolated from the water system at any concentration. Or • Descriptive epidemiology suggests that the case/outbreak is related to the recreational water and excludes obvious alternative explanations; and • *Legionella* spp. are isolated from the water system at any concentration and environmental isolates show identical genotype profiles of clinical isolates.
Probable	• An analytical epidemiological study demonstrates a significant association between case/outbreak of legionellosis and exposure to the recreational water; and • *Legionella* spp. are not isolated from the recreational water. Or • Descriptive epidemiology suggests that the case/outbreak is related to the recreational water and excludes obvious alternative explanations; and • the same species and serogroups of *Legionella* spp. are isolated from the water system at any concentration.
Possible	• Descriptive epidemiology suggests that the case/outbreak is related to exposure to the recreational water and excludes obvious alternative explanations; and • *Legionella* spp. are not isolated from the recreational water.

Data were analysed as the frequency distribution of the different variables included.

3. Results

Of the 326 articles retrieved from Medline, 259 were excluded for the following reasons: 99 investigations did not refer to recreational water, 82 were environmental studies without cases, 4 were not primary studies, 68 articles were focused only on clinical and laboratory aspects, and 6 publications were in a language other than English and did not have an exhaustive English abstract, as shown in Figure 1.

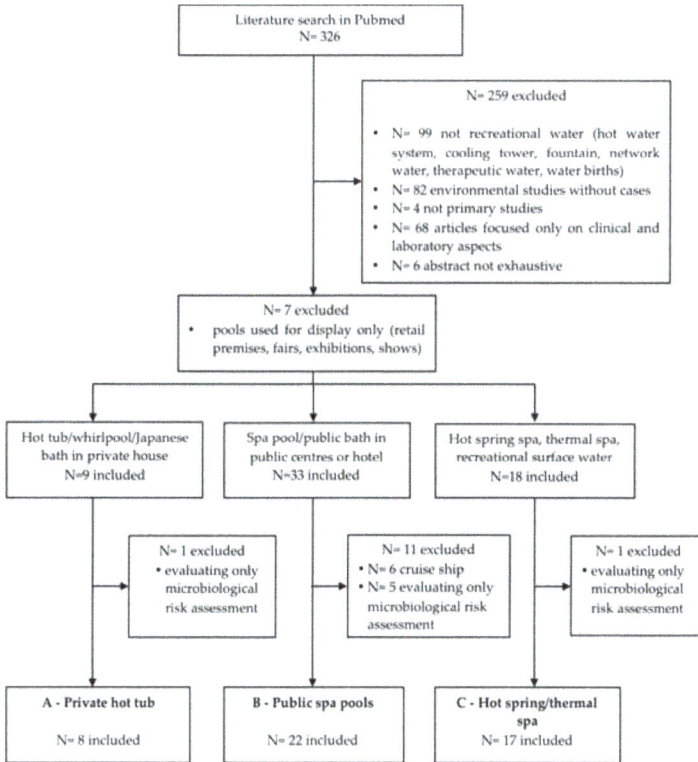

Figure 1. Flow chart of the selection process of articles.

At the end of the selection process, 47 articles were considered eligible for inclusion in the present review, corresponding to 42 events. In four cases, different articles described varying aspects of the same event, while two articles reported two and three different events, respectively. Among the 42 events of legionellosis, eight were linked to a hot tub/whirlpool/Japanese bath used in private houses (Category A in Figure 1, in brief "private hot tub"), 22 were related to whirlpool spa/baths in public centres and hotels (Category B in Figure 2, in brief "public spa pools"), and 12 to hot spring/thermal spa pools (Category C in Figure 1, in brief "hot spring/thermal spa").

The selected articles were published: Four in the 1980s, 16 in the 1990s, 19 in the 2000s, and three from 2010 to 2018. In 11 articles, the authors did not report the date of onset. The events occurred in different countries across the world, with the highest frequency of hot spring related events in Japan (83.3%) and an overall highest frequency in Japan (18 events: 42.9%), followed by the USA (11 events: 26.2%), and the United Kingdom (4 events: 9.5%).

3.1. Legionellosis in Relation to Recreational Water Source

Table 2 shows all events and cases of legionellosis associated with recreational water systems, distinguished per facility category. Of the 1079 total cases included in the 42 events, 57.5% were diagnosed as PF, without any deaths, and 42.5% were of LD, with a fatality rate of 6.3%.

Table 2. Events of Pontiac fever (PF) and Legionnaires' disease (LD) associated with recreational water.

Characteristics of the Events	Hot Tub/Whirlpool/Japanese Bath in Private House (8 Events)	Spa Pools/Public Baths in Public Centres or Hotels (22 Events)	Hot Spring Spa, Thermal Spa, Recreational Surface Water (12 Events)	Total Recreational Waters (42 Events)
Number of events with single cases	5	2	10	17
Number of outbreaks or events with repeated cases [a]	3	20	2	25
Number of total cases	28	744	307	1079
Median number of cases per outbreak (range)	6 (4–13)	23.5 (3–170)	148.5 (2–295)	23 (2–295)
Total number of PF cases (fatal cases)	22 (0)	598 (0)	0	620 (0)
Total number of LD cases (fatal cases)	6 (1)	146 (16)	307 (12)	459 (29)
Fatality rate on total cases (on LD cases)	3.6% (16.7%)	2.2% (11.0%)	3.9% (3.9%)	2.7% (6.3%)
Analytical epidemiology in outbreak investigation (% of total outbreaks)	0 (0%)	8 (40.0%)	1 (50.0%)	9 (36.0%)
Events with environmental investigation (% of total events)	6 (75.0%)	20 (90.9%)	9 (75.0%)	35 (83.3%)
Legionella spp. detected in environmental water samples (% of total events)	4 (50.0%)	20 (90.9%)	8 (66.7%)	32 (76.2%)
Identical Legionella genotype in clinical and environmental isolates (% of total events)	1 (12.5%)	6 (27.3%)	7 (58.3%)	14 (33.3%)
Strength of evidence				
Strong (%)	1 (12.5%)	15 (68.2%)	7 (58.3%)	23 (52.4%)
Probable (%)	3 (37.5%)	5 (22.7%)	1 (8.3%)	9 (21.4%)
Possible (%)	4 (50.0%)	2 (9.1%)	4 (33.3%)	10 (23.9%)

[a] 22 outbreaks and three events with repeated cases or cluster.

The private hot tubs were all supplied by municipal network water and were subjected to a supplementary disinfection system only in two of the eight facilities involved in the legionellosis events. Single cases occurred in five events (62.5%) corresponding to 17.9% of cases, while the remaining three events were outbreaks with a low number of persons involved (from four to 13). LD represented 21.4% of the cases, with a fatality rate of 16.7%.

Public spa pools were generally supplied by municipal network water and only three out of 22 facilities had their own supply system from groundwater (two spa pools) and mountain spring water (one spa pool). In 54.5% of the facilities, water treatment included recycling, filtering, and chemical disinfection with bromine (seven spa pools) or chlorine (five spa pools). In the remaining public spa pools, water disinfection was not mentioned. Public spa pools were responsible for the highest number of events (22), cases (744), and deaths (16). A sporadic case only occurred in 9.1% of the events, while the remaining events were outbreaks often involving a high number of cases of up to 170 [19]. The LD cases formed 19.6% of the total cases, with a fatality rate of 11.0%.

Hot spring/thermal spas were supplied by natural waters, i.e., hot springs and thermal waters. This group also includes the only LD case associated with bathing in surface water. This was a fatal case in a 27-year-old woman who had nearly drowned in estuarine water [20]. Water treatment and chlorine disinfection were reported in only three out of the 11 hot spring/thermal water facilities (27.3%), while, in one case, the authors specified that national regulations (France) precluded the addition of chemicals to thermal spas to preserve the characteristics of the mineral water [21]. All cases linked to this recreational water category were diagnosed as LD, with a fatality rate of 3.9%. Single cases occurred in 83.3% of the events and only two outbreaks were reported. However, one of these was the largest outbreak of LD associated with a hot spring bathhouse in Japan, with 295 cases, including confirmed and probable cases [22].

3.2. Epidemiological Investigations

All the events with sporadic cases were studied by descriptive epidemiology. The epidemiological investigations included an analytical study in 36.0% of outbreaks, with higher percentages in events linked to public spa pools (40.0%) and hot spring/thermal water (50%), compared to private hot tubs (no events with an analytical study). An environmental investigation was carried out in 83.3% of events (private hot tubs and hot spring/thermal water: 75%; public spa pools: 90.9%) and allowed the detection of *Legionella* spp. in 76.2% of the incriminated water sources and to evidence identical molecular profiles of both clinical and environmental isolates in 33.3% of the events. Based on the epidemiological and microbiological criteria specified in Table 1, the strength of evidence linking the case/outbreak of legionellosis with the recreational water system was strong in 23 events (52.4%), with percentages higher for public spa pools (68.2%) and hot spring/thermal water (58.3%) compared to private hot tubs (12.5%). This was a consequence of the previously mentioned differences regarding both the implementation of analytic epidemiology and the detection of environmental *Legionella* spp., which were carried out less frequently in private hot tub related events.

3.3. Events with Sporadic Cases of Legionellosis

Sporadic cases of legionellosis occurred in 17 distinct events, only one of PF [23] and 16 of LD (Table 3), with a fatality rate of 29.4% (31.2% for LD cases). Most cases occurred in Japan (70.6%) [24–35], and hot spring/thermal waters (56.2%) were the facilities most involved, followed by private hot tubs (25%). Only two cases occurred in spa centres/public baths [35,36]. Four cases, three of which fatal, were consequent to near drowning [20,32,35,37] and one case involved a 10-year-old girl, subjected to immunosuppressive therapy for hemosiderosis after being exposed several times to the hot tub in her maternal home [38].

Etiological diagnosis was confirmed by culture of clinical specimens in 75.0% of LD cases and *L. pneumophila* was the species most frequently involved, in particular *L. pneumophila* SG 6 (31.2% of LD cases). No differences were observed on the onset of cases in relation to the different concentrations of legionellae detected from the suspected water sources. Genotyping of clinical and environmental isolates was performed in seven out of 17 events. In accordance with the microbiological criteria specified in Table 1, the strength of evidence linking the cases with the recreational water system was strong in all the cases confirmed by molecular typing (43.7% of LD cases).

Table 3. Events with sporadic cases of Pontiac fever (PF) and Legionnaires' disease (LD) associated with recreational water.

	Pontiac Fever (1 Event) [a]	Legionnaires' Disease (16 Events) [b]
Number of cases (fatal cases)	1 (0)	16 (5)
Gender		
Males		9
Females		6
Not reported	1	1
Median age (range)	37	56.5 (10–88)
Confirmation by culture in clinical specimen	0	12 (75.0%)
Legionella species and serogroup		
L. pneumophila SG 1	0	3 (18.7%)
L. pneumophila SG 2	0	1 (6.2%)
L. pneumophila SG 3	0	2 (12.5%)
L. pneumophila SG 4	0	1 (6.2%)
L. pneumophila SG 6	0	5 (31.2%)
L. pneumophila SG 13	0	2 (12.5%)
L. pneumophila (SG not reported)	1 (100%)	1 (6.2%)
L. rubrilucens	0	1 (6.2%)

Table 3. *Cont.*

	Pontiac Fever (1 Event) [a]	Legionnaires' Disease (16 Events) [b]
Environmental source		
Private hot tub	1	4 (25.0%)
Public and hotel spa	0	2 (12.5%)
Hot spring/thermal spa	0	9 (56.2%)
Estuarine water	0	1 (6.2%)
Legionella colonization		
<1000 cfu/L	0	2 (12.5%)
1000–10,000 cfu/L	0	2 (12.5%)
>10,000 cfu/L	0	2 (12.5%)
Not reported	1 (100%)	11 (68.7%)
Identical *Legionella* genotype in clinical and environmental isolates	0	7 (43.7%)
Strength of evidence		
Strong (%)	0	7 (43.7%)
Probable (%)	1 (100%)	2 (12.5%)
Possible (%)	0	7 (43.7%)

[a] [23]; [b] [20,24–38].

3.4. Outbreaks of Legionellosis

A total of 25 outbreaks of legionellosis were found: 7 outbreaks of PF (Table 4), 11 outbreaks of LD (Table 5), and 7 mixed events of PF and LD (Table 6). Among the LD events, two were repeated cases on the same site, which occurred in different time periods (No. 2, 3 in Table 6), and one was a long-lasting outbreak with three consecutive clusters (No. 10 in Table 6).

The total number of outbreak cases was 1062, of which 619 were PF cases (58.3%) and 443 were LD cases (41.7%), with 24 deaths (total fatality rate: 2.3%, for LD: 5.4%). Most events occurred in public spas (20/25 outbreaks, 80%), particularly in whirlpool spas of hotels or similar residential facilities, such as inns and holiday resorts (11 of 25 outbreaks, 44%). The attack rate varied from 29.8% to 86.7% for PF outbreaks and from 0.13% to 1.9% for LD outbreaks.

Etiological diagnosis was confirmed by culture of clinical specimens in 10 out of 11 outbreaks of LD and in one out of seven mixed events of PF and LD (61.1% of total events with LD cases), while it was never performed in PF outbreaks. *L. pneumophila* was the species most frequently involved, in particular *L. pneumophila* SG 1 in 68% of total outbreaks (83.3% of outbreaks with LD cases) and SG 6 in 24% of total outbreaks (27.8% of outbreaks with LD cases). In three events, various species or serogroups were identified as responsible for the disease by culture and/or serological assay.

Environmental isolates of *Legionella* spp. were obtained in 22 outbreaks (88%), in seven of which various species or serogroups were detected (28%). Genotyping of clinical and environmental isolates was performed in 10 events (40% of total outbreaks, 55.5% of outbreaks with LD cases). In accordance with the epidemiological and microbiological criteria specified in Table 1, the strength of evidence linking the outbreak with the recreational water system was strong in 16 events (64%).

Table 4. Outbreaks of Pontiac fever (PF) associated with recreational water.

Event No. Country, Year (Reference)	Water System	*Legionella* spp. (Confirmed Diagnosis Based on)	No. of Cases (Fatal Cases)	Attack Rate	Proportion of Males	Median Age (Range)	Environmental Isolates (cfu/L)	Strength of Evidence
1 Vermont, US, 1981 [39]	Inn whirlpool spa	*L. pneumophila* SG 6 (antibody titre)	34 (0)	45.9%	53.0%	27.9	*L. pneumophila* SG 1,6 *L. dumoffii*	Strong
2 Michigan, US, 1982 [40]	Public whirlpool spa (women's pool)	*L. pneumophila* SG 6 (antibody titre)	14 (0)	29.8%	0	32 (25–39)	*L. pneumophila* SG 6	Strong
3 Colorado, US, 1992 [41]	Resort indoor whirlpool	*L. pneumophila* SG 6 (antibody titre)	13 (0)	38.0%	na	na	*L. pneumophila* SG 6 (>1,000,000)	Strong
4 Denmark, 1995 [42]	Private summerhouse whirlpool	*L. pneumophila* SG 1 (culture, antibody titre) *L. micdadei* (antibody titre)	13 (0)	86.7%	na	na	negative samples (after whirlpool cleaning)	Possible
5 Wisconsin, US, 1998 [43]	Hotel whirlpool spa	*L. micdadei* (antibody titre)	45 (0)	whirlpool area: 66.0% whirlpool users: 71.0%	na	na	*L. micdadei* (90,000/L)	Strong
6 Sweden, 1999 [44]	Hotel whirlpool spa	*L. micdadei* (antibody titre)	29 (0)	whirlpool area: 71.0% whirlpool users: 88.9%	37.9%	41 (21–57)	negative samples	Probable
7 England, 2008 [45]	Resort whirlpool spa	*L. pneumophila* SG 1 (antibody titre, urinary antigen)	6 (0)	86.0%	0	(24–37)	*Legionella* non *pneumophila* (100/L)	Probable

na: Not available; clinical and environmental isolates were never compared by molecular typing.

Table 5. Outbreaks of Legionnaires' disease (LD) associated with recreational water.

Event No. Country, Year (Reference)	Water System	Legionella spp. (Diagnosis Based on)	Number of Cases (Fatal Cases)	Attack Rate	Proportion of Males	Median Age (Range)	Environmental Isolates (cfu/L)	Strength of Evidence
1 Vermont, US, 1987 [46]	Inn whirlpool spa	L. pneumophila SG 1 (culture, antibody titre)	3 (0)	na	na	na	L. pneumophila SG 1,4	Strong
2 Netherlands 1992–96 [47]	Public spa sauna's footbath	L. pneumophila SG 1 (culture)	6 repeated cases (2)	na	83.3%	males: 50 females: 28	L. pneumophila SG 1	Strong
3 France 1994–97 [21]	Thermal spa	L. pneumophila SG 1 (culture)	2 repeated cases (1)	na	50%	54.5 (40–69)	L. pneumophila SG 1,2,3,6,9,13 L. dumoffii	Strong
4 Japan, 1996 [48]	Public Japanese spa	L. pneumophila SG 1 (antibody titre)	3 (0)	na	na	na	L. pneumophila SG 1	Probable
5 Japan, 2000 [27]	Public bath house	L. pneumophila SG 1,6 (culture, antibody titre, urinary antigen)	23 (2)	0.13%	91.3%	67 (50–86)	L. pneumophila SG 1 (880,000)	Strong
6 Japan, 2000 [49,50]	Public bath house	L. pneumophila SG 1 (culture, antibody titre, urinary antigen)	34 (20 confirmed) (3)	0.20%	65.0% (only confirmed)	62.2 (27–85)	L. pneumophila SG 1,3,5,6 (11400–842000)	Strong
7 Japan, 2002 [22,51–55]	Hot spring bath	L. pneumophila SG 1 (culture, antibody titre, urinary antigen)	295 including suspected cases (7)	1.5%	64.5% (of 76 examined)	65 (9–95)	L. pneumophila SG 1,8 (1,600,000) L. dumoffii (5,200,000) L. londiniensis (15,000,000)	Strong
8 Japan, 2003 [27]	Public bath house	L. pneumophila SG 1 (culture)	9 (1)	0.13%	na	65 (52–82)	L. pneumophila SG 1 (1,300,000)	Probable
9 France, 2010 [56]	Public whirlpool spa	L. pneumophila SG 1 (culture, urinary antigen)	3 (1)	na	33.3%	50 (30–70)	L. pneumophila SG 1 (150,000)	Strong
10 Spain, 2011–12 [57]	Hotel spa pool	L. pneumophila SG 1 (culture)	Total: 44 (6) Cluster1: 21 Cluster2: 2 Cluster3: 3 Cluster4: 18	na	na	tourists: 71.5 hotel workers: 49.5	L. pneumophila SG 1 L. micdadei	Strong
11 Japan, 2015 [58]	Spa house (men's pool)	L. pneumophila SG 1,13 (culture)	7 (0)	na	100%	66.3	L. pneumophila SG 1,13	Strong

na: Not available; clinical and environmental isolates showed correlated molecular profiles in events No. 1, 2, 3, 5, 6, 7, 9, 10, and 11.

Table 6. Outbreaks of Pontiac fever (PF)/Legionnaires' disease (LD) associated with recreational water.

Event No. Country, Year (Reference)	Water System	Legionella spp. (Diagnosis Based on)	Number of Cases PF + LD (Fatal Cases)	Attack Rate	Proportion of Males	Median Age (Range)	Environmental Isolates (cfu/L)	Strength of Evidence
1 Scotland, 1987–88 [19,59]	Hotel whirlpool spa	L. micdadei (antibody titre)	169 + 1 (0)	90.9% (LD: 0.5%)	48.8%	32 (2–72)	L. micdadei	Probable
2 Vermont US, 1991 [60]	Private hot tub in holiday home	L. pneumophila SG 1 (antibody titre)	5 + 1 (0)	na	na	na	not investigated	Possible
3 Georgia US, 1999 [61]	Hotel whirlpool spa	L. pneumophila SG 6 (culture, antibody titre, urinary antigen)	22 + 2 (0)	22.0% (LD: 1.8%)	na	PF: 12 (5–31) LD: 66 (61–71)	L. pneumophila SG 6	Strong
4 Illinois US, 2002 [62]	Hotel spa area	L. micdadei L. maceachernii (antibody titre)	49 + 1 (0)	62.7% (LD: 1.2%)	46%	20 (2–58)	L. micdadei L. maceachernii L. dumoffii	Strong
5 Oklaoma US, 2004 [63]	Hotel pool and hot tub area	L. pneumophila SG 1 (antibody titre, urinary antigen)	101 + 6 (0)	33.7% (LD: 1.9%)	PF: 43.6% LD: 100%	PF: 15 (2–65) LD: 6.5 (2–44)	L. pneumophila SG 1	Strong
6 England, 2006 [64]	Leisure club spa pool	L. pneumophila SG 1 (antibody titre, urinary antigen)	116 + 2 (0)	na	PF: 41.4% LD: 100%	(18–85)	L. pneumophila SG 1	Probable
7 Netherlands, 2009 [65]	Private outdoor whirlpool spa	L. pneumophila SG 1 (antibody titre, urinary antigen)	3 + 1 (1 LD)	na	PF: 66.7% LD: 0%	PF: 54 (52–83) LD: 78	L. pneumophila SG 1	Probable

na: Not available; clinical and environmental isolates showed correlated molecular profiles in the event No. 3.

3.5. Patient Contributing Factors

PF cases showed no evidence of underlying risk factors. The median age of the PF patients, when reported, varied from 12 to 54 years and, overall, males and females were affected with a similar frequency.

LD patients were males in 60% of sporadic cases (Table 3) and in 71.9% of outbreaks, considering only the events reporting gender distribution. The median age was 56.5 years (range: 10–88) in sporadic cases and over 60 years in nine of the 13 LD outbreaks in which the age data was reported. Patient risk factors and underlying medical conditions were specified in 24 of the 34 LD events (71.3%), for a total of 155 cases. Figure 2 shows the occurrence of contributing factors and underlying medical conditions in these patients. Heavy smoking was the most frequent risk factor (58.7% of patients) and, among the underlying medical conditions, cardiovascular diseases (23.9%) and diabetes (11.0%) had the highest prevalence. Four cases of *Legionella* pneumonia occurred after near drowning, one in estuarine water and three in hot spring spas and public baths.

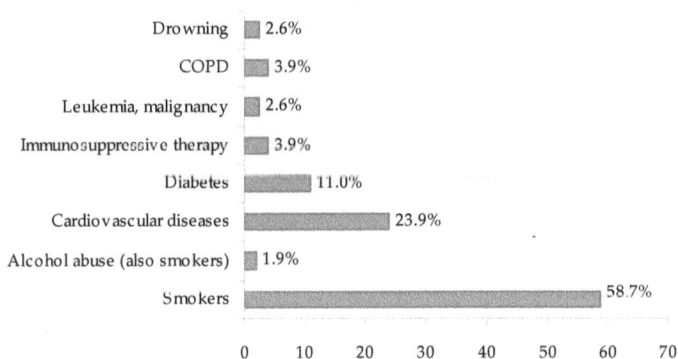

Figure 2. Distribution of underlying medical conditions and risk factors in 155 cases of Legionnaires' disease.

3.6. Environmental Contributing Factors

Excluding the only sporadic case related to estuarine water, environmental contributing factors were investigated in 22 out of 41 events. In only one of these, no contributing environmental conditions were found. In the other 21 events, inadequate water treatment and residual disinfectant below the recommended levels were the most frequent factors that could have favoured the onset of cases or outbreaks. The water temperature was reported in only four events and in three of these the temperature was above 40 °C (Figure 3). In PF events, the most frequent environmental contributing factors were those related to plant maintenance and chemical treatment management (i.e., inappropriate residual disinfectant concentration), while the inadequacy or absence of the treatment system was observed only for LD cases or outbreaks. This could be explained by the fact that many LD events occurred in private hot tubs not subjected to a supplementary disinfection system.

Legionella spp. were isolated from the environmental samples of 32 facilities, at concentrations higher than 10^3 cfu/L in water samples obtained from 11 of them (34.4%).

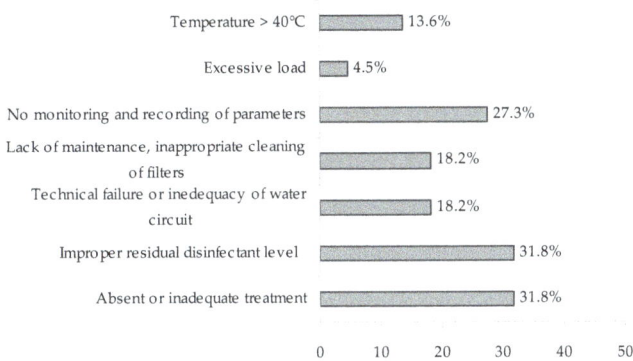

Figure 3. Distribution of environmental contributing factors in 22 recreational facilities associated with legionellosis events.

4. Discussion

This review aimed to evaluate the cases and outbreaks of legionellosis associated with exposure to recreational water since the disease was first described in 1976. Both sporadic cases and outbreaks of LD and PF, described in the scientific literature, were included. Relevant findings from 47 articles were synthesized, including 42 legionellosis events (17 sporadic cases and 25 outbreaks).

4.1. Temporal and Geographical Distribution

The events of legionellosis correlated with exposure to recreational water showed a non-homogeneous distribution over time. In the 1980s, only four events were reported, probably because, in these first years, there was a lower awareness of the problem and many cases were not identified or associated with exposure to recreational water. In the 1990s and 2000s, the number increased (16 and 19 events, respectively) and then declined in the years from 2010 until today (only three reported in the literature). It could be hypothesized that the increase in knowledge and awareness of risks associated with recreational water led to an improvement in the management and maintenance and control measures, also after the issuing of international guidelines on the control of legionellosis in recreational facilities. In 2006, the WHO Guidelines for safe recreational water environments recommended the implementation of safety plans and adequate control measures in pools and hot tubs [17]. Moreover, from 2005, the European Legionnaires' Disease Surveillance Network (ELDSNet, previously EWGLI), with respect to *Legionella* risk reduction in whirlpool spas, recommended continuous treatment with 2–3 mg/L of chlorine or bromine, the checking of these levels almost three times a day, the replacement of at least half of the water each day, sand filters backwashed daily, and cleaning and disinfection of the whole system every day [66]. The implementation of these measures could explain the reduction in the number of events in the most recent period.

The reported events of legionellosis involved 10 countries, with the highest number of events (18) and cases (385) in Japan, where the habit of frequenting hot spring spas and public baths is very widespread, following a long-established tradition in Japanese culture. Moreover, the average water temperature in hot tubs in Japan usually ranges from 40 °C to 43 °C, which is higher than in Europe (30–40 °C) [27].

4.2. Clinical Features and Laboratory Evidence

This review includes both PF and LD events. PF cases totalled 620, only one of which was sporadic, the others being included in 14 outbreaks. The number of PF cases related to recreational water is probably underestimated: The benign nature of the disease, which often presents as an influenza-like illness, means that the cases, especially when sporadic, are not identified as legionellosis and are, therefore, not subjected to laboratory diagnosis. In the selected PF events, laboratory diagnosis was performed only in outbreaks, and *Legionella* spp. were never culturally isolated. On the contrary, in the events involving LD cases, cultural isolation from patients' specimens allowed the species to be identified in 75% of the sporadic cases and in 11 of the 18 outbreaks with LD cases (61.1%).

Among the different species and serogroups, *L. pneumophila* SG 1 (three sporadic cases and 15 outbreaks of LD) and SG 6 (five sporadic cases and two outbreaks of LD) were the agents most frequently responsible, while, among the other species, *L. micdadei* was implicated in three outbreaks of PF and two outbreaks of mixed PF and LD. In five events, various species or serogroups were involved [27,30,42,58,62], one of which was the first case where the same genotype of *L. rubrilucens* was isolated from the LD patient's sputum and the hot spring water [30].

This review confirms certain known characteristics of the epidemiology of legionellosis. PF cases showed no evidence of underlying risk factors and PF outbreaks had a high attack rate, with no difference between males and females. On the contrary, LD cases prevalently involved males and individuals presenting risk factors, such as smoking and all the underlying medical conditions that reduce immune defenses. In LD outbreaks, the attack rate is low and the fatality rate is high (on average, 6.3%, but up to 31.2% in events related to private hot tubs).

4.3. Recreational Water Facilities and Risk Assessment

Most events occurred in public spa pools (22 events, 744 cases). Of these, 10 were associated with hotels or similar residential facilities and, therefore, fall within the surveillance system for legionellosis linked to travel, which in Europe is carried out by the ELDSNet and coordinated by ECDC. The recreational facilities supplied by natural water (hot spring, thermal water) were the setting for 12 events, 10 of which with a single case. Most studies referring to hot spring/thermal spas (seven out of 11) did not specify if the water was treated or untreated and how the facility was managed; this is a limitation that makes it difficult to draw conclusions about the environmental conditions contributing to these infections.

The recommended standards for *Legionella* spp. in hot tub water range from 0/100 mL to 1000/L in different countries [67]. In the selected studies, the environmental isolates of *Legionella* spp. are reported in 32 events, but only 13 specify the level of contamination, which ranges between 100 cfu/L and >10^6 cfu/L. However, it should be noted that the isolation of *Legionella* spp. from environmental samples was carried out after the legionellosis event had occurred and so the environmental conditions may have changed. The lack of data on the *Legionella* concentrations in the water, and on the frequency and duration of exposure, makes it difficult to perform a risk assessment. Various studies tried to estimate the risk for *Legionella* infection due to spa pool use. Bouwknegt et al., (2013) estimated that the infection risk for sitting in an active whirlpool for 15 min ranged from around 3% for a concentration of 10 *L. pneumophila* cfu/L to up to 95% for >1000 cfu/L [68]. These findings suggest that a risk cannot be excluded even in the presence of very low concentrations, and stricter requirements may be needed to ensure adequate protection for users. Azima et al. (2013) suggested a reference value of <1 cfu/L, which is less than the current detection limit [69].

4.4. Epidemiological Investigation and Strength of Evidence

The epidemiological investigation included an analytical study in nine outbreaks, four with a case-control study and five with a retrospective cohort study. In all the events related to private hot tubs, only descriptive epidemiology was carried out. This is justified by the difficulty in such events to find a control group not exposed to the private hot tub. Also, sporadic cases were studied only through descriptive epidemiology (case reports).

The environmental investigation was often delayed with respect to the event onset and, in some cases, was made after control measures had already been adopted. These measures are specified only in a limited number of articles and information is lacking on the follow-up procedures in almost all the articles. Many studies do not report the environmental conditions that could have favoured such infections. In 19 events, no information is available on the type of water treatment, the level of residual disinfectant, or the state of maintenance of the facility. Only in three events is the water temperature specified, a factor that, in these types of recreational facilities, plays a fundamental role in the development of *Legionella* spp. and was probably co-responsible for three LD cases associated with near drowning in hot spring spas and public baths [32,35,37]. Lying in or sitting up to the neck in hot water (above 40 °C), especially in combination with alcohol consumption, may cause drowsiness, which may then lead to unconsciousness and, consequently, drowning [70].

Based on the selected criteria, the strength of evidence linking the cases/outbreaks to the recreational water facilities was strong in 52.4% of events, probable in 21.4%, and possible in 23.9%. Strong evidence was principally attributable to the results of analytical study in nine events, and to the match of environmental and clinical isolates in 17 events. The comparison between strains of environmental and clinical origin using molecular biology techniques was carried out at a very high level of frequency, especially in cases concerning LD (43.7% of sporadic cases and 81.8% of LD outbreaks).

4.5. Limitations

The present study was limited to articles published in English or with an exhaustive abstract in English, and only peer-reviewed literature was considered. Furthermore, the legionellosis events that are published represent only part of the overall number of cases: Larger LD outbreaks are more likely to be published than sporadic cases and smaller events, especially of Pontiac fever. Also, the review does not include cruise ship cases [18] and cases associated with display spa pools in retail premises, fairs, exhibitions, and shows [71,72], which represent another important source of infection. Therefore, the role of the recreational facilities as a source of infection is underestimated, also considering that in many LD and PF cases the source of *Legionella* remains unknown [3,16].

The heterogeneity of epidemiological investigations, in terms of study design, sample size, and information about the duration of exposure and environmental contributing factors, limited the comparison of results. In particular, the lack of information about the treatment and management of recreational facilities makes it difficult to exhaustively evaluate the role of environmental conditions.

5. Conclusions

Data extracted from the articles in this systematic review show that hot tubs, whirlpools, and spa pools represent an important source of infection of *Legionella* spp., given the number of cases involved (1079 from 1981 to 2015), the number of deaths (29), and the high percentage of events with strong evidence of an association. On the contrary, the risk related to the natural recreational water of rivers and lakes appears negligible: The only sporadic case reported is a case consequent to a near-drowning in estuarine water [20].

Among the cases included in this review, PF cases were the most numerous and were caused by a variety of species and serogroups: *L. pneumopghila* SG 6 and *L. micdadei* were the most often responsible agents, while *L. pneumophila* SG 1 was responsible for most LD cases. Unlike PF cases, LD cases prevalently involved individuals presenting risk factors, such as smoking, and underlying medical conditions that reduce immune defenses.

Certain operating conditions that facilitate the formation of aerosol, such as the high temperature of the water and the presence of hydromassage systems, are risk factors inherent to this kind of recreational water. In hot tubs and similar facilities, it is impractical to maintain a water temperature outside the range considered at risk. Therefore, other management strategies need to be implemented, which may include appropriate design and adequate disinfection residual and proper maintenance and cleaning of equipment as well as adequate ventilation. Features, such as water sprays, should be periodically cleaned and flushed with a level of disinfectant adequate to eliminate *Legionella* spp. [3,17,67]. In this review, the environmental conditions were described for

22 events, and in 21 of these (95.5%) at least one of the preventive measures recommended by the various guidelines was not respected. Therefore, it seems important to increase collaboration between the different professionals involved (public health experts, policy makers, facility managers, technical staff, equipment manufacturers) to improve the knowledge of the operators and their awareness of the risk and to favour compliance with control measures.

Author Contributions: E.L.: conception, design and supervision of the study; F.C., S.M., L.D.: selection and analysis of the articles, collection of data of interest in a structured form. E.L. and L.D. drafted the manuscript. All authors approved the final version of the manuscript.

Acknowledgments: The authors would like to thank Maria Cristina Labanti, Document Delivery Service, Biblioteca Interdipartimentale di Medicina, Biblioteca Biomedica, Bologna University, who provided the full text of some articles of interest.

Conflicts of Interest: The authors declare no conflict of interest.

Abbreviations

The following abbreviations are used in this manuscript:

LD	Legionnaires' Disease
PF	Pontiac Fever
cfu	colony forming unit

References

1. Muder, R.R.; You, V.L.; Woo, A.H. Mode of transmission of *Legionella pneumophila*: A critical review. *Arch. Int. Med.* **1986**, *146*, 1607–1612. [CrossRef]
2. Springston, J.P.; Yocavitch, L. Existence and control of *Legionella* bacteria in building water systems: A review. *J. Occup. Environ. Hyg.* **2017**, *14*, 124–134. [CrossRef] [PubMed]
3. ECDC. European Technical Guidelines for the Prevention, Control and Investigation of Infections Caused by *Legionella* Species. June 2017. Available online: https://ecdc.europa.eu/sites/portal/files/documents/Legionella%20GuidelinesFinal%20updated%20for%20ECDC%20corrections.pdf (accessed on 9 July 2018).
4. Cunha, B.A.; Cunha, C.B. Legionnaire's Disease and its mimics: A clinical perspective. *Infect. Dis. Clin. N. Am.* **2017**, *31*, 95–109. [CrossRef] [PubMed]
5. Borella, P.; Montagna, M.T.; Stampi, S.; Stancanelli, G.; Romano Spica, V.; Triassi, M.; Marchesi, I.; Bargellini, A.; Tato, D.; Napoli, C.; et al. *Legionella* contamination in hot water of Italian hotels. *Appl. Environ. Microbiol.* **2005**, *71*, 5805–5813. [CrossRef] [PubMed]
6. Leoni, E.; De Luca, G.; Legnani, P.; Sacchetti, R.; Stampi, S.; Zanetti, F. *Legionella* waterline colonization: Detection of *Legionella* species in domestic, hotel and hospital hot water systems. *J. Appl. Microbiol.* **2005**, *98*, 373–379. [PubMed]
7. Walser, S.M.; Gerstner, D.G.; Brenner, B.; Höller, C.; Liebl, B.; Herr, C.E. Assessing the environmental health relevance of cooling towers—A systematic review of legionellosis outbreaks. *Int. J. Hyg. Environ. Health* **2014**, *217*, 145–154. [CrossRef] [PubMed]
8. Dallolio, L.; Scuderi, A.; Rini, M.S.; Valente, S.; Farruggia, P.; Bucci Sabattini, M.A.; Pasquinelli, G.; Acacci, A.; Roncarati, G.; Leoni, E. Effect of different disinfection protocols on microbial and biofilm contamination of dental unit waterlines in community dental practices. *Int. J. Environ. Res. Public Health* **2014**, *11*, 2064–2076. [CrossRef] [PubMed]
9. Ricci, M.L.; Fontana, S.; Pinci, F.; Fiumana, E.; Pedna, M.F.; Farolfi, P.; Sabattini, M.A.; Scaturro, M. Pneumonia associated with a dental unit waterline. *Lancet* **2012**, *379*, 684. [CrossRef]
10. Donati, M.; Cremonini, E.; Di Francesco, A.; Dallolio, L.; Biondi, R.; Muthusamy, R.; Leoni, E. Prevalence of *Simkania negevensis* in chlorinated water from spa swimming pools and domestic supplies. *J. Appl. Microbiol.* **2015**, *118*, 1076–1082. [PubMed]
11. Leoni, E.; Legnani, P.; Bucci Sabattini, M.A.; Righi, F. Prevalence of *Legionella* spp. in swimming pool environment. *Water Res.* **2001**, *35*, 3749–3753. [CrossRef]

12. Leoni, E.; Sacchetti, R.; Zanetti, F.; Legnani, P.P. Control of *Legionella pneumophila* contamination in a system for respiratory hydrotherapy with sulphurous spa water. *Inf. Control Hosp. Epidemiol.* **2006**, *27*, 716–721. [CrossRef] [PubMed]

13. Leoni, E.; Sanna, T.; Zanetti, F.; Dallolio, L. Controlling *Legionella* and *Pseudomonas aeruginosa* re-growth in therapeutic spas: Implementation of physical disinfection treatments, including UV/ultrafiltration, in a respiratory hydrotherapy system. *J. Water Health* **2015**, *13*, 996–1005. [CrossRef] [PubMed]

14. Fields, B.S.; Benson, R.F.; Besser, R.E. *Legionella* and Legionnaire's disease: 25 year of investigation. *Clin. Microbiol. Rev.* **2002**, *15*, 506–526. [CrossRef] [PubMed]

15. Leoni, E.; Dallolio, L.; Sanna, T.; Stagni, F.; D'Alessandro, G.; Piana, G. Impact of a risk management plan on *Legionella* contamination of dental unit water. *Int. J. Environ. Res. Public Health* **2015**, *12*, 2344–2358. [CrossRef] [PubMed]

16. Hamilton, K.A.; Prussin, A.J.; Ahmed, W.; Haas, C.N. Outbreaks of Legionnaires' Disease and Pontiac Fever 2006–2017. *Curr. Environ. Health Rep.* **2018**, *5*, 263–271.

17. WHO. *Guidelines for Safe Recreational Water Environments. Volume 2, Swimming Pools and Similar Environments*; WHO: Geneva, Switzerland, 2006. Available online: http://www.who.int/water_sanitation_health/bathing/srwe2full.pdf (accessed on 9 July 2018).

18. Mouchtouri, V.A.; Rudge, J.W. Legionnaires' Disease in hotels and passenger ships: A systematic review of evidence, sources, and contributing factors. *J. Travel Med.* **2015**, *22*, 325–337. [PubMed]

19. Goldberg, D.J.; Wrench, J.G.; Collier, P.W.; Emslie, J.A.; Fallon, R.J.; Forbes, G.I.; McKay, T.M.; Macpherson, A.C.; Markwick, T.A.; Reid, D. Lochgoilhead fever: Outbreak of non-pneumonic legionellosis due to *Legionella micdadei*. *Lancet* **1989**, *1*, 316–318. [CrossRef]

20. Faris, B.; Faris, C.; Schousboe, M.; Heath, C.H. Legionellosis from *Legionella pneumophila* serogroup 13. *Emerg. Infect. Dis.* **2005**, *11*, 1405–1409. [CrossRef] [PubMed]

21. Molmeret, M.; Jarraud, S.; Mori, J.P.; Pernin, P.; Forey, F.; Reyrolle, M.; Vandenesch, F.; Etienne, J.; Farge, P. Different growth rates in amoeba of genotypically related environmental and clinical *Legionella pneumophila* strains isolated from a thermal spa. *Epidemiol. Infect.* **2001**, *126*, 231–239. [CrossRef] [PubMed]

22. Yabuuchi, E.; Agata, K. An outbreak of legionellosis in a new facility of hot spring bath in Hiuga City. *Kansenshogaku Zasshi* **2004**, *78*, 90–98. [CrossRef] [PubMed]

23. Tolentino, A.; Ahkee, S.; Ramirez, J. Hot tub legionellosis. *J. Ky. Med. Assoc.* **1996**, *94*, 393–994. [PubMed]

24. Chiba, Y.; Okamoto, H.; Nagatomo, A.; Kunikane, H.; Watanabe, K. Legionnaires' disease diagnosed by bronchoalveolar lavage. *Intern. Med.* **1998**, *37*, 153–156. [CrossRef] [PubMed]

25. Ishikawa, A.; Okada, J.; Kondo, H.; Takayama, Y.; Sunagawa, K.; Enari, T.; Ishii, Y. *Legionella* pneumonia which occurred in a private whirlpool bath user. *Kansenshogaku Zasshi* **2004**, *78*, 898–904. [CrossRef] [PubMed]

26. Ito, I.; Naito, J.; Kadowaki, S.; Mishima, M.; Ishida, T.; Hongo, T.; Ma, L.; Ishii, Y.; Matsumoto, T.; Yamaguchi, K. Hot spring bath and *Legionella* pneumonia: An association confirmed by genomic identification. *Intern. Med.* **2002**, *41*, 859–863. [CrossRef] [PubMed]

27. Kuroki, T.; Ishihara, T.; Ito, K.; Kura, F. Bathwater-associated cases of legionellosis in Japan, with a special focus on *Legionella* concentrations in water. *Jpn. J. Infect. Dis.* **2009**, *62*, 201–205. [PubMed]

28. Kurosawa, H.; Fujita, M.; Kobatake, S.; Kimura, H.; Ohshima, M.; Nagai, A.; Kaneko, S.; Iwasaki, Y.; Kozawa, K. A case of *Legionella* pneumonia linked to a hot spring facility in Gunma Prefecture, Japan. *Jpn. J. Infect. Dis.* **2010**, *63*, 78–79. [PubMed]

29. Mashiba, K.; Hamamoto, T.; Torikai, K. A case of Legionnaires' disease due to aspiration of hot spring water and isolation of *Legionella pneumophila* from hot spring water. *Kansenshogaku Zasshi* **1993**, *67*, 163–166. [CrossRef] [PubMed]

30. Matsui, M.; Fujii, S.; Shiroiwa, R.; Amemura-Maekawa, J.; Chang, B.; Kura, F.; Yamauchi, K. Isolation of *Legionella rubrilucens* from a pneumonia patient co-infected with *Legionella pneumophila*. *J. Med. Microbiol.* **2010**, *59*, 1242–1246. [CrossRef] [PubMed]

31. Miyamoto, H.; Jitsurong, S.; Shiota, R.; Maruta, K.; Yoshida, S.; Yabuuchi, E. Molecular determination of infection source of a sporadic *Legionella* pneumonia case associated with a hot spring bath. *Microbiol. Immunol.* **1997**, *41*, 197–202. [CrossRef] [PubMed]

32. Nozue, T.; Chikazawa, H.; Miyanishi, S.; Shimazaki, T.; Oka, R.; Shimazaki, S.; Miyamoto, S. *Legionella* pneumonia associated with adult respiratory distress syndrome caused by *Legionella pneumophila* serogroup 3. *Intern. Med.* **2005**, *44*, 73–78. [CrossRef] [PubMed]

33. Sasaki, E.; Kaida, H.; Izumikawa, K.; Izumikawa, K.; Hara, K.; Hirakata, Y.; Tomono, K.; Kohno, S. Two cases of *Legionella pneumophila* pneumonia improved by parenteral ciprofloxacin administration. *Nihon Kokyuki Gakkai Zasshi* **2003**, *41*, 211–218. [PubMed]

34. Shimizu, Y.; Nagase, K.; Kadono, K.N.; Funayama, Y.; Tsurushima, Y.; Hibino, T.; Kikuchi, H.; Nagase, S.; Koyama, A. The haemodialysis patient who developed acute respiratory distress syndrome after a trip to a hot spring spa. *Nephrol. Dial. Transplant.* **1999**, *14*, 455–457. [CrossRef] [PubMed]

35. Tokuda, H.; Yahagi, N.; Kasai, S.; Kitamura, S.; Otsuka, Y. A case of fatal pneumonia caused by *Legionella pneumophila* serogroup 6 developed after drowning in a public bath. *Kansenshogaku Zasshi* **1997**, *71*, 169–174. [CrossRef] [PubMed]

36. Su, H.P.; Tseng, L.R.; Tzeng, S.C.; Chou, C.Y.; Chung, T.C. A legionellosis case due to contaminated spa water and confirmed by genomic identification in Taiwan. *Microbiol. Immunol.* **2006**, *50*, 371–377. [CrossRef] [PubMed]

37. Shiota, R.; Takeshita, K.; Yamamoto, K.; Imada, K.; Yabuuchi, E.; Wang, L. *Legionella pneumophila* serogroup 3 isolated from a patient of pneumonia developed after drowning in bathtub of a hot spring spa. *Kansenshogaku Zasshi* **1995**, *69*, 1356–1364. [PubMed]

38. Watson, A.M.; Boyce, T.G.; Wylam, M.E. *Legionella* pneumonia: Infection during immunosuppressive therapy for idiopathic pulmonary hemosiderosis. *Pediatr. Infect. Dis. J.* **2004**, *23*, 82–84. [CrossRef] [PubMed]

39. Spitalny, K.C.; Vogt, R.L.; Orciari, L.A.; Witherell, L.E.; Etkind, P.; Novick, L.F. Pontiac fever associated with a whirlpool spa. *Am. J. Epidemiol.* **1984**, *120*, 809–817. [CrossRef] [PubMed]

40. Mangione, E.J.; Remis, R.S.; Tait, K.A.; McGee, H.B.; Gorman, G.W.; Wentworth, B.B.; Baron, P.A.; Hightower, A.W.; Barbaree, J.M.; Broome, C.V. An outbreak of Pontiac fever related to whirlpool use, Michigan 1982. *JAMA* **1985**, *253*, 535–539. [CrossRef] [PubMed]

41. Miller, L.A.; Beebe, J.L.; Butler, J.C.; Martin, W.; Benson, R.; Hoffman, R.E.; Fields, B.S. Use of polymerase chain reaction in an epidemiologic investigation of Pontiac fever. *J. Infect. Dis.* **1993**, *168*, 769–772. [CrossRef] [PubMed]

42. Lüttichau, H.R.; Vinther, C.; Uldum, S.A.; Møller, J.; Faber, M.; Jensen, J.S. An outbreak of Pontiac fever among children following use of a whirlpool. *Clin. Infect. Dis.* **1998**, *26*, 1374–1378. [PubMed]

43. Fields, B.S.; Haupt, T.; Davis, J.P.; Arduino, M.J.; Miller, P.H.; Butler, J.C. Pontiac fever due to *Legionella micdadei* from a whirlpool spa: Possible role of bacterial endotoxin. *J. Infect. Dis.* **2001**, *184*, 1289–1292. [CrossRef] [PubMed]

44. Götz, H.M.; Tegnell, A.; De Jong, B.; Broholm, K.A.; Kuusi, M.; Kallings, I.; Ekdahl, K.A. Whirlpool associated outbreak of Pontiac fever at a hotel in Northern Sweden. *Epidemiol. Infect.* **2001**, *126*, 241–247. [CrossRef] [PubMed]

45. Modi, A.; Gardner, J.; Lighton, L.; Coetzee, N. Pontiac fever outbreak associated with a spa-pool, United Kingdom, April 2008. *Euro Surveill.* **2008**, *13*, 18934. [PubMed]

46. Vogt, R.L.; Hudson, P.J.; Orciari, L.; Heun, E.M.; Woods, T.C. Legionnaires' disease and whirlpool-spa. *Ann. Intern. Med.* **1987**, *107*, 596. [CrossRef] [PubMed]

47. Den Boer, J.W.; Yzerman, E.; Van Belkum, A.; Vlaspolder, F.; Van Breukelen, F.J. Legionnaire's disease and saunas. *Lancet* **1998**, *351*, 114. [CrossRef]

48. Nakadate, T.; Yamauchi, K.; Inoue, H. An outbreak of Legionnaire's disease associated with a Japanese spa. *Nihon Kokyuki Gakkai Zasshi* **1999**, *37*, 601–607. [PubMed]

49. Nakamura, H.; Yagyu, H.; Kishi, K.; Tsuchida, F.; Oh-Ishi, S.; Yamaguchi, K.; Matsuoka, T. A large outbreak of Legionnaires' disease due to an inadequate circulating and filtration system for bath water, epidemiologic manifestations. *Intern. Med.* **2003**, *42*, 806–811. [CrossRef] [PubMed]

50. Nakamura, H.; Yagyu, H.; Tsuchida, F.; Sudou, A.; Watanabe, O.; Kioi, K.; Kishi, K.; Oh-ishi, S.; Kiguchi, T.; Yamaguchi, K.; et al. A major outbreak of Legionnaire's disease due to a public bathhouse, clinical examination. *Nihon Kokyuki Gakkai Zasshi* **2003**, *41*, 325–330. [PubMed]

51. Kawano, K.; Okada, M.; Kura, F.; Amemura-Maekawa, J.; Watanabe, H. Largest outbreak of legionellosis associated with spa baths, comparison of diagnostic tests. *Kansenshogaku Zasshi* **2007**, *81*, 173–182. [CrossRef] [PubMed]

52. Matsumoto, N.; Matsumoto, Y.; Ashitani, J.; Katoh, S.; Nakazato, M. An outbreak of Legionnaires' disease associated with a circulating bath water system at a public bathhouse. *Nihon Kokyuki Gakkai Zasshi* **2004**, *42*, 75–79. [PubMed]

53. Matsumoto, N.; Sasaki, T.; Nakao, H.; Katoh, T.; Fukuda, Y.; Nakazato, M.; Okayama, A. An outbreak of Legionnaires' disease associated with a circulating bathwater system at a public bathhouse. II: Radiological findings of pneumonia. *J. Infect. Chemother.* **2008**, *14*, 123–129. [CrossRef] [PubMed]

54. Okada, M.; Kawano, K.; Kura, F.; Amemura-Maekawa, J.; Watanabe, H.; Yagita, K.; Endo, T.; Suzuki, S. The largest outbreak of legionellosis in Japan associated with spa baths, epidemic curve and environmental investigation. *Kansenshogaku Zasshi* **2005**, *79*, 365–374. [CrossRef] [PubMed]

55. Sasaki, T.; Matsumoto, N.; Nakao, H.; Katoh, T.; Fukuda, Y.; Nakazato, M.; Okayama, A. An outbreak of Legionnaires' disease associated with a circulating bathwater system at a public bathhouse. I: A clinical analysis. *J. Infect. Chemother.* **2008**, *14*, 117–122. [PubMed]

56. Campese, C.; Roche, D.; Clément, C.; Fierobe, F.; Jarraud, S.; de Waelle, P.; Perrin, H.; Che, D. Cluster of Legionnaires' disease associated with a public whirlpool spa, France, April–May 2010. *Euro Surveill.* **2010**, *15*, 19602. [PubMed]

57. Sánchez-Busó, L.; Guiral, S.; Crespi, S.; Moya, V.; Camaró, M.L.; Olmos, M.P.; Adrián, F.; Morera, V.; González-Morán, F.; Vanaclocha, H.; et al. Genomic investigation of a Legionellosis outbreak in a persistently colonized hotel. *Front. Microbiol.* **2016**, *6*, 1556. [CrossRef] [PubMed]

58. Kuroki, T.; Amemura-Maekawa, J.; Ohya, H.; Furukawa, I.; Suzuki, M.; Masaoka, T.; Aikawa, K.; Hibi, K.; Morita, M.; Lee, K.I.; et al. Outbreak of Legionnaire's Disease caused by *Legionella pneumophila* serogroups 1 and 13. *Emerg. Infect. Dis.* **2017**, *23*, 349–351. [CrossRef] [PubMed]

59. Fallon, R.J.; Rowbotham, T.J. Microbiological investigations into an outbreak of Pontiac fever due to *Legionella micdadei* associated with use of a whirlpool. *J. Clin. Pathol.* **1990**, *43*, 479–483. [CrossRef] [PubMed]

60. Thomas, D.L.; Mundy, L.M.; Tucer, P.C. Hot tub legionellosis. Legionnaires' Disease and Pontiac Fever after a point-source exposure to *Legionella pneumophila*. *Arch. Intern. Med.* **1993**, *153*, 2597–2599. [CrossRef] [PubMed]

61. Benin, A.L.; Benson, R.F.; Arnold, K.E.; Fiore, A.E.; Cook, P.G.; Williams, L.K.; Fields, B.; Besser, R.E. An outbreak of travel-associated Legionnaires disease and Pontiac fever, the need for enhanced surveillance of travel-associated legionellosis in the United States. *J. Infect. Dis.* **2002**, *185*, 237–243. [CrossRef] [PubMed]

62. Huhn, G.D.; Adam, B.; Ruden, R.; Hilliard, L.; Kirkpatrick, P.; Todd, J.; Crafts, W.; Passaro, D.; Dworkin, M.S. Outbreak of travel-related Pontiac fever among hotel guests illustrating the need for better diagnostic tests. *J. Travel Med.* **2005**, *12*, 173–179. [PubMed]

63. Burnsed, L.J.; Hicks, L.A.; Smithee, L.M.; Fields, B.S.; Bradley, K.K.; Pascoe, N.; Richards, S.M.; Mallonee, S.; Littrell, L.; Benson, R.F.; et al. Legionellosis outbreak investigation team. A large, travel-associated outbreak of legionellosis among hotel guests, utility of the urine antigen assay in confirming Pontiac fever. *Clin. Infect. Dis.* **2007**, *44*, 222–228. [CrossRef] [PubMed]

64. Foster, K.; Gorton, R.; Waller, J. Outbreak of legionellosis associated with a spa pool, United Kingdom. *Euro Surveill.* **2006**, *11*, E060921.2. [CrossRef]

65. Euser, S.M.; Pelgrim, M.; den Boer, J.W. Legionnaires' disease and Pontiac fever after using a private outdoor whirlpool spa. *Scand. J. Infect. Dis.* **2010**, *42*, 910–916. [CrossRef] [PubMed]

66. Josef, C.A.; Lee, J.; van Wijngaarden, J.; Draser, V.; Castellanis Pastoris, M. European Guidelines for Control and Prevention of Travel Associated Legionnaires' Disease. The European Working Group for Legionella Infections (EWGLI), 2005. Available online: http://www.legionellaonline.it/linee_guidaEWGLI_gen2005.pdf (accessed on 9 July 2018).

67. WHO. *Legionella and the Prevention of Legionellosis*; WHO: Geneva, Switzerland, 2007; Available online: http://www.who.int/water_sanitation_health/emerging/legionella.pdf (accessed on 9 July 2018).

68. Bouwknegt, M.; Schijven, J.F.; Schalk, J.A.; de Roda Husman, A.M. Quantitative risk estimation for a *Legionella pneumophila* infection due to whirlpool use. *Risk Anal.* **2013**, *33*, 1228–1236. [PubMed]

69. Azuma, K.; Uchiyama, I.; Okumura, J. Assessing the risk of Legionnaires' disease: The inhalation exposure model and the estimated risk in residential bathrooms. *Regul. Toxicol. Pharmacol.* **2013**, *65*, 1–6. [CrossRef] [PubMed]

70. Press, E. The health hazards of saunas and spas and how to minimize them. *Am. J. Public Health* **1991**, *81*, 1034–1037. [CrossRef] [PubMed]

71. Coetzee, N.; Duggal, H.; Hawker, J.; Ibbotson, S.; Harrison, T.G.; Phin, N.; Laza-Stanca, V.; Johnston, R.; Iqbal, Z.; Rehman, Y.; et al. An outbreak of Legionnaires' disease associated with a display spa pool in retail premises, Stoke-on-Trent, United Kingdom, July 2012. *Euro Surveill.* **2012**, *17*, 20271. [PubMed]
72. Den Boer, J.W.; Yzerman, E.P.; Schellekens, J.; Lettinga, K.D.; Boshuizen, H.C.; Van Steenbergen, J.E.; Bosman, A.; Van den Hof, S.; Van Vliet, H.A.; Peeters, M.F.; et al. A large outbreak of Legionnaires' disease at a flower show, the Netherland, 1999. *Emerg. Infect. Dis.* **2002**, *8*, 37–43. [CrossRef] [PubMed]

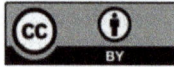

International Journal of
*Environmental Research
and Public Health*

MDPI

Article

Norovirus Outbreak Associated with Swimming in a Recreational Lake Not Influenced by External Human Fecal Sources in The Netherlands, August 2012

Franciska M. Schets [1,*], Harold H. J. L. van den Berg [1], Harry Vennema [1], Manon T. M. Pelgrim [2], Cees Collé [3], Saskia A. Rutjes [1] and Willemijn J. Lodder [1]

[1] National Institute for Public Health and the Environment, P.O. Box 1, 3720 BA Bilthoven, The Netherlands; harold.van.den.berg@rivm.nl (H.H.J.L.v.d.B.); harry.vennema@rivm.nl (H.V.); saskia.rutjes@rivm.nl (S.A.R.); willemijn.lodder@rivm.nl (W.J.L.)
[2] Public Health Service Veiligheids-en Gezondheidsregio Gelderland-Midden, Postbus 5364, 6802 EJ Arnhem, The Netherlands; manon.pelgrim@vggm.nl
[3] Province of Gelderland, Postbus 9090, 6800 GX Arnhem, The Netherlands; c.colle@gelderland.nl
* Correspondence: ciska.schets@rivm.nl; Tel.: +31-302743929

Received: 28 September 2018; Accepted: 9 November 2018; Published: 14 November 2018

Abstract: Swimming in fecally contaminated recreational water may lead to gastrointestinal illness. A recreational water-associated outbreak of norovirus (NoV) infections affecting at least 100 people in The Netherlands occurred in August 2012. Questionnaire responses from patients indicated swimming in recreational lake Zeumeren as the most likely cause of illness. Most patients visited the lake during the weekend of 18–19 August, during which the weather was exceptionally warm (maximum temperatures 32–33 °C), and visitor numbers elevated. Patients, mostly children, became ill with gastroenteritis 1–6 days (median 2 days) after exposure. Four stool samples from patients were NoV GI positive. Subsurface sandy soil from one of the beaches where most patients swam was NoV GI positive; the water sample was negative. The epidemiological curve and the timeline of investigation based on reported symptoms demonstrate the difficulty in discovering the source in recreational water outbreaks. A NoV outbreak in a recreational lake that is not subjected to external fecal contamination sources shows the need for active communication about human shedding of viruses during and after diarrheal episodes and the advice to refrain from swimming, even a few weeks after the symptoms have resolved.

Keywords: outbreak; recreational water; norovirus; swimming

1. Introduction

Noroviruses (NoV) are the leading cause of diarrhea in all age groups worldwide and they are primarily transmitted through the fecal-oral route [1]. The viruses are extremely contagious, with an estimated 50% infectious dose (ID_{50}) as low as 2.6 (aggregated) viral particles [2]. Primary cases often result from exposure to contaminated food or water, whereas person-to-person contact results in further spread of the infection. Infected persons shed large numbers of viral particles into the environment, and (low level) shedding may continue after symptoms have resolved [1,3]. Symptoms of NoV infections are mainly projectile vomiting and watery non-bloody diarrhoea, but fever, abdominal cramping and nausea do also occur. The incubation period is 10 to 51 h and illness is generally self-limiting, normally lasting 2–3 days [1,4], but the duration of illness can be prolonged to 4–6 days in children younger than 11 years of age [5].

NoV have been genetically classified into five genogroups (G) [6]. GI and GII are primarily associated with human disease [1]. The GII.4 cluster is responsible for most human norovirus outbreaks [7]; for example, over 80% of the outbreaks in the United States (1994–2006) were caused by strains from this cluster [4]. GI strains are more often associated with waterborne outbreaks than other genogroups [8]. NoV have been the cause of outbreaks related to contaminated municipal water supplies, e.g., in Sweden [9], drinking water wells, e.g., in The Netherlands [10], ground water, e.g., in South Korea [11], and various recreational water settings [12], including a fountain in Belgium, where Dutch school children became ill during a school trip [13], a swimming pool [14] and a fresh water lake in the United States [15], and a recreational lake in Finland [16]. A survey of recreational water associated viral disease outbreaks, occurring between 1977 and 2006, identified noroviruses as the cause of the illness in 45% (*n* = 25) of the outbreaks [12]. The majority of these outbreaks resulted from exposure to lakes (56%, *n* = 14). In a recently published study of bathing water related outbreaks in Finland that all occurred in 2014, epidemiological and microbiological data showed that NoV was the main causative agent [17].

This paper describes the occurrence and investigation of a recreational water associated outbreak of NoV infections affecting at least 100 people in The Netherlands in August 2012.

2. Materials and Methods

2.1. Outbreak Description

On Monday, 20 August 2012, over 20 people reported gastro-intestinal complaints to the province of Gelderland after swimming in recreational lake Zeumeren in Barneveld, The Netherlands. During the week of 20–24 August, over 100 people reported the same with Public Health Service Veiligheids-en Gezondheidsregio Gelderland-Midden (VGGM). All patients, who were mainly children, had visited the lake during the previous weekend of 18 and 19 August. During that weekend, the weather in The Netherlands was exceptionally warm with maximum temperatures of 32–33 °C (at weather station De Bilt, the station closest to Zeumeren) (www.knmi.nl). Because of the warm weather, several thousands of people swam at Zeumeren during the weekend. Most patients became ill one to one-and-a-half day after exposure to the lake water, and had swum at two of the ten possible beaches surrounding the lake (Figure 1). The majority of the patients reported short-term symptoms and recovered rapidly.

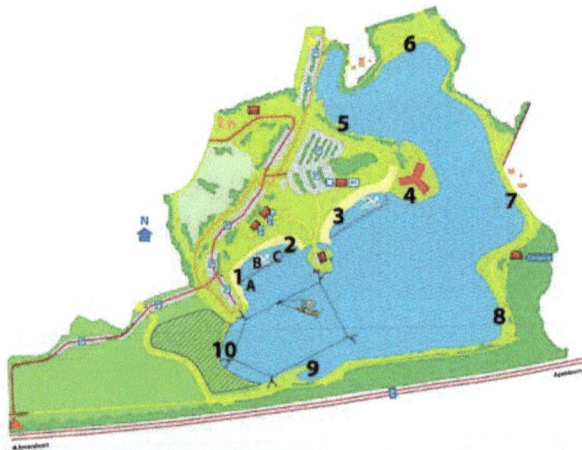

Figure 1. Recreational water lake Zeumeren, The Netherlands, with beaches 1—10 and sampling points. A—C. Beaches 1—2 and 3 are the official beaches, which are sampled for monitoring according to the EU BWD [18]. Sampling points for the outbreak investigation: A—water and subsurface sandy soil sample taken, B and C—subsurface sandy soil samples taken.

Investigation of the outbreak started on Monday, 20 August 2012; as a precaution, an advice against bathing in lake Zeumeren was set at the end of the afternoon on that same day. The advice against bathing was removed on 14 September 2012 (Figure 2). Since occasionally swimmers were observed in the lake after setting the advice against bathing, the case definition was defined as: all people that visited lake Zeumeren between 15 August and 24 August 2012, and subsequently developed gastro-intestinal symptoms.

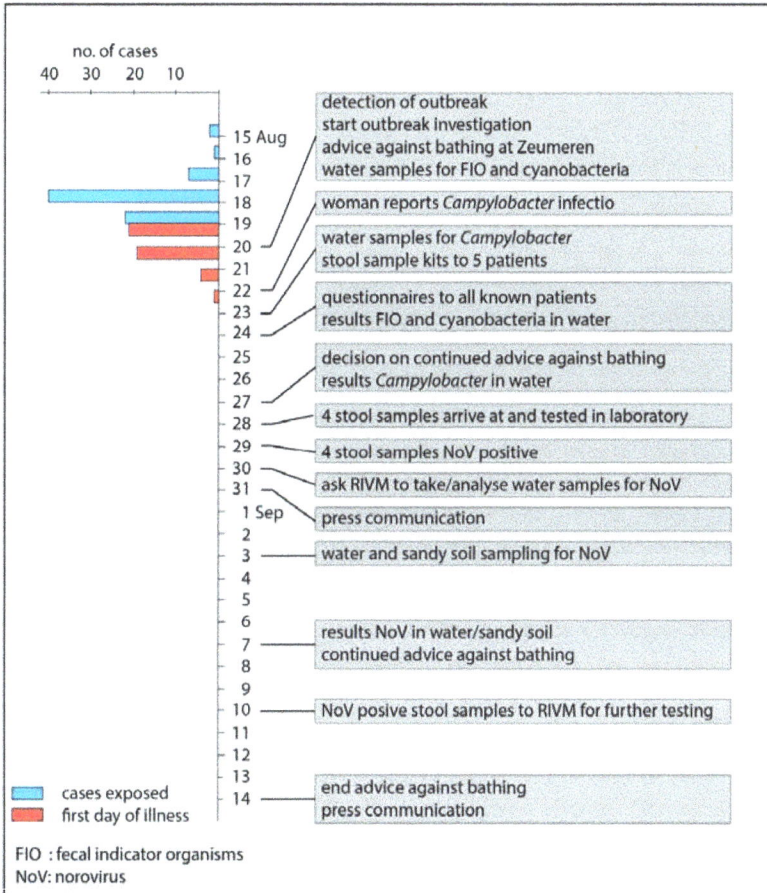

Figure 2. Epidemiological curve, indicating the days on which the cases (n_{total} = 45) were exposed and their first day of illness, and the timeline of the outbreak investigation.

2.2. Site Description

Lake Zeumeren is located in a rural area (community Barneveld) in the center of The Netherlands. It is a 32-hectare isolated fresh water lake with stagnant water, with groundwater and rainwater as sources. The maximum water depth is 17 m and it has a sandy soil. Lake Zeumeren is an official bathing site, where the water quality is monitored for fecal indicator parameters *Escherichia coli* and intestinal enterococci, according to the European Bathing Water Directive (EU BWD) [18] with a fortnightly frequency during the bathing season (1 May–1 October). The lake is surrounded by beaches, two of which are identified as the official beaches, with demarcated bathing areas. At the two official beaches, regular samples are taken for monitoring according to the EU BWD (Figure 1). The bathing zone has a surface of 1.7 hectare, a maximum water depth of 1.5 m, and a total beach length of 530 m. On-site facilities include toilets, showers, waste bins, and play equipment; the play equipment is located on the dry land of beach 4 (Figure 1). Dogs are not allowed at the location during the bathing season. The bathing water profile indicates that there is no connection to other water bodies, and that the water quality is not influenced by wastewater treatment plants or run-off from agricultural land. A substantial seagull population foraging at the lake may however occasionally influence the water quality. According to the EU BWD, water quality at lake Zeumeren is classified as 'excellent'.

2.3. Epidemiological Investigation

The province of Gelderland and the Public Health Service VGGM sent questionnaires by email on 24 August 2012 to all patients with whom they had primary contact and for whom they had kept records ($n = 36$). The patients were asked to answer the questions and to forward the questionnaire to anyone they knew who had swum at the same site during the same period and had become ill with the same symptoms. This approach was chosen in an attempt to rapidly identify the source of the outbreak. Since there was no aim at performing a full case-control study, no matching controls were sought. By allowing questionnaires to be forwarded, no records were (or could be) kept of the number of questionnaires distributed. Apart from demographic questions about age and gender, questionnaires included information requests about having visited lake Zeumeren (date between 15 August and 24 August 2012), having entered the water (including specification of beaches visited), having swum (including duration of swimming), health conditions (choose from diarrhea, vomiting, fever, fatigue, skin conditions, other), using the on-site toilets, and having bought and consumed food and beverages on-site. Analysis of questionnaire responses was done by using SPSS (IBM, Armonk, NY, USA, version 22).

2.4. Microbiological Investigation of Clinical Samples

Five patients were asked to send in stool samples; samples from four patients were received and analyzed for the bacterial enteropathogens *Salmonella*, *Shigella*, *Campylobacter*, shiga toxin-producing *Escherichia coli* (STEC) and *Yersinia*, and NoV at the medical microbiological laboratory of the Rijnstate Hospital in Arnhem, The Netherlands, by using routine PCR. Later, the four samples were sent to the National Institute for Public Health and the Environment (RIVM) for further testing. At RIVM, the samples were analyzed for the presence of NoV by using a real-time RT-PCR assay, with primers, probes and PCR conditions as previously described [19].

2.5. Environmental Investigation

In order to narrow down the outbreak and to identify the source, several leads were followed. In response to the reported cases of gastroenteritis, water samples were taken from lake Zeumeren at the two official beaches (Figure 1) on 20 August 2012 and were analyzed for fecal indicator parameters *E. coli* and intestinal enterococci, by using the most probable number methods specified in the EU BWD [18].

Although lake Zeumeren does not have a history of problems with cyanobacteria, the presence of a faint greenish colouring of the water led to visual inspection for the presence of cyanobacteria and sampling of the water at beach 4 (Figure 1) for determination of the dominant cyanobacterium genus by microscopy and toxin levels by ELISA on Monday, 20 August 2012.

On Wednesday, 22 August, a woman reported to the province of Gelderland having fallen ill after swimming in lake Zeumeren during the weekend prior to the outbreak weekend (11–12 August). She attended a physician and had blood, urine and feces examined, which revealed a *Campylobacter jejuni* infection that was treated with antibiotics. Although the woman did not meet the case definition, it was decided to follow this lead because of the known nuisance caused by gulls at lake Zeumeren that take over the beaches after the bathers have left. Water samples were taken at the two official beaches on 23 August and analyzed for the presence of *Campylobacter* spp. by using a membrane filtration method with incubation on Karmali Agar at 42 ± 0.5 °C for 48 ± 2 h (in house method of Het Waterlaboratorium, Haarlem, The Netherlands).

When the four analyzed stool samples appeared to be NoV positive, RIVM was contacted on 30 August and asked to take environmental samples for NoV analysis at lake Zeumeren. Sampling was done on 3 September 2012. Water and subsurface sandy soil samples were only taken from the beaches where most of the patients had stayed or swum during the weekend of 18 and 19 August as was pointed out by the questionnaire results. One water sample was taken at sampling point A, and one subsurface sandy soil sample was taken at each of the sampling points A–C (Figure 1).

The water sample (600 L) was taken by using an on-site filtration adsorption-elution procedure for concentration of the sample [20,21]. The eluate was further concentrated by ultrafiltration under high pressure (three bars) using a cellulose-acetate filter with a nominal molecular weight limit of 10,000 (Sartorius). The ultrafilter was rinsed with 3% beef extract (pH 9.0) resulting in the final concentrate of approximately 40 mL which was stored at −70°C until further analysis. RNA extraction was performed on 0.2, 1 and 5 mL of the concentrate as described by Rutjes et al. [21].

Subsurface sandy soil samples of approximately 50 g were taken by using a tubular soil sampler. Subsequently, 10 mL 0.05 M glycine buffer pH 9.0 was added to 5.0 g of each sandy soil sample and mixed at 500 rpm for 35 min at 4°C, after which it was allowed to settle for 10 min (in house method RIVM). RNA extraction was done according to Rutjes et al. [21], by adding 20 and then 9 mL of lysis buffer (Biomerieux, Boxtel, The Netherlands) to 5 mL and 1 mL volumes, respectively, of the supernatant. Purification of the RNA extract was done by using a Qiagen RNeasy kit according to the manufacturers' instructions.

A real time reverse transcriptase PCR (RT-PCR) assay as described by Verhaelen et al. [19] was performed to detect the presence of norovirus GI and GII RNA. The sequence of the detected norovirus strain was determined by directly sequencing the purified RT-PCR product, which was 86 nucleotides long.

3. Results

3.1. Epidemiological Investigation

Public Health Service VGGM received 45 filled-in questionnaires that met the case definition. Of the respondents, 56% ($n = 25$) were female. The age of the respondents ranged between 0 and 59 years of age, with more than half being children of 0–12 years of age (53%, $n = 24$), while the others were adults of 18–59 years of age (47%, $n = 21$). All respondents visited lake Zeumeren between 15 and 19 August, but the majority were at the site on 18 August (89%, $n = 40$) and/or 19 August (49%, $n = 22$). In total, 27 cases were exposed on more than one day during the specified period. All cases went into the water for swimming and became ill afterwards, with health complaints starting 1–6 days (average and median 2 days) after exposure to the bathing water and beaches at Lake Zeumeren and lasting for 0.5–6 days (average and median 2 days). Reported health conditions were (multiple answers per case allowed): diarrhea (84%, $n = 38$), vomiting (82%, $n = 37$), fatigue (49%, $n = 22$), and fever (16%, $n = 7$). None of the cases reported skin conditions, and eight cases reported other complaints than those indicated above, of which seven were related to gastro-intestinal discomfort. One case reported a headache.

Forty-four of the cases indicated at which beach they had swum (multiple answers per case were allowed), showing that most cases swam at beach 1 (70%, $n = 31$) and/or beach 2 (32%, $n = 14$). Most cases (82%, $n = 37$) were in the water for 30 min to over an hour.

Fifty-eight percent ($n = 26$) of the cases used the permanent on-site toilets, the others did not. Buying and consuming on-site sold food and beverages were not very common: 87% ($n = 39$) did not buy or consume food and 98% ($n = 44$) did not buy or consume beverages.

3.2. Microbiological Investigation of Clinical Samples

The four investigated stool samples were positive with NoV GI, and not with any of the other aetiologies. The fecal samples contained NoV genotype GI.Pd-GI.3. The partial genomic sequence of the strain was submitted to Genbank under accession number MH828423. The size of the PCR product was 1116 base pairs, including the primers. Sequence analysis yielded 1007 nucleotides, 733 overlapping with the typing region of open reading frame 1 (ORF1), and 275 overlapping with the typing region of ORF2. Genotype assignment by phylogenetic analysis was supported by 100% and 99% bootstrap analysis, for ORF1 and ORF2, respectively. Typing from RT-PCR products is reliable if the fragment has >100 nucleotides overlapping with both of the typing regions of ORF1 and ORF2.

3.3. Environmental Investigation

Water samples taken on 20 August 2012 showed levels of *E. coli* at the official beaches of 16 most probable number (mpn)/100 mL at beach 1–2 and 6 mpn/100 mL at beach 3. Compared to previous and later routine samplings during the same bathing season, slightly elevated levels of intestinal enterococci at both beaches, 230 mpn/100 mL and 160 mpn/100 mL, respectively, were observed.

Examination of the samples taken for cyanobacteria analyses by microscopy demonstrated the presence of *Microcystis* spp. at beach 4; intracellular microcystin levels were very low (<2 µg/L).

Campylobacter spp. were present in the water samples taken at the official beaches (one sample per beach) on 23 August. Numbers appeared to be low, but could not be exactly determined due to overgrowth of the culture medium. Further identification to the species level was not done.

NoV GI was detected in the subsurface sandy soil sample taken at sampling point A (beach 1). The other subsurface sandy soil samples and the water sample were NoV negative. Sequencing of the RT-PCR product from the subsurface sandy soil sample was impossible because the method for typing of RT-PCR products is less sensitive than the detection method, and the amount of RNA in the subsurface sandy soil sample appeared to be too low.

4. Discussion

Following the reporting of many cases of gastroenteritis that seemed related to exposure to a recreational lake in The Netherlands during an exceptionally warm weekend in August 2012, several leads were investigated in order to discover the etiological agent and the source of the outbreak. Although the epidemiological investigation implicated the recreational lake as the most likely location of contracting illness, the different directions in which the investigation went, based on reported symptoms, demonstrate the difficulty in narrowing down the possible cause of recreational water related outbreaks. The results of the examination of patient material can ease the search for the etiological agent and the source; however, in this case, the reporting of a patient with a *Campylobacter* infection in combination with the presence of a large seagull population resulted in choosing, what later appeared to be, the wrong direction. Following several leads and having various patient and environmental samples examined takes time, and in this case, led to the examination of water and subsurface sandy soil samples only over two weeks after the outbreak presumably started, thus diminishing the chances of detecting the etiological agent. Due to of the time gap between the onset of the outbreak and the environmental sampling, subsurface sandy soil sampling was performed in addition to the normal procedure of water sampling because sedimentation of virus particles during the delay period could have resulted in the presence of virus particles in the subsurface sandy soil [22]. In this outbreak investigation, this appeared to be true and therefore subsurface sandy soil sampling could be considered while environmental sampling in outbreak situations is delayed. However, even if environmental samples are taken sooner, factors such as dispersion, dilution, sedimentation and inactivation of the microorganisms in the water body may result in the inability to detect the microorganisms that caused the outbreak [23]. The detection of NoV GI in the stool samples of outbreak related patients and the detection of NoV GI in the subsurface sandy soil of the beach where most patients swam support the probability that exposure to the lake resulted in the outbreak. NoV G I strains have a stronger association with waterborne transmission than GII strains [8,24], possibly because they are more stable in water than GII strains [8]. In a survey of recreational waters in Europe, 9.4% of 1440 samples were positive with NoV GI and GII [25], thus demonstrating the presence of NoV in randomly selected recreational waters.

The epidemiological investigation showed that most of the patients were children. It has been demonstrated that, while swimming, compared to adults, children spend more time in the water and ingest a larger volume of water, thus increasing their exposure [26,27] and resulting in a higher infection risk and attributable disease burden [28]. High exposure of children in combination with the low infectious dose of NoV [2] and the incompletely developed immune system in young children explain the high number of affected children. A possible bias is that parents are more likely to report health complaints and sooner when their children are involved.

The detection of the same NoV genogroup in subsurface sandy soil and in patients two weeks after the onset of the outbreak shows that NoV may be present in the environment for prolonged time through accumulation in sediment [22], and may even be re-dispersed when bathers whirl the soil. Although only RNA from virus particles was detected and no information about their infectivity was available, these results indicate the value of a prolonged advice against bathing. Lake Zeumeren is an isolated lake that is not subject to external sources of fecal contamination that may introduce NoV, such as sewage water treatment plants, and the majority of the cases did not buy or consume on-site sold food and beverages. Therefore, a food-related cause of the outbreak is unlikely and the most plausible cause of contamination of the water is an infected human. Evidence of a single person being responsible for contamination of the water was, however, not discovered, as is often the case [8,24]. Prevention of outbreaks that have an infected human as the source can be done by active communication of the long-standing advice of not to swim while having diarrhea, combined with the information that viral shedding continues even after symptoms have resolved, although this does not prevent occasional asymptomatic shedding [29].

5. Conclusions

An outbreak of gastrointestinal illness among over 100 visitors of a recreational lake in The Netherlands during an exceptionally warm weekend was caused by NoV. The results of the epidemiological investigation, combined with the detection of NoV GI in the stool samples of outbreak related patients and in the subsurface sandy soil of the beach where most patients swam, suggest that exposure to the recreational lake resulted in the outbreak. Although the primary contamination source has not been discovered, the most likely cause of contamination of the water is an infected human, because the lake is an isolated water body that is not subject to external sources of fecal contamination. An outbreak like this warrants active communication about human shedding of viruses during and after diarrheal episodes and the advice to refrain from swimming. The epidemiological curve and the timeline of investigation based on reported symptoms demonstrate the difficulty in discovering the source in recreational water outbreaks.

Author Contributions: Conceptualization, M.T.M.P., C.C. and F.M.S.; Methodology, H.H.J.L.v.d.B., W.J.L. and H.V.; Investigation, F.M.S., H.H.J.L.v.d.B., M.T.M.P., W.J.L. and S.A.R.; Data Analysis, M.T.M.P., F.M.S., W.J.L. and H.V.; Writing—Original Draft Preparation, F.M.S.; Writing—Review & Editing, F.M.S., H.H.J.L.v.d.B., H.V., M.T.M.P., C.C., S.A.R. and W.J.L.; Visualization, F.M.S. and M.T.M.P.; Supervision, F.M.S.

Funding: This research received no external funding.

Acknowledgments: The authors thank the location manager of lake Zeumeren and the colleagues from the province of Gelderland and Public Health Service VGGM involved in this outbreak investigation for their contribution, Ana Maria de Roda Husman (RIVM) for critically reading of the manuscript and Leonard Bik for his help with the figures.

Conflicts of Interest: The authors declare no conflict of interest.

References

1. Patel, M.M.; Hall, A.J.; Vinjé, J.; Parashar, U.D. Noroviruses: A comprehensive review. *J. Clin. Virol.* **2009**, *44*, 1–8. [CrossRef] [PubMed]
2. Teunis, P.F.M.; Moe, C.L.; Liu, P.; Miller, S.E.; Lindesmith, L.; Baric, R.S.; Le Pendu, J.; Calderon, R.L. Norwalk virus: How infectious is it? *J. Med. Virol.* **2008**, *80*, 1468–1476. [CrossRef] [PubMed]
3. Atmar, R.L.; Opekum, A.R.; Gilger, M.A.; Estes, M.K.; Crawford, S.E.; Neill, F.H.; Graham, D.Y. Norwalk virus shedding after experimental human infection. *Emerg. Infect. Dis.* **2008**, *14*, 1553–1557. [CrossRef] [PubMed]
4. Glass, R.I.; Parashar, U.D.; Estes, M.K. Norovirus gastroenteritis. *N. Engl. J. Med.* **2009**, *361*, 1776–1785. [CrossRef] [PubMed]
5. Rockx, B.; De Wit, M.; Vennema, H.; Vinjé, J.; De Bruin, E.; Van Duynhoven, Y.; Koopmans, M. Natural history of human calicivirus infection: A prospective cohort study. *Clin. Infect. Dis.* **2002**, *35*, 246–253. [CrossRef] [PubMed]
6. Zheng, D.P.; Ando, T.; Fankhauser, R.L.; Beard, R.S.; Glass, R.I.; Monroe, S.S. Norovirus classification and proposed strain nomenclature. *Virology* **2006**, *346*, 312–323. [CrossRef] [PubMed]
7. Atmar, R.L.; Ramani, S.; Estes, M.K. Human noroviruses: recent advances in a 50-year history. *Curr. Opin. Infect. Dis.* **2018**, *31*, 422–432. [CrossRef] [PubMed]
8. Matthews, J.E.; Dickey, B.W.; Miller, R.D.; Felzer, J.R.; Dawson, B.P.; Lee, A.S.; Rocks, J.J.; Kiel, J.; Montes, J.S.; Moe, C.L.; et al. The epidemiology of published norovirus outbreaks: A review of risk factors associated with attack rate and genogroup. *Epidemiol. Infect.* **2012**, *140*, 1161–1172. [CrossRef]
9. Riera-Montes, M.; Sjölander, K.B.; Allestam, G.; Hallin, E.; Hedlund, K.O.; Löfdahl, M. Waterborne norovirus outbreak in a municipal drinking-water supply in Sweden. *Epidemiol. Infect.* **2011**, *139*, 1928–1935. [CrossRef] [PubMed]
10. Ter Waarbeek, H.L.; Dukers-Muijrers, N.H.; Vennema, H.; Hoebe, C.J. Waterborne gastroenteritis outbreak at a scouting camp caused by two norovirus genogroups: GI and GII. *J. Clin. Virol.* **2010**, *47*, 268–272. [CrossRef] [PubMed]
11. Cho, H.G.; Lee, S.G.; Kim, W.H.; Lee, J.S.; Park, P.H.; Cheon, D.S.; Jheong, W.H.; Jho, E.H.; Lee, J.B.; Paik, S.Y. Acute gastroenteritis outbreaks associated with ground-waterborne norovirus in South Korea during 2008–2012. *Epidemiol. Infect.* **2014**, *142*, 2604–2609. [CrossRef] [PubMed]
12. Sinclair, R.G.; Jones, E.L.; Gerba, C.P. Viruses in recreational water-borne disease outbreaks: A review. *J. Appl. Microbiol.* **2009**, *107*, 1769–1780. [CrossRef] [PubMed]
13. Hoebe, C.J.; Vennema, H.; De Roda Husman, A.M.; Van Duynhoven, Y.T. Norovirus outbreak among primary schoolchildren who had played in a recreational water fountain. *J. Infect. Dis.* **2004**, *189*, 699–705. [CrossRef] [PubMed]
14. Podewils, L.J.; Zanardi Blevins, L.; Hagenbuch, M.; Itani, D.; Burns, A.; Otto, C.; Blanton, L.; Adams, A.; Monroe, S.S.; Beach, M.J.; et al. Outbreak of norovirus illness associated with a swimming pool. *Epidemiol. Infect.* **2007**, *135*, 827–833. [CrossRef] [PubMed]
15. Zlot, A.; Simckes, M.; Vines, J.; Reynolds, L.; Sullivan, A.; Scott, M.K.; McLuckie, J.M.; Kromer, D.; Hill, V.R.; Yoder, J.S.; et al. Norovirus outbreak associated with a natural lake used for recreation–Oregon, 2014. *Am. J. Transplant.* **2015**, *15*, 2001–2005. [CrossRef] [PubMed]
16. Polkowska, A.; Räsänen, S.; Al-Hello, H.; Bojang, M.; Lyytikäinen, O.; Nuorti, J.P.; Jalava, K. An outbreak of norovirus infections associated with recreational lake water in Western Finland, 2014. *Epidemiol. Infect.* **2018**, *146*, 544–550. [CrossRef] [PubMed]
17. Kauppinen, A.; Al-Hello, H.; Zacheus, O.; Kilponen, J.; Maunula, L.; Huusko, S.; Lappalainen, M.; Miettinen, I.; Blomqvist, S.; Rimhanen-Finne, R. Increase in outbreaks of gastroenteritis linked to bathing water in Finland in summer 2014. *Euro Surveill.* **2017**, *22*, 30470. [CrossRef] [PubMed]
18. The European Parliament and the Council of the European Union. Directive 2006/7/EC of the European Parliament and of the Council of 15 February 2006 concerning the management of bathing water quality and repealing Directive 76/160/EEC. *Off. J. Europ. Union* **2006**, *L64*, 37–51.
19. Verhaelen, K.; Bouwknegt, M.; Lodder-Verschoor, F.; Rutjes, S.A.; De Roda Husman, A.M. Persistence of human norovirus GII.4 and GI.4, murine norovirus, and human adenovirus on soft berries as compared with PBS at commonly applied storage conditions. *Int. J. Food Microbiol.* **2012**, *160*, 137–144. [CrossRef] [PubMed]

20. Van Olphen, M.; Kapsenberg, J.G.; Van de Baan, E.; Kroon, W.A. Removal of enteric viruses from surface water at eight waterworks in The Netherlands. *Appl. Environ. Microbiol.* **1984**, *47*, 927–932. [PubMed]

21. Rutjes, S.A.; Italiaander, R.; Van den Berg, H.H.; Lodder, W.J.; De Roda Husman, A.M. Isolation and detection of enterovirus RNA from large-volume water samples by using the NucliSens miniMAG system and real-time nucleic acid sequence-based amplification. *Appl. Environ. Microbiol.* **2005**, *71*, 3734–3740. [CrossRef] [PubMed]

22. Skraber, S.; Schijven, J.; Italiaander, R.; De Roda Husman, A.M. Accumulation of enteric bacteriophage in fresh water sediments. *J. Water Health* **2009**, *7*, 372–379. [CrossRef] [PubMed]

23. Schets, F.M.; De Roda Husman, A.M.; Havelaar, A.H. Disease outbreaks associated with untreated recreational water use. *Epidemiol. Infect.* **2011**, *139*, 1114–1125. [CrossRef] [PubMed]

24. Bitler, E.J.; Matthews, J.E.; Dickey, B.W.; Eisenberg, J.N.; Leon, J.S. Norovirus outbreaks: a systematic review of commonly implicated transmission routes and vehicles. *Epidemiol. Infect.* **2013**, *141*, 1563–1571. [CrossRef] [PubMed]

25. Wyn-Jones, A.P.; Carducci, A.; Cook, N.; D'Agostino, M.; Divizia, M.; Fleischer, J.; Gantzer, C.; Gawler, A.; Girones, R.; Höller, C.; et al. Surveillance of adenoviruses and noroviruses in European recreational waters. *Water Res.* **2011**, *45*, 1025–1038. [CrossRef] [PubMed]

26. Schets, F.M.; Schijven, J.F.; De Roda Husman, A.M. Exposure assessment for swimmers in bathing waters and swimming pools. *Water Res.* **2011**, *45*, 2392–2400. [CrossRef] [PubMed]

27. DeFlorio-Barker, S.; Arnold, B.F.; Sams, E.A.; Dufour, A.P.; Colford, J.M., Jr.; Weisberg, S.B.; Schiff, K.C.; Wade, T.J. 2017 Child environmental exposures to water and sand at the beach: Findings from studies of over 68,000 subjects at 12 beaches. *J. Expo. Sci. Environ. Epidemiol.* **2017**, *28*, 93–100. [CrossRef] [PubMed]

28. Arnold, B.F.; Wade, T.J.; Benjamin-Chung, J.; Schiff, K.C.; Griffith, J.F.; Dufour, A.P.; Weisberg, S.B.; Colford, J.M., Jr. Acute gastroenteritis and recreational water: highest burden among young US children. *Am. J. Public Health* **2016**, *106*, 1690–1697. [CrossRef] [PubMed]

29. Teunis, P.F.; Sukhrie, F.H.; Vennema, H.; Bogerman, J.; Beersma, M.F.; Koopmans, M.P. Shedding of norovirus in symptomatic and asymptomatic infections. *Epidemiol. Infect.* **2015**, *143*, 1710–1717. [CrossRef] [PubMed]

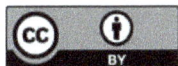

International Journal of
*Environmental Research
and Public Health*

MDPI

Article

Assessment of Microbiological Safety of Water in Public Swimming Pools in Guangzhou, China

Xiaohong Wei [1,2,†], Juntao Li [1,†], Shuiping Hou [1], Conghui Xu [1], Hao Zhang [1], Edward Robert Atwill [3,4], Xunde Li [3,4], Zhicong Yang [1,*] and Shouyi Chen [1,*] (iD)

[1] Guangzhou Center for Disease Control and Prevention, Guangzhou 510440, China; weijuanwo@163.com (X.W.); jtwl1011@163.com (J.L.); gzcdc367@163.com (S.H.); yeast-27@163.com (C.X.); haozsu@163.com (H.Z.)

[2] School of Public Health, Sun Yat-Sen University, Guangzhou 510030, China

[3] Department of Population Health and Reproduction, University of California Davis, California, CA 95616, USA; ratwill@ucdavis.edu (E.R.A.); xdli@ucdavis.edu (X.L.)

[4] Western Institute for Food Safety and Security, University of California Davis, California, CA 95616, USA

[*] Correspondence: yangzc@gzcdc.org.cn (Z.Y.); Shouyi_chen@163.com (S.C.); Tel.: +86-138-2614-0717 (Z.Y.)

[†] These authors contributed equally to this article.

Received: 15 June 2018; Accepted: 3 July 2018; Published: 5 July 2018

Abstract: This study assessed microbiological safety of water from public swimming pools in Guangzhou, China. Water samples from 39 outdoor municipal swimming pools were collected from late June to early September, 2013 and subjected to detection of protozoa (*Giardia* and *Cryptosporidium*) and bacteria (*Pseudomonas aeruginos*, total coliforms, *E. coli*, *E. coli* O157, *Shigella*, and *Salmonella*). *Cryptosporidium* and *Giardia* were both detected in 5 (12.8%) swimming pools. Total coliforms were detected in 4 (10.3%) samples with concentrations ranging from 1.3 to 154.0 MPN/100 mL while *E. coli* was detected in 4 (10.3%) samples with concentrations ranging from 0.5 to 5.3 MPN/100 mL. *P. aeruginosa* was detected in 27 (69.2%) samples but *E. coli* O157, *Shigella* and *Salmonella* were not detected. Among these swimming pools, 9 (23%) met the Chinese National Standard of residual chlorine levels and 24 (62%) were tested free of residual chlorine at least once. The multi-locus sequence typing (MLST) analysis showed that all *P. aeruginosa* isolates belonged to new sequence types (STs) with dominant ST-1764 and ST-D distributed in different locations within the area. Some *P. aeruginosa* strains were resistant to medically important antibiotics. Results indicate potential public health risks due to the presence of microbiological pathogens in public swimming pools in this area.

Keywords: swimming pool; water; *Giardia*; *Cryptosporidium*; *P. aeruginosa*; antibiotic resistance; multi-locus sequence typing

1. Introduction

Many microbiological pathogens, including bacteria, viruses, and parasites can cause waterborne disease [1]. Waterborne disease is estimated to cause more than 2.2 million deaths per year and many cases of illness every day, including diarrhea, gastrointestinal diseases and other systemic illnesses [2,3]. Waterborne disease can have a significant impact locally and globally [4]. Waterborne infections are transmitted in numerous ways, including but not limited to ingestion, airborne or contact with contaminated water by a variety of infectious agents.

In addition to drinking water, which serves as a route for waterborne illness worldwide, especially in developing countries [5], exposure to recreational water also frequently causes outbreaks of waterborne diseases in both developed and developing countries [6–9]. For examples of recreational water related outbreaks in developed countries, there have been reports of waterborne disease associated with swimming pools in Australia [10], England and Wales [11] and other countries [12]. Most countries have programs for monitoring microbiological safety of swimming pool water. However, diverse public health and economic conditions among countries result in different microbiological and physical-chemical standards for swimming pool water even within countries of the European Union [13]. In China, a National Standard for swimming pool water quality, entitled "Hygienic Standard for Swimming Places" has been established (GB9667-1996). Major parameters in the National Standard are water temperature (22–26 °C), pH (6.5–8.5), turbidity ($\leq$5 NTU), urea ($\leq$3.5 mg/L), free residual chlorine levels (0.3–0.5 mg/L), total bacteria count ($\leq$1000 cfu/mL), total coliforms ($\leq$18 cfu/L). Although some recent works have studied water quality of swimming pools in China, most of these studies have primarily focused on the basic parameters that are highlighted in the National Standards, including pH, turbidity, urea content and total coliforms [14–16]. Literature on the microbiological safety of swimming pool water in China has been notably sparse. Furthermore, from a public health perspective it remains unknown if swimming pool water transmits antibiotic resistant bacteria. By detection and analysis of key waterborne protozoa and bacteria, this study evaluated the microbiological safety of water in outdoor public swimming pools in Guangzhou, which is a large metropolitan area in southern China.

2. Materials and Methods

2.1. Swimming Pools Selection and Water Sample Collection

This survey was conducted between 20 June and 4 September 2013. Due to the potential differences in public health conditions between suburban and urban districts within the Guangzhou area [17], the suburban Baiyun district and the urban Haizhu district were chosen for sampling. In total 39 pools, including 27 pools from the Baiyun district (21 residential pools, 6 pools from two water parks) and 12 pools from the Haizhu district (5 residential pools, 3 school pools, and 4 pools from one water park) were enrolled in the study. All enrolled pools were outdoor public swimming pools. Three swimming pools were exclusively for children while the remaining 36 pools were for both adults and children. Water samples were collected between 10:00 a.m. and noon, a period prior to the pools being open to swimmers. Using a submersible pump, 50 L water samples were pumped 10 cm from the bottom of the pool into two sterile 25 L carboys. Four hundred milligrams of sodium thiosulfate ($Na_2S_2O_3$, XK13-001-00008, GB/T-637 standard, Guangzhou, China) was added to each carboy for dechlorination of water. Carboys were placed in containers with ice and transported to the laboratory within two hours and stored in a cold room (4 °C) upon arrival at the laboratory and before processing.

A questionnaire was filled out for each swimming pool in order to support the microbiological analysis. The questionnaires contained three sections that include general data on the swimming pools (type, location, dimensions and depth), levels of residual chlorine, and management information (opening time, hours of operation, availability of swimming-suit rentals, whether toddlers were required to wear diapers during swimming, methods used to refresh water, frequency of testing residual chlorine levels).

2.2. Detection of Microbiological Pathogens from Water

With the aid of hollow fiber ultrafiltration as described by Rhodes et al. [18], the 50 L water sample was filtered no later than 24 h after collection and concentrated to approximately 700 mL (retentate). To test for *Giardia* and *Cryptosporidium*, 500 mL of the retentate was centrifuged at 4000 rcf at 25 °C for 15 min without breaking. Supernatant was discarded by aspiration and approximately 3 mL of residual pellet was harvested. An immunomagnetic separation (IMS) procedure was carried out to separate (oo) cysts from concentrated water samples using the Dynabeads GC-Combo kit (Invitrogen Dynal AS, Oslo, Norway) according to the manufacturer's instructions. The IMS was carried out using a Bead Retriever with the procedure of 'GC Combo' (Invitrogen, Finland). Immunofluorescent staining of final IMS products (approximately 50 μL) was performed using the Aqua-Glo G/C Direct kit (Waterborne, New Orleans, LA, USA) according to the manufacturer's instructions. Slides were examined for (oo) cysts using an immunofluorescent microscope (Leica DM6000B).

All bacteria were detected according to China's National Standard (GB) protocols. Specifically, *P. aeruginosa* was detected using methods described in the Hygienic Standard for Cosmetics (GB7918.4-2007, Ministry of Health, China). The methods used for detection of other bacteria were based on the National Food Safety Standard (Ministry of Health, China), i.e., GB4789.3-2010 for total coliforms, GB4789.38-2012 for *E. coli*, GB4789.36-2008 for *E. coli* O157, GB4789.5-2012 for *Shigella* and GB4789.4-2010 for *Salmonella*, respectively. The procedures for detection of these bacteria are described below.

To detect *P. aeruginosa*, 10 mL of retentate was resuspended in 90 mL of Soya Casein Digest Lecithin Polysorbate (SCDLP) broth and incubated at 37 °C for 24 h. Then, 100 μL of the culture was streaked on cetrimide agar and incubated at 37 °C for 24 h. For total coliforms, triplication of serially diluted retentate (1, 0.1 and 0.01 mL) were resuspended in tubes of LST (Lauryl Sulfate Tryptose) broth and incubated at 37 °C for 48 h. The most probable number (MPN) was calculated according to the number of tubes that generated positive reactions (generating bubbles). Similarly, triplication of serially diluted culture (1, 0.1, and 0.01 mL) of LST broth generating bubbles were transferred into *E. coli* broth and incubated at 44.5 °C for 48 h for calculating MPN of *E. coli*. To detect *E. coli* O157, 25 mL of retentate was added to 225 mL of modified *E. coli* broth and incubated at 37 °C for 24 h. An aliquot of the culture was streaked onto *E. coli* O157 chromogenic medium and incubated at 37 °C for 24 h. Red or purple colonies were chosen to cultivate on TSI (Triple Sugar Iron) agar medium at 37 °C for 24 h. For detection of *Shigella*, 25 mL of retentate was added to 225 mL of *Shigella* broth and incubated at 42 °C for 20 h. Then, an aliquot of the culture was streaked onto *Shigella* chromogenic medium and incubated at 37 °C for 48 h. Typical colonies were selected for cultivation on TSI (Triple Sugar Iron) agar medium at 37 °C for 24 h. For detection of *Salmonella*, 25 mL of retentate was added to 225 mL of Buffered Peptone Water (BPW) and incubated at 37 °C for 18 h. An aliquot of the BPW culture was added to 10 mL of TTB (Tatrathionate Broth) and incubated at 42 °C for 24 h. The culture in TTB was then streaked onto *Salmonella* chromogenic medium and incubated at 37 °C for 24 h. Purple or red colonies were selected for incubation on TSI (Triple Sugar Iron) agar medium at 37 °C for 24 h. Isolates of *P. aeruginosa*, *Shigella* and *Salmonella* were confirmed biochemically and phenotypically using the VITEK2 GN method (bioMériux, Marcy d'Etoile, France).

2.3. Testing P. aeruginosa Susceptibility to Antibiotics

P. aeruginosa susceptibility to antibiotics was tested using the VITEK2 AST-GN04 method (bioMériux, Marcy d'Etoile, France). The selection of antimicrobial agents and interpretation of minimum inhibitory concentration (MIC) (S = susceptible, IR = intermediate resistant, R = resistant) were based on the Clinical and Laboratory Standards Institute [19]. The antimicrobial agents tested are of medical importance, including piperacillin, piperacillin-tazobactam, ticarcillin-clavulanic acid, ceftazidime, cefepime, imipenem, gentamicin, tobramycin, amikacin, levofloxacin and ciprofloxacin.

2.4. Multilocus Sequence Typing (MLST) of P. aeruginosa

Two or three typical *P. aeruginosa* colonies were picked and homogenized in 100 μL autoclaved deionized water. The bacterial solutions were incubated at 100 °C for 10 min followed by cooling at 4 °C for 3 min, then centrifuging at 12,000× *g* for 3 min. The primer pairs used for PCR and sequencing are shown in Table 1. The amplification reactions and conditions for MLST of *P. aeruginosa* were performed as described in the PubMLST (http://pubmlst.org/paeruginosa/info/primers.shtml). Because the original temperature could not successfully amplify mutL, ppsA and trpE alleles, slightly modified conditions (primer annealing temperature) were used to optimize amplification in each reaction. The following adjusted PCR protocol was used: denaturing at 95 °C for 1 min, 35 cycles of 1 min at 95 °C (denaturing), 1 min at 55–57 °C (primer annealing, 57 °C for mutL and ppsA, 55 °C for trpE) and 1 min at 72 °C (primer extension), and a final elongation step at 72 °C for 10 min. Sequencing of all the genes were performed by Life Biological Technology Company (Shanghai,

China). Sequences from the study and alleles and STs from the PubMLST (http://pubmlst.org/) were used to construct a phylogenetic tree of *P. aeruginosa* isolates using MLST Data Analysis-Tree drawing (https://pubmlst.org/paeruginosa/). A population snapshot was operated using the software eBRUST V3 available at the website of http://eburst.mlst.net/v3/enter_data/comparative/.

Table 1. Primers used for multi-locus sequence typing (MLST) of *P. aeruginosa* isolates.

Locus and Functions		Primers Sequence (5′—3′)		Size (bp)
		Forward	Reverse	
acsA	Amplification	ACCTGGTGTACGCCTCGCTGAC	GACATAGATGCCCTGCCCCTTGAT	842
	Sequencing	GCCACACCTACATCGTCTAT	GTGGACAACCTCGGCAACCT	390
aroE	Amplification	TGGGGCTATGACTGGAAACC	TAACCCGGTTTTGTGATTCCTACA	825
	Sequencing	ATGTCACCGTGCCGTTCAAG	TGAAGGCAGTCGGTTCCTTG	495
guaA	Amplification	CGGCCTCGACGTGTGGATGA	GAACGCCTGGCTGGTCTTGTGGTA	940
	Sequencing	AGGTCGGTTCCTCCAAGGTC	TCAAGTCGCACCACAACGTC	372
mutL	Amplification	CCAGATCGCCGCCGGTGAGGTG	CAGGGTGCCATAGAGGAAGTC	940
	Sequencing	AGAAGACCGAGTTCGACCAT	ATGACTTCCTCTATGGCACC	441
nuoD	Amplification	ACCGCCACCCGTACTG	TCTCGCCCATCTTGACCA	1042
	Sequencing	ACGGCGAGAACGAGGACTAC	TTCACCTTCACCGACCGCCA	366
ppsA	Amplification	GGTCGCTCGGTCAAGGTAGTGG	GGGTTCTCTTCTTCCGGCTCGTAG	989
	Sequencing	GGTGACGACGGCAAGCTGTA	TCCTGTGCCGAAGGCGATAC	369
trpE	Amplification	GCGGCCCAGGGTCGTGAG	CCCGGCGCTTGTTGATGGTT	811
	Sequencing	TTCAACTTCGGCGACTTCCA	GGTGTCCATGTTGCCGTTCC	441

2.5. Statistical Analysis

The Chi-square (χ^2) test was applied to assess the potential differences in *Giardia* and *Cryptosporidium* presence in water between suburban and urban swimming pools, because we found the prevalence of *Cryptosporidium* was significantly higher in children hospitalized in suburban hospitals than in urban hospitals in the same area in a previous study [17]. Logistic correlation was applied to analyze whether the presence of *P. aeruginosa* was associated with the levels of free residual chlorine in water.

3. Results

3.1. Characteristics of Swimming Pools

Outdoor swimming pools in the Guangzhou area mostly open between June and September. The swimming water of all enrolled pools is refreshed by refilling the pools with tap water as needed. No swimming suit rental was available in any of the surveyed swimming pools. Swimmers brought their own swimming suits and children were not required to wear diapers when swimming. The studied swimming pools had a diversity of shapes and surface areas that ranged from 100 to 1000 m². The depth of these pools ranged from 0.3 m to 2.0 m with 1.0 to 1.3 m for the majority of the enrolled pools. All swimming pools used standard chlorination to disinfect water, and no further treatment of the water had taken place. Among the pools, 24 (62%) checked free residual chlorine levels once per day; 8 (20%) check twice per day; and 7 (18%) check 3–5 times per day. Free residual chlorine levels were >0.5 mg/L in 18 (46%) swimming pools and <0.3 mg/L in 12 (31%) of the swimming pools. The highest free chlorine level was 2.0 mg/L and the lowest free chlorine level was 0 mg/L. According to the Chinese National Standard, 'Hygienic Standard for Swimming Places' (GB9667-1996, China) the free residual chlorine level in swimming water should be between 0.3 mg/L and 0.5 mg/L. Our survey results showed that only 9 (23%) of the studied swimming pools had free residual chlorine levels that met this criteria.

3.2. Occurrence of Protozoa in Swimming Pool Water

Cryptosporidium and *Giardia* were both detected in 12.8% (5/39) of the enrolled swimming pools. Among these positive pools, 2 pools were positive for *Giardia* only, another 2 were positive for *Cryptosporidium* only, and 1 was positive for both *Giardia* and *Cryptosporidium*. Concentrations of (oo) cysts in positive pool water were 0.03 cysts/L of *Giardia* and 0.03–0.14 oocysts/L of *Cryptosporidium*. The proportional occurrences of both *Giardia* and *Cryptosporidium* were 25% (3/12) and 7.4% (2/27) in pools in the Baiyun district (suburban) and the Haizhu district (urban), respectively. There was no significant difference in the occurrence of *Giardia* and *Cryptosporidium* in swimming pools between suburban and urban areas ($p = 0.159$).

3.3. Occurrence of Bacteria in Swimming Pool Water

Total coliforms were detected in 4 (10.3%) of 39 swimming pools, with concentrations of 1.3, 3.2, 154.0, and 154.0 MPN/100 mL, respectively. Concentrations of total coliform in 2 of the positive pools were lower while that of the other 2 pools were higher than the 18 cfu/L specified in the Chinese Standard. *E. coli* was also detected in the same 4 (10.3%) of 39 swimming pools, with concentrations of 0.5, 1.3, 3.2, and 5.3 MPN/100 mL. Using the standard methods stated above, pathogenic *E. coli* O157, *Shigella* and *Salmonella* were not detected in any of the enrolled swimming pools. *P. aeruginosa* was detected in 27 (69.2%) of the swimming pools. Based on the Chinese National Standard, the free residual chlorine levels in water of these swimming pools were divided into three groups: <0.3 mg/L, 0.3–0.5 mg/L, and >0.5 mg/L. The proportional occurrence of *P. aeruginosa* in each group is shown in Table 2. As shown in the table, the results of logistic correlation analysis using <0.3 mg/L as the control group indicated that there was no significant relationship between the level of free residual chlorine and the presence of *P. aeruginosa*. ($p = 0.55$ and 1.00, respectively).

Table 2. Occurrence of *P. aeruginosa* in swimming pool water with different residual levels of free chlorine.

Residual Levels of Free Chlorine (mg/L)	% (Positive/Total) Occurrence of *P. aeruginosa*	*p*	OR (95% CI)
<0.3	66.7 (8/12)	-	-
0.3 to 0.5	77.8 (7/9)	1.00	1.00 (0.21, 4.71)
>0.5	66.7 (12/18)	0.55	1.75 (0.28, 11.15)
Total	69.2 (27/39)	-	-

Note: OR = odds ratio, CI = confidence interval. <0.3 mg/L was used as control group.

3.4. MLST of P. aeruginosa

Among the 27 *P. aeruginosa* isolates, 17 isolates were positive for all the seven housekeeping genes, therefore they were analyzed using MLST. One or more housekeeping genes in each isolate could not be amplified or sequenced, as a result, 6 alleles of acsA, ppsA and trpE; 5 alleles of aroE, mutL and nuoD; and 7 alleles of guaA were successfully sequenced (Table 3). The MLST analysis identified 11 STs from the tested isolates, all were distinct from existing STs at (http://pubmlst.org/) and therefore were novel STs. Using the curator Ellie Pinnock of PubMLST (http://pubmlst.org/), three ST types have been named as ST-1764, ST-1765 and ST-1766 and the remaining types are designated as ST-A, ST-B, ST-C, ST-D, ST-E, ST-F, ST-G and ST-H. According to the most stringent definition by the eBURST, a ST group was defined as isolates sharing identical alleles at ≥6 of the 7 loci among isolates in a group that belonged to a clonal complex. Otherwise it was singleton. Isolates stemming from a group were considered as belonging to a single clonal complex. The STs with one and two distinct loci compared to the founder strain were named single-locus variants (SLV) and double-locus variants (DLV), respectively (Table 3). Phylogenetic analysis indicated that these STs from different pools and different districts fell into the same branches with the exceptions of ST-D and ST-E in one branch, ST-C and ST-1766 in one branch, and ST-A, ST-B, and ST-1764 in one branch (Figure 1). The type and locations of these samples are listed in Table 3. To further explore the associations between the *P. aeruginosa* isolates from current study and *P. aeruginosa* isolates from the database of PubMLST, a population structure of *P. aeruginosa* isolates was created (Figure 2). As shown in the figure, STs and isolates of *P. aeruginosa* from the current study were distinct from the 1833 STs at the PubMLST, which supports the assertion of the existence of unique and novel STs of *P. aeruginosa* in swimming pool water in the Guangzhou area.

Table 3. List of the alleles and bioinformatics analysis of STs of *P. aeruginosa* isolates from public swimming pools in Guangzhou, 2013.

acsA	aroE	guaA	mutL	nuoD	ppsA	trpE	Group	STs	SLV	DLV	Freq	Pool Type	District
81	11	112	5	73	20	139	1	ST-A	1	1	1	Residential	Haizhu
81	11	112	5	13	20	139	1	ST-B	2	0	2	Residential	Baiyun
81	11	57	5	13	20	139	1	ST-1764	1	1	3	Residential	Baiyun
5	3	95	5	93	6	47	2	ST-1766	1	0	2	Residential; Water park	Baiyun; Haizhu
5	3	95	5	13	6	47	2	ST-C	1	0	3	Residential; Water park *	Baiyun; Haizhu
70	5	72	2	3	20	26	3	ST-D	1	0	1	School	Haizhu
70	5	72	2	3	4	26	3	ST-E	1	0	1	Water park	Baiyun
5	5	57	13	13	74	3	Singleton	ST-F	-	-	1	Water park	Haizhu
83	5	9	3	13	10	3	Singleton	ST-G	-	-	1	Residential	Baiyun
32	13	24	13	13	6	25	Singleton	ST-H	-	-	1	Water park	Baiyun
39	6	4	14	61	15	2	Singleton	ST-1765	-	-	1	Residential	Baiyun

* Represents two pools from the water park located in Haizhu district.

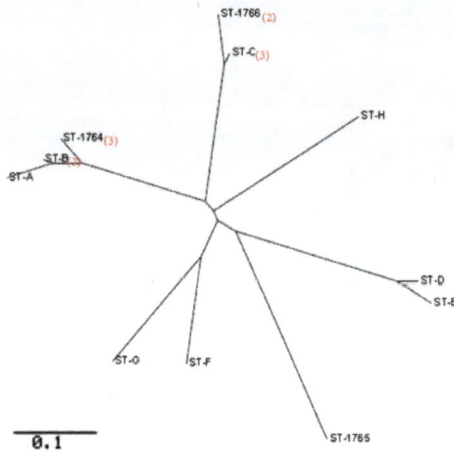

Figure 1. Phylogenetic tree of MLSTs of 17 *P. aeruginosa* isolates each from different swimming pools. The red digits in the parentheses denote the numbers of the STs. The number of unmarked STs was 1.

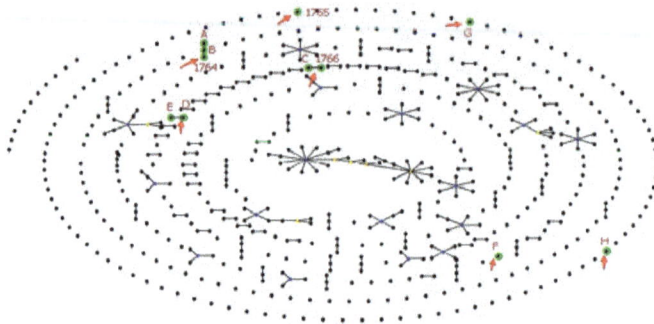

Figure 2. Population structure of the 1833 STs listed in the *P. aeruginosa* PubMLST database and the 11 STs from this study. Note: The figure shows all BURST groups (connected STs), singleton STs, ancestral founders (blue STs), and subgroup founders (yellow STs). Dots represent STs and lines connect single-locus variants. Purple letters and digits represent STs of *P. aeruginosa* from the current study and STs with green halos represent STs detected only in the current study. Line length and singleton ST placement is arbitrary.

3.5. P. aeruginosa Susceptibility to Antibiotics

Susceptibility tests were performed on all the 27 *P. aeruginosa* isolates, each from different pools. Six isolates (ID# 2, 16, 17, 32, 33 and 37) exhibited different levels of susceptibility (R, IR, or S) to tested antibiotics while all the other isolates (IDs not provided) were susceptible to all tested drugs (Table 4). Among the tested drugs, 2 isolates (#2 and #37) were resistant to piperacillin, 2 isolates (#17 and #33) were resistant to imipenem, and 1 isolate (#17) was resistant to gentamicin (Table 4). The isolates #2, #16, #17 and #37 corresponded to the MLST groups of ST-A, ST-1765, ST-1766, and ST-D, respectively. All the rest of the isolates (not listed in Table 4) were susceptible to all tested drugs.

Table 4. Phenotypic antibiotic resistance traits of *P. aeruginosa* from public swimming pools in Guangzhou, 2013.

Isolates ID	PENICILLINS	B-LACTAM		Cephems		Carbapenems	Aminoglycosides			Fluoroquinolones	
	Piperacillin	Ticarcillin-Clavulanic Acid	Tazobactam	Ceftazidime	Cefepime	Imipenem	Gentamicin	Tobramycin	Amikacin	Ciprofloxacin	Levofloxacin
2	R *	S	S	S	S	S	S	S	S	S	S
16	IR **	S	S	S	S	S	IR	S	S	S	S
17	S ***	S	S	S	S	R	R	S	S	S	S
32	IR	S	S	S	S	S	IR	S	S	S	S
33	S	S	S	S	S	R	S	S	S	S	S
37	R	S	S	S	S	S	S	S	S	S	S
All other isolates	S	S	S	S	S	S	S	S	S	S	S

* R = Resistant; ** IR = Intermediate Resistant; *** S = Susceptible.

4. Discussion

According to our observations during the survey and the survey results, overall there is a lack of good practices in pool management, including water disinfection. The free residual chlorine levels of 18 (46%) swimming pools were greater than 0.5 mg/L, which is higher than that of China's National Standard for swimming pools. However, the standards for free residual chlorine for swimming pool water in some European countries [13] are higher than the Chinese standard, which may increase the efficiency of water disinfection. On the other hand, the pools open in June through September which is the warmest season of the whole year in Guangzhou. UV radiation can lead to the formation of chlorate in the water, which reduces the concentration of free chlorine available in water and subsequently impacts the effects of chlorine disinfection. Also, because children were not required to wear diapers when swimming, there was a potential of pool water contamination by children with diarrhea, which is a reported route for swimming pool contamination with *Cryptosporidium* [20]. Finally, the manner of refreshing pool water (adding water when necessary instead of replacing water completely) could facilitate the accumulation of pathogens in water.

The overall prevalence of *Giardia* and *Cryptosporidium* were both 12.8% in swimming pools during the study period. No significant differences in the occurrence of the two protozoal parasites were found between pools in urban and suburban areas. This is converse to our previous findings that prevalence of *Cryptosporidium* was significantly higher in children hospitalized in suburban hospitals than in urban hospitals in the same area [17]. This is probably because of the different transmission routes of *Cryptosporidium* in children patients living in urban and suburban areas. Due to limited numbers of (oo) cysts detected from pool water we did not characterize the two parasites by genotyping, hence the genotypes and zoonotic potential of the two parasites in pool water were unknown. In our previous study we found that the dominant species of *Cryptosporidium* in children hospitalized for diarrhea in the same area was *C. parvum*, a species that infects humans and a wide range of animals [17]. Also, because of the limited numbers of oocysts detected in samples, we did not assess the viability of oocysts, therefore, it was unknown if the oocysts detected in pool water were infective. However, it is known that oocysts are resistant to chlorine and cause waterborne illness associated with swimming pools [21,22]. *Cryptosporidium* and *Giardia* are infectious to people, especially children, the elderly, others with weakened immunity (such as AIDS patients) and travelers, and may cause severe diarrhea and even death [23,24]. The two parasites are major causes of waterborne parasitic infections all over the world, including developed countries such as New Zealand, Australia and USA [25]. A challenge to control these waterborne parasites is that chlorination is ineffective against (oo) cysts [25]. Although UV irradiation [26] and ozone [27] show promising effects against (oo) cysts, these methods have not been practical for disinfection of swimming pool water. As a result, waterborne *Cryptosporidium* and *Giardia* associated with swimming occur frequently [28,29]. Therefore, it was not a surprise to detect *Cryptosporidium* and *Giardia* in swimming pool water in the area, and the results demonstrated that control of the two most common waterborne protozoa is a continuous task in Guangzhou area, as it is elsewhere.

With respect to bacterial pathogens, both total coliform and *E. coli* were detected in approximately 10% of the enrolled swimming pools. These indicator organisms can potentially cause various diseases, particularly in children under five years old and the elderly [6]. Presence of these organisms in water often indicates the ineffectiveness of water disinfection [30], especially the pools with total coliform concentrations higher than the National Standard in this study. The good news is that pathogenic bacteria, *E. coli* O157, *Shigella* and *Salmonella* were not detected in all swimming pools, including those 10% of pools that were positive for total coliforms and *E. coli*. However, another pathogenic bacterium, *P. aeruginosa* was found to be highly prevalent (69%) in studied swimming pools.

P. aeruginosa is ubiquitous in water and is resistant to chemical disinfectants such as chlorine [31]. *P. aeruginosa* cause a variety of disease including folliculitis, external otitis, keratitis, urinary infections and gastrointestinal infections through exposure to skin, ears, eyes, urinary track, lungs and the gut [12,30,32]. Seventy-nine percent of ear infections in swimmers were ascribed to *P. aeruginosa* with symptoms ranging from earache to hearing loss [33]. According to a survey of waterborne diseases in the USA between 1999 and 2008, *P. aeruginosa* was the second most common waterborne pathogenic micro-organism after *Cryptosporidium* [6]. A study reported that *P. aeruginosa* was detected in 95 (59%) of 161 samples of swimming pool filter backwash in Atlanta, Georgia, GA, USA [34]. In the present study we detected similarly high occurrence (69%) of *P. aeruginosa* in public swimming pools in the Guangzhou area. Also, the same STs or the same group of STs of *P. aeruginosa* were distributed among different types of pools in different complexes, and in different locations (Table 3). Our MLST (Figure 1) and population structure analysis (Figure 2) showed that STs of *P. aeruginosa* from swimming pools in the studied area were distinct from strains from other areas and other types of samples, indicating that unique *P. aeruginosa* strains were present in the aquatic environment in the area. Although our study did not determine the routes of transmission of *P. aeruginosa* in the area, *P. aeruginosa* can be carried on the equipment of swimmers [33]. Finally, several isolates of *P. aeruginosa* from swimming pools were resistant to some medically important antibiotics such as piperacillin, imipenem, and gentamicin (Table 4). This result is consistent with reports that *P. aeruginosa* isolates from water environments have lower antibiotic resistance than those of clinical specimens [35]. However, the presence of antibiotic resistant *P. aeruginosa* in swimming pool water indicates that swimming pool water can serve as a route for transmitting antibiotic resistant bacteria and genes, hence presenting additional risks to swimmers who use public swimming pools and workers who perform maintenance of the pools.

Waterborne illness associated with swimming pools is commonly attributed to fecal contamination of water either by swimmers or animals that have access to outdoor pools [36,37]. Other non-fecal substances, such as vomit, mucus, saliva and skin can also serve as sources of pathogenic micro-organisms in swimming pools [38]. Although there are microbiological standards using total bacteria count and total coliform for swimming water, research on microbiological safety associated with pathogens in swimming pool water has been sparse in China. Our study showed the presence of pathogens such as *Cryptosporidium*, *Giardia* and antibiotic resistant *P. aeruginosa* in public swimming pools that potentially pose risks to public health. Data from our study and future similar studies will provide a background for public health agencies and communities to improve the management of public swimming pools in order to prevent waterborne illness associated with swimming pools.

5. Conclusions

This is the initial work of assessing microbiological safety of water in public swimming pools in Guangzhou, China. The presence of *Cryptosporidium*, *Giardia* and antibiotic resistant *P. aeruginosa* in swimming water indicate potential risks to public health in this area. Results suggest the need of updating management of swimming pool facilities and treatment of swimming water in order to prevent waterborne illness associated with swimming in the area.

Author Contributions: Conceptualization, E.R.A., X.L. and S.C.; Methodology, S.H. and C.X.; Data Curation, X.W., J.L. and H.Z.; Data Analysis X.W. and X.L.; Draft Preparation, X.W.; Writing-Review & Editing, X.L. E.R.A. and S.C.; Supervision, E.R.A., Z.Y., and S.C.

Funding: This work was supported by the University Outreach and International Programs (UOIP) Seed Grant (2012) of University of California Davis and the Project for Key Medicine Discipline Construction of Guangzhou Municipality (2013-2015-07).

Acknowledgments: The authors thank the Guangzhou Center for Disease Control and Prevention for its' kind support of this study.

Conflicts of Interest: The authors declare no conflict of interest.

References

1. Leclerc, H.; Schwartzbrod, L.; Dei-Cas, E. Microbial agents associated with waterborne diseases. *Crit. Rev. Microbiol.* **2002**, *28*, 371–409. [CrossRef] [PubMed]
2. Bitton, G. *Microbiology of Drinking Water Production and Distribution*, 1st ed.; John Wiley & Sons, Inc.: Hoboken, NJ, USA, 2014; p. 312.

3. WHO. Water Sanitation Hygiene. Available online: http://www.who.int/water_sanitation_health/en/ (accessed on 6 June 2018).

4. Alhamlan, F.S.; Al-Qahtani, A.A.; Al-Ahdal, M.N. Recommended advanced techniques for waterborne pathogen detection in developing countries. *J. Infect. Dev. Ctries.* **2015**, *9*, 128–135. [CrossRef] [PubMed]

5. WHO. Global Water Supply and Sanitation Assessment 2000 Report. Available online: http://www.who.int/water_sanitation_health/monitoring/jmp2000.pdf (accessed on 30 May 2018).

6. Barna, Z.; Kadar, M. The risk of contracting infectious diseases in public swimming pools. A review. *Ann. Ist. Super. Sanita* **2012**, *48*, 374–386. [CrossRef] [PubMed]

7. WHO. Water Recreation and Disease. 2005. Available online: http://www.who.int/water_sanitation_health/bathing/recreadis.pdf (accessed on 28 May 2018).

8. Giampaoli, S.; Romano Spica, V. Health and safety in recreational waters. *Bull. World Health Organ.* **2014**, *92*, 79. [CrossRef] [PubMed]

9. Mavridou, A.; Pappa, O.; Papatzitze, O.; Blougoura, A.; Drossos, P. An overview of pool and SPA regulations in Mediterranean countries with a focus on the tourist industry. *J. Water Health* **2014**, *12*, 359–371. [CrossRef] [PubMed]

10. Waldron, L.S.; Ferrari, B.C.; Cheung-Kwok-Sang, C.; Beggs, P.J.; Stephens, N.; Power, M.L. Molecular epidemiology and spatial distribution of a waterborne cryptosporidiosis outbreak in Australia. *Appl. Environ. Microbiol.* **2011**, *77*, 7766–7771. [CrossRef] [PubMed]

11. Smith, A.; Reacher, M.; Smerdon, W.; Adak, G.K.; Nichols, G.; Chalmers, R.M. Outbreaks of waterborne infectious intestinal disease in England and Wales, 1992–2003. *Epidemiol. Infect.* **2006**, *134*, 1141–1149. [CrossRef] [PubMed]

12. Rice, S.A.; van den Akker, B.; Pomati, F.; Roser, D. A risk assessment of Pseudomonas aeruginosa in swimming pools: A review. *J. Water Health* **2012**, *10*, 181–196. [CrossRef] [PubMed]

13. Dallolio, L.; Belletti, M.; Agostini, A.; Teggi, M.; Bertelli, M.; Bergamini, C.; Chetti, L.; Leoni, E. Hygienic Surveillance in Swimming pools: Assessment of the Water Quality in Bologna Facilities in the Period 2010–2012. *Microchem. J.* **2013**, *110*, 624–628. [CrossRef]

14. Zhang, L.Y.; Chen, R.Y.; Li, Y. Investigation of various pathogenic bacteria in indoor swimming pool water. *Chin. J. Health Lab. Technol.* **2008**, *18*, 335–337.

15. Zhang, H.X.; Li, D.; Guo, Q. Monitoring results of water quality of swimming pools in Dalian city during 2009–2010. *Occup. Health* **2011**, *27*, 2–3.

16. Zhou, W.M.; Han, R.P.; Qiu, Y.R. Detection result of water quality of swimming pools in Kunming City from 2009–2011. *Occup. Health* **2013**, *29*, 990–991.

17. Chen, X.; Atwill, E.R.; Zhong, F.; Wei, Y.; Hou, S.; Li, J.; Xu, C.; Xiao, C.; Yang, Z.; Li, X. Prevalence and risk factors of Cryptosporidium infection in children with clinical diarrhea in Guangzhou, China. *J. Bacteriol. Parasitol.* **2017**, *8*, 1–8. [CrossRef]

18. Rhodes, E.R.; Villegas, L.F.; Shaw, N.J.; Miller, C.; Villegas, E.N. A modified EPA Method 1623 that uses tangential flow hollow-fiber ultrafiltration and heat dissociation steps to detect waterborne Cryptosporidium and Giardia spp. *J. Vis. Exp.* **2012**, *3791*–4177. [CrossRef] [PubMed]

19. CLSI. *Performance Standards for Antimicrobial Susceptibility Testing*; 23th Informational Supplement (Document M100-S23); CLSI: Wayne, PA, USA, 2013.

20. Causer, L.M.; Handzel, T.; Welch, P.; Carr, M.; Culp, D.; Lucht, R.; Mudahar, K.; Robinson, D.; Neavear, E.; Fenton, S.; et al. An outbreak of Cryptosporidium hominis infection at an Illinois recreational waterpark. *Epidemiol. Infect.* **2006**, *134*, 147–156. [CrossRef] [PubMed]

21. MacKenzie, W.R.; Kazmierczak, J.J.; Davis, J.P. An outbreak of cryptosporidiosis associated with a resort swimming pool. *Epidemiol. Infect.* **1995**, *115*, 545–553. [CrossRef] [PubMed]

22. Takagi, M.; Toriumi, H.; Endo, T.; Yamamoto, N.; Kuroki, T. An outbreak of cryptosporidiosis associated with swimming pools. *Kansenshogaku zasshi J. Jpn. Assoc. Infect. Dis.* **2008**, *82*, 14–19. [CrossRef]

23. Gao, J.Z. *Clinical Laboratory Parasitology*; People's Health Publishing House: Beijing, China, 2009.

24. White, G.C. *Handbook of Chlorination and Alternative Disinfectants*, 4th ed.; John Wiley & Sons Inc.: New York, NY, USA, 1999.

25. Baldursson, S.; Karanis, P. Waterborne transmission of protozoan parasites: Review of worldwide outbreaks—An update 2004–2010. *Water Res.* **2011**, *45*, 6603–6614. [CrossRef] [PubMed]

26. Hijnen, W.A.; Beerendonk, E.F.; Medema, G.J. Inactivation credit of UV radiation for viruses, bacteria and protozoan (oo)cysts in water: A review. *Water Res.* **2006**, *40*, 3–22. [CrossRef] [PubMed]

27. Korich, D.G.; Mead, J.R.; Madore, M.S.; Sinclair, N.A.; Sterling, C.R. Effects of ozone, chlorine dioxide, chlorine, and monochloramine on Cryptosporidium parvum oocyst viability. *Appl. Environ. Microbiol.* **1990**, *56*, 1423–1428. [PubMed]

28. Hall, V.; Taye, A.; Walsh, B.; Maguire, H.; Dave, J.; Wright, A.; Anderson, C.; Crook, P. A large outbreak of gastrointestinal illness at an open-water swimming event in the River Thames, London. *Epidemiol. Infect.* **2017**, *145*, 1246–1255. [CrossRef] [PubMed]

29. Levy, D.A.; Bens, M.S.; Craun, G.F.; Calderon, R.L.; Herwaldt, B.L. Surveillance for waterborne-disease outbreaks—United States, 1995–1996. *MMWR CDC Surveill. Summ. Morb. Mortal. Wkly. Rep. CDC Surveill. Summ.* **1998**, *47*, 1–34.

30. McFeters, G.A.; Kippin, J.S.; LeChevallier, M.W. Injured coliforms in drinking water. *Appl. Environ. Microbiol.* **1986**, *51*, 1–5. [PubMed]

31. Craun, G.F.; Calderon, R.L.; Craun, M.F. Outbreaks associated with recreational water in the United States. *Int. J. Environ. Health Res.* **2005**, *15*, 243–262. [CrossRef] [PubMed]

32. Mena, K.D.; Gerba, C.P. Risk assessment of Pseudomonas aeruginosa in water. *Rev. Environ. Contam. Toxicol.* **2009**, *201*, 71–115. [PubMed]

33. Hajjartabar, M. Poor-quality water in swimming pools associated with a substantial risk of otitis externa due to Pseudomonas Aeruginosa. *Water Sci. Technol. J. Int. Assoc. Water Pollut. Res.* **2004**, *50*, 63–67. [CrossRef]

34. Hutcheson, C.; Cira, R.; Gaines, S.L.; Jones, K.R.; Howard, W.; Hornsby, D.; Redmond, M.; Rustin, C.; Hlavsa, M.C.; Murphy, J.L.; et al. Microbes in Pool Filter Backwash as Evidence of the Need for Improved Swimmer Hygiene—Metro-Atlanta, Georgia, 2012. *MMWR-Morbid. Mortal. Wkly. Rep.* **2013**, *62*, 385–388.

35. Reali, D.; Rosati, S. Antibiotic susceptibility and serotyping of Pseudomonas aeruginosa strains isolated from surface waters, thermomineral waters and clinical specimens. *Zent. Hyg. Umweltmed.* **1994**, *196*, 75–80.

36. WHO. Microbial hazards. In *Guidelines for Safe Recreational Water Environments. Swimming Pools and Similar Environments*; WHO Press: Geneva, Switzerland, 2006.

37. Nichols, G. Infection risks from water in natural and man-made environments. *Euro Surveill. Bull. Eur. Mal. Transm. Eur. Commun. Dis. Bull.* **2006**, *11*, 76–78. [CrossRef]

38. Papadopoulou, C.; Economou, V.; Sakkas, H.; Gousia, P.; Giannakopoulos, X.; Dontorou, C.; Filioussis, G.; Gessouli, H.; Karanis, P.; Leveidiotou, S. Microbiological quality of indoor and outdoor swimming pools in Greece: Investigation of the antibiotic resistance of the bacterial isolates. *Int. J. Hyg. Environ. Health* **2008**, *211*, 385–397. [CrossRef] [PubMed]

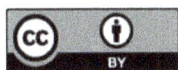

International Journal of
*Environmental Research
and Public Health*

MDPI

Article

Legionella spp. Risk Assessment in Recreational and Garden Areas of Hotels

Antonios Papadakis [1,2,†] [iD], Dimosthenis Chochlakis [1,3,†], Vassilios Sandalakis [1], Maria Keramarou [1], Yannis Tselentis [1] and Anna Psaroulaki [1,3,*]

[1]   Department of Clinical Microbiology and Microbial Pathogenesis, School of Medicine, University of Crete, Voutes—Staurakia, 71110 Heraklion, Crete, Greece; medp2011758@med.uoc.gr (A.P.); d.chochlakis@uoc.gr (D.C.); v.sandalakis@uoc.gr (V.S.); keramarou@gmail.com (M.K.); tselendi@med.uoc.gr (Y.T.)
[2]   Public Health Authority of Heraklion, 71201 Heraklion, Crete, Greece
[3]   Regional Laboratory of Public Health, School of Medicine, 71110 Heraklion, Crete, Greece
*   Correspondence: psaroulaki@uoc.gr; Tel.: +30-2810-039-4743
†   These authors contributed equally to this work.

Received: 7 February 2018; Accepted: 22 March 2018; Published: 26 March 2018

Abstract: Several Travel-associated Legionnaires' disease (TALD) cases occur annually in Europe. Except from the most obvious sites (cooling towers and hot water systems), infections can also be associated with recreational, water feature, and garden areas of hotels. This argument is of great interest to better comprehend the colonization and to calculate the risk to human health of these sites. From July 2000–November 2017, the public health authorities of the Island of Crete (Greece) inspected 119 hotels associated with TALD, as reported through the European Legionnaires' Disease Surveillance Network. Five hundred and eighteen samples were collected from decorative fountain ponds, showers near pools and spas, swimming pools, spa pools, garden sprinklers, drip irrigation systems (reclaimed water) and soil. Of those, 67 (12.93%), originating from 43 (35.83%) hotels, tested positive for *Legionella* (*Legionella pneumophila* serogroups 1, 2, 3, 6, 7, 8, 13, 14, 15 and non-pneumophila species (*L. anisa*, *L. erythra*, *L. taurinensis*, *L. birminghamensis*, *L. rubrilucens*). A Relative Risk (R.R.) > 1 ($p < 0.0001$) was calculated for chlorine concentrations of less than 0.2 mg/L (R.R.: 54.78), star classification (<4) (R.R.: 4.75) and absence of Water Safety Plan implementation (R.R.: 3.96). High risk ($\geq 10^4$ CFU/L) was estimated for pool showers (16.42%), garden sprinklers (7.46%) and pool water (5.97%).

Keywords: *Legionella*; recreational water systems; risk; water safety plan; hotel

---

1. Introduction

Legionella bacteria live naturally in fresh water, as well as in artificial water systems such as hot water tanks, hot tubs or spas, cooling towers, plumbing systems, and decorative pools or fountains [1,2]. Hotel gardens are, also, frequently irrigated with sprinklers and these may present an additional risk, particularly if they utilize recycled grey-water or sewage-based water [3]. *Legionella* species are able to reproduce at 25–43 °C and able to survive at temperatures of up to 55–60 °C, making it possible for them to thrive even in hot water systems [4].

Two forms of legionellosis are caused by the *Legionella* pathogens: Legionnaires' disease (LD), presenting with pneumonia-like symptoms, and Pontiac fever, presenting with influenza-like symptoms [5]. Legionnaires' disease, a serious form of pneumonia, may be caused by any type of *Legionella* bacteria, although *L. pneumophila* serogroup 1 is considered the most virulent of all species and serogroups, causing approximately 75% of all *Legionella* infections [2,6,7]. Until now, more than 52 different species of *Legionella* with at least 73 different serogroups have been described, of which

IJERPH **2018**, *15*, 598; doi:10.3390/ijerph15040598

72

approximately 20 species have been associated with human disease [8–11]. The case-fatality ratio of LD has been recorded in the order of 10–15%. Usually the incubation period ranges from two to 10 days, but in rare cases it may be longer, for up to 16–20 days after exposure [12,13]. Since LD is normally acquired through the respiratory system by inhaling air that contains *Legionella* bacteria in an aerosol, droplets with a diameter of less than 5 μm (~90% showers aerosols) may come into contact with the lower human airways [8,14–16].

Travel-associated Legionnaires' disease (TALD) corresponds to the cases of travelers who get infected in the country they visit, but usually get diagnosed and/or report their infection back in the country of their residence. These human cases do not include domestic ones, that is, cases in which humans travel within their own country. Due to the long incubation period (2–10 days), travelers may be exposed to *Legionella* bacteria in one country but develop symptoms and seek medical attention in another (such as their home) country [17]. According to the 2015 report by the European Centre for Disease Prevention and Control (ECDC), a total of 1141 human cases related to TALD were reported during that year at the 28 EU Member States and Norway, with the number being 20% higher than that in 2014; in 2014, a total of 953 human cases were reported (21% higher than the corresponding ones of 2013) [3]. The average risk to TALD ranged from 0.02 cases/million nights in the United Kingdom to 0.88 cases/million nights in Greece, according to a study carried out in 2009. In Greece, the pooled risk of 1.68 cases/million nights when travelling to the country was the highest among the 10 European countries [18,19].

Since 2004, the World Health Organization (WHO) has developed a Water Safety Plan (WSP) approach according to its Guidelines for Drinking Water Quality, which is based on risk assessment and risk management principles [20]. Together with the standard EN 15975-2 (concerning security of drinking water supply), these guidelines are an internationally recognized principle on which the production, distribution, monitoring and analysis of parameters in drinking water is based upon. In Europe, the Commission Directive Council 98/83/EC (EU) and 2015/1787 align with the principles and needs of the quality of water intended for human consumption. The WSP approach includes, also, supporting programs such as verification monitoring, appropriate documentation and record-keeping, training and communication [21,22].

The aims of the present study were: (1) culture and identify *L. pneumophila* and *Legionella* species in environmental samples obtained from recreational areas and determine the frequency and severity of colonization of *Legionella* in these sites; (2) estimate the risk factors associated with *Legionella* colonization of recreational systems and (3) evaluate the implementation of WSPs to limit *Legionella* colonization.

2. Materials and Methods

2.1. Inspections—Sample Collection

During the period of 2000–2017, the Local Public Health Authorities of the Island of Crete in Greece inspected 119 hotels associated with TALD. Environmental samples from decorative fountain ponds, showers near pools and spas, swimming pools, spa pools, garden sprinklers, drip irrigation systems (reclaimed water) and soil were collected from each hotel, where applicable.

Specifically, as regards the reclaimed water from the drip irrigation systems, in all sample cases it consisted of a product of secondary biological treatment followed by advanced treatment and disinfection. According to the National legislation "Common Ministerial Decision (CMD) No 145116: Measures, limits and procedures for reuse of treated wastewater (Issuing Institutions: Ministry of Environment, Energy and Climate Change)", this kind of water can be used unrestrictedly in irrigation of gardens and in recreational areas of hotels provided that it fulfills the following criteria: (1) Total coliforms (TC) (cfu/100 mL) ≤ 2 in 80% of samples and ≤ 20 in 95% of samples; (2) Biochemical oxygen demand (BOD$_5$) (mg/L) ≤ 10 in 80% of samples; (3) Total suspended solids (TSS) (mg/L) ≤ 2 in 80% of samples; (4) Turbidity (NTU) ≤2 median. The above criteria are met following secondary biological treatment followed by advanced treatment and disinfection.

The sample sites were chosen based on the sites that could produce aerosols and on the sites (rooms, areas and so on) potentially associated with a TALD case. The samples were collected according to: (a) the guidelines for drinking-water quality (second edition) and (b) ISO 5667-2:1982—Part 2: guidance on sampling techniques; since 2006, samples were collected following the ISO 19458:2006 Water quality—Sampling for microbiological analysis methodology. The samples were labeled and temporarily stored in a cool box at a temperature of up to 5 (±3) °C protected from direct light, before being delivered to the laboratory immediately after the sampling (no more than 24 h).

2.2. Data Collection

Data on water temperature, pH, chlorine concentration, disinfection methodology, hotel star rating, number of rooms/beds, implementation of a WSP, season and water supply were recorded. Inspections were conducted following a checklist developed with some information such as name, address of building, type of hot water production system, water disinfection system, periodicity and type of water system maintenance and cleaning, water supplying and number of rooms and beds. The temperatures were measured (two minutes after flushing) using a calibrated thermometer, placed in the middle of the water stream. Free chlorine and pH were measured using a calibrated portable, microprocessor based meter. Samples were collected in 1 L sterile containers containing sufficient sodium thiosulphate (20 mg) to neutralize any chlorine or other oxidizing biocides.

2.3. Plate Culture Method

The isolation of *Legionella* from water samples was performed by culture according to the International Standard method ISO 11731 (1998) and ISO 11731-2 (2004). The latter ISO was implemented from 2004 onwards. Briefly, water samples were concentrated by filtration and were re-suspended in Distilled Deionized water. A volume of the suspension (200 μL) was spread on BCYE (Buffered Charcoal Yeast Extract), BCY (Buffered Charcoal Yeast Extract without L-cysteine) and GVPC (Glycine Vancomycin Polymyxin Cycloheximide) (Biomérieux, Craponne, France) Petri dishes: (a) directly after filtration; (b) after incubation at 50 °C for 30 min and (c) after the addition of an acid buffer (0.2 mol/L solution of HCL, pH 2.2). The detection limit of the procedure was 50 CFU/L. The inoculated plates were incubated for 10 days at 36 ± 1 °C in 2.5% CO_2 with increased humidity. Suspected colonies were randomly chosen for subculture on BCY, BCYE and GVPC agar.

2.4. Typing of Legionella Isolates

Up until 2010, the isolated colonies were identified using an agglutination test (SLIDEX *Legionella*-Kit, Biomérieux, Craponne, France), which allows for the discrimination of *L. pneumophila* serogroup 1 from serogroups 2–14 and of *L. anisa*, while for the exact detection of each *L. pneumophila* serogroup, individual latex polyclonal reagents were used (Pro-lab, Richmond Hill, ON, Canada).

2.5. Identification—MALDI-TOF Mass Spectrometry

From 2010 onwards, a MALDI Biotyper (Microflex LT MALDI-TOF mass spectrometer) (Bruker Daltonics, Leipzig, Germany) equipped with a microSCOUT ion source was used for the identification of individual *Legionella* colonies against its microbial database (v 3.1.2.0). Spectra were recorded using the flexControl software with the default parameters for optimization set by the manufacturer (Bruker Daltonics, Leipzig, Germany). For each spectrum, 240 laser shots were collected and analyzed (6 × 40 laser shots from 120 different positions of the target spot). All identifications were evaluated according to the manufacturer scoring scheme.

2.6. Risk Assessment of Legionella Presence in Water Distribution Systems

To better calculate the risk, we used two different approaches. The first one was in accordance with the recommendations of the European Legionnaires' disease Surveillance Network (ELDSNet), at which the microbiological results of the water samples were analytically and statistically analyzed according to the number of *Legionella* bacteria in the water sample, which could represent a particular risk to the human health. In particular, an insignificant risk was noted at $\leq 10^3$ CFU/L, medium risk at $>10^3$ CFU/L but $<10^4$ CFU/L, and high risk at $\geq 10^4$ CFU/L. Especially for spa pools, the recommendations point to the risk of legionellosis following *Legionella* sampling to low risk ($>10^2$ but $<10^3$) and to high risk ($\geq 10^3$ CFU/L) [23]. A second inspection was performed at a hotel when the *Legionella* count was $\geq 10^4$ CFU/L in at least one sample or between $>10^3$ and $\leq 10^4$ CFU/L in more than two samples or between $>10^3$ and $\leq 10^4$ CFU/L in at least one sample in concordance with an aerobic count higher than 10^5 CFU/L.

The second approach for the assessment of the risk was based on a semi-quantitative risk matrix approach, which was used to implement the water supply system risk assessment (Table 1). The risk levels were divided into: high (≥ 20), medium (10–19), and low (<10). The risk (R) was evaluated based on the following parameters: Likelihood (L) or the occurrence of accidents/damage, frequency of the risk exposure, consequence or severity (S). The level of the risk was calculated as follows: R = L × S [24,25].

Table 1. Presentation of the semi-quantitative risk matrix approach that was used to implement the water supply system risk assessment. The risk levels were divided into: high (≥ 20), medium (10–19), and low (<10). The risk (R) was evaluated based on the following parameters: Likelihood (L) or the occurrence of accidents/damage, frequency of the risk exposure, consequence or severity (S). The level of the risk was calculated as follows: R = L × S.

		Severity or Consequence				
		Insignificant (Wholesome water) Rating: 1	Minor (Short term or localised, not health related non-compliance or aesthetic) Rating: 2	Moderate (Widespread aesthetic issues or long-term non-compliance, not heath related) Rating: 4	Major (Potential long-term health effects) Rating: 8	Catastrophic (Potential illness) Rating: 16
Likelihood or Frequency	Most unlikely (Has not taken place in the past and it is highly improbable that it will occur in the future) Rating: 1	1	2	4	8	16
	Unlikely (Is possible and cannot be ruled out completely) Rating: 2	2	4	8	16	32
	Foreseeable (Is possible and under certain circumstances could occur) Rating: 3	3	6	12	24	48
	Very likely (Has occurred in the past and has the potential to occur again) Rating: 4	4	8	16	32	64
	Almost certain (Has occurred in the past and could occur again) Rating: 5	5	10	20	40	80

2.7. Instructions Given in Case of Positive Samples

According to the national guidelines, in samples which met the criteria of $>10^3$ to $<10^4$, either: (i) if a small proportion of samples (10–20%) were positive, the system was re-sampled. If a similar count was recorded again, then a review of the control measures and risk assessment was carried out to identify any remedial actions; (ii) if the majority of samples were positive, the system was considered as colonized, even at a low level, with *Legionella*. Disinfection of the system was considered but an immediate review of control measures and a risk assessment was carried out to identify any other remedial actions required. In samples which met the criteria of $\geq 10^4$: The system was re-sampled and an immediate review of the control measures and risk assessment was carried out to identify any remedial actions, including whether a disinfection of the whole system or affected area was necessary.

2.8. Implementation of a Water Safety Plan

As from 2005, a detailed standardized questionnaire (checklist, Appendix A) was used to evaluate the risk associated with the non-implementation of a WSP. The checklist consisted of 42 scoring items (11 of which were designated as "critical"), which were classified into seven categories: construction and maintenance; cleaning and disinfection; cold-water distribution system; hot-water distribution system; system protection cross-connections and backflow; record keeping; and on-site manually conducted tests. The total negative score was calculated and classified qualitatively in the following three categories: satisfactory result (0–7 points, <10% of the total negative score, no critical violation), relatively satisfactory result (8–14 points, 11–20% of the total negative score, or a critical violation), and unsatisfactory result (more than 14 points, >20% of the total negative score).

2.9. Statistical Analysis

All statistical analyses were conducted using the IBM SPSS Statistics Version 24 statistical package, the Epi-Info 2000 version 7.2.0.1 (Centers for Disease Control and Prevention, Atlanta, GA, USA) and the MedCalc relative risk calculator statistical software free online version; Relative risk (R.R.) at a 95% confidence interval (CI). The analyses were calculated to assess categorical risk variables from water distribution systems and hotel characteristics, associated with *Legionellae*-positive test results. The results were considered statistically significant when the *p* value was <0.05 and highly significant when the *p* value was <0.0001.

3. Results

3.1. Descriptive Data

Of the 518 samples collected, 67 (12.93%) originated from 43 (35.83%) hotels that tested positive for *Legionella* species. The mean positivity was 9.41% (standard deviation of 11.91, max of 33.33% min 0.00%) (Table 2). A second inspection was required for 49 hotels, a third for 16 hotels, a fourth for five (5) hotels, while a fifth inspection was required for two (2) hotels. The repetitive inspections were carried out in cases where the implementation of measures did not deliver the expected results in terms of the presence of *Legionella* species at the sites tested and/or the risk factors (as these are explained below) were repeatedly tested out of the limits.

In 14/119 (28.57%) of the hotels inspected, a cluster was noted (clusters were defined as the presence of two or more cases having stayed overnight at the same accommodation site in the 14 days before onset of illness and whose illness was within say the same two-year period) [23].

3.2. Isolation and Identification of L. pneumophila and Legionella Species in Environmental Samples Obtained from Recreational Systems

Legionella was isolated from swimming pool showers, garden sprinklers, reclaimed water, swimming pool water, decorative fountain, spa water and spa showers. On the contrary, no *Legionella* species were isolated from shower heads, from Jacuzzis and from garden soil. All results are summarized in Table 2.

Legionella pneumophila serogroups 1, 2, 3, 6, 7, 8, 13, 14, 15 and 2–15 were detected. Of the non-pneumophila species, *L. anisa*, *L. erythra*, *L. taurinensis*, *L. birminghamensis*, *L. rubrilucens* and *Legionella* species were identified, the majority of which, belonged to the human pathogenic species *L. anisa*. The CFU/L ranged from 50–350,000. The lowest CFU/L were detected in spa waters, while the highest ones were identified in swimming pool showers and in garden sprinklers. All results are summarized in Table 3.

Table 2. Collection sites and sites where *Legionella* species were detected. The percentages of the positive samples have been calculated based on the total number of collected samples. The ranges have been assigned based on the European Centre for Disease Prevention and Control recommendations. The numbers at the left side of the slash (/) correspond to the sample findings and the numbers at the right side of the slash (/) correspond to the hotel findings.

Original Sample Description	Samples/Hotels		Range (CFU/L)		
	Total No	Positive	$\leq 10^3$	$>10^3$ and $<10^4$	$\geq 10^4$
Reclaimed Water	13/9	3 (23.08%)/2 (2.22%)	2 (66.67%)/2 (22.22%)	1 (33.33%)/1 (11,11%)	-
Decorative Fountains	45/24	3 (6.67%)/3 (12.50%)	1 (33.33%)/1 (4.17%)	2 (66.67%)/2 (8.33%)	-
Shower Heads	2/1	0	-	-	-
Garden Sprinklers	37/21	15 (40.54%)/11 (52.38%)	6 (40%)/6 (28.57%)	4 (26.67%)/4 (19.05%)	5 (33.33%)/5 (23.81%)
Jacuzzi Water	15/10	0	-	-	-
Pool Water	107/61	5 (4.67%)/4 (6.56%)	1 (20%)/1 (1.64%)	-	4 (80%)/3 (4.92%)
Spa Water	10/7	1 (10%)/1 (14.29%)	1/1 (100%)	-	-
Swimming pool Showers	271/104	38 (14.02%)/30 (28.85%)	17 (44.74%)/15 (50%)	10 (26.32%)/9 (30%)	11(28.95%)/10 (33.33%)
Spa Showers	16/7	2 (12.50%)/2 (28.57%)	2 (100%)/2 (28.57%)	-	-
Garden Soil	2/1	0	-	-	-
Total	518/119	67 (12.98%)/43 (36.13%)	30 (44.78%)/25 (21.01%)	17 (25.37%)/4 (11.76%)	20 (29.85%)/14 (11.76%)

Table 3. *Legionella* serogroups and species isolated and identified from recreational waters (Ranges as CFU/L).

Legionella Serogroups/Species	Swimming Pool Water		Spa		Swimming Pool Shower		Spa Shower		Fresh Water from Garden Sprinklers		Decoration Fountain		Reclaimed Water	
	Pos.	Range	Pos.	Range	Pos.	Range	Pos.	Range	Pos.	Range	Pos.	Range	Pos.	Range
L.p. sg 1	1	700			5	350–1150			1	26,000				
L.p. sg 2					4	100–2050								
L.p. sg 3									3	50–650				
L.p. sg 6					1	150								
L.p. sg 7					5	200–3350	2	150–600						
L.p. sg 8					2	50			1	300				
L.p. sg 13									1	32,500				
L.p. sg 14					3	150–100,000	1/1	150	3	250–13,000				
L.p. sg 15														
L.p. sg 2–15			1	50	8	50–100,000			4	13,500–200,000			1	1000
L. anisa	2	19,500–26,500	1	650	9	250–350,000			3	50–13,000	1	2500		
L. erythra					3	400–13,000			1	200	1	1500		
L. taurinensis					2	50			1	6500	1	2000		
L. birminghamensis					1	650–8250			1	65,000				
L. rubrilucens	1	26,000			3	50–6500								
L. species	1	200,000			4	50–1000					1	1000	3	1000

Pos.: positive. *L.p.*: *Legionella pneumophila*. sg: serogroup.

3.3. Univariate Examination of Risk Factors

The presence of *Legionella* was possibly associated (statistically significant correlation together with a relative risk of >1) with: (a) the implementation of a WSP; (b) free chlorine <0.2 mg/L; (c) hotel star classification of <4; (d) seasonal operation; (e) municipality hosting hotels population of <10^4 people and (f) absence of an automated chlorination system together with free chlorine out of range. The number of beds of >200, the number of rooms of >80 and the use of groundwater as a source of water supply showed a statistically significant correlation in the absence of a relative risk >1. On the other hand, no statistically significant correlation was calculated for cold water temperature of >25 °C, temperature of >20 °C, the absence of an automated chlorination system, pH out of limits value (pH within limits 7.0–7.8), the opening/closing period and the high season period (June–August). All results are summarized in Table 4.

Table 4. Association of water distribution systems and hotel characteristics with *Legionella* colonization. The terminology number needed to treat (NNT) has been used as proposed at the free online relative risk calculator statistical software, MedCalc (Altman 1998). In our case, the term benefit is associated with the number of additional inputs required for each parameter tested to get a positive association with this parameter.

Risk Factors	R.R.	95% CI	z Statistic Statistic	p Value	NNT
Free chlorine <0.2 mg/L	54.78	20.47–148.04	7.94	<0.0001	(Harm) 1.85
No Water Safety Plan	3.96	2.32–6.75	5.04	<0.0001	(Harm) 6.06
Wrong implementation of WSP	3.78	1.42–10.08	2.66	0.0077	(Harm) 7.33
Number of rooms >80	0.29	0.17–0.47	4.83	<0.0001	(Benefit) 6.25
Number of beds >200	0.22	0.12–0.40	5.08	<0.0001	(Benefit) 5.89
Star classification <4	4.75	2.80–8.06	5.78	<0.0001	(Harm) 4.95
Groundwater as a source of water supply	0.27	0.13–0.58	3.34	0.0008	(Benefit) 5.70
No automated chlorination system and free chlorine <0.2 mg/L	5.16	2.58–10.31	4.65	<0.0001	(Harm) 3.60
pH out of limits and free chlorine <0.2 mg/L	4.52	1.71–11.96	3.04	0.0024	(Harm) 3.08
Population < 10,000	1.61	1.03–2.58	2.11	0.02	(Harm) 15.78
No automated chlorination system	1.93	0.71–5.25	1.29	0.04	(Harm) 12.57
Closing period	1.56	0.87–2.78	1.51	0.07	(Harm) 14.59
Seasonal operation	1.47	0.66–3.28	0.94	0.17	(Harm) 23.93
Cold water >25 °C	1.38	0.82–2.64	1.29	0.14	(Harm) 18.17
Cold water >20 °C	1.21	0.70–2.08	0.70	0.35	(Harm) 39.29
pH out of limits	0.68	0.2–1.98	0.69	0.25	(Benefit) 18.59
High season months	1.10	0.70–1.730	0.44	0.65	(Harm) 76.27
Opening period	1.03	0.35–3.05	0.06	0.45	(Harm) 214.76

Based on the risk assessment according to the guidelines of ECDC (low, medium and high for CFU/L < 10^3, 10^3–10^3 and >10^4 respectively) a corresponding Figure 1 was built to demonstrate the risk for each site tested. According to the semi-quantitative risk assessment a number of areas were designated as low, medium and high according to the likelihood of any species been present, the severity caused in the presence of any *Legionella* and the total risk (as a factor taking these two parameters into consideration). Of the total sites tested, the garden sprinklers and the swimming pool showers presented a higher risk when all three hazardous events were considered. As regards the pool water, a high risk was calculated for the event of finding *Legionella* in the water system, only. All results are summarized in Table 5.

Table 5. Risk assessment of the sites based on the likelihood for the presence of *Legionella* (*), the severity raised if *Legionella* is present (ˆ) and the final risk score calculated (#). The final risk score was calculated based on the findings of the previous two parameters.

Area	Hazard and Hazardous Event	Likelihood or Frequency *	Severity or Consequence ˆ	Risk Score #	Risk Rating #
Reclaimed Water	Event of finding *Legionella* in the water system	3	4	12	Medium
	Inadequate disinfection method	3	4	12	Medium
	Low chlorine residual in distribution systems	3	4	12	Medium
Decorative Fountains	Event of finding *Legionella* in the water system	3	4	12	Medium
	Inadequate disinfection method	3	4	12	Medium
	Low chlorine residual in distribution systems	3	4	12	Medium
Shower Heads	Event of finding *Legionella* in the water system	2	4	8	Low
Garden Sprinklers	Event of finding *Legionella* in the water system	5	8	40	High
	Inadequate disinfection method	5	8	40	High
	Low chlorine residual in distribution systems	5	8	40	High

Table 5. *Cont.*

Area	Hazard and Hazardous Event	Likelihood or Frequency *	Severity or Consequence ^	Risk Score #	Risk Rating #
	Event of finding *Legionella* in the water system	2	4	8	Low
Jacuzzis Water	Inadequate disinfection method	2	4	8	Low
	Low chlorine residual in distribution systems	2	4	8	Low
	Event of finding *Legionella* in the water system	3	8	24	High
Pool Water	Inadequate disinfection method	2	8	16	Medium
	Low chlorine residual in distribution systems	2	8	16	Medium
	Event of finding *Legionella* in the water system	2	4	8	Low
Spa Water	Inadequate disinfection method	2	4	8	Low
	Low chlorine residual in distribution systems	2	4	8	Low
	Event of finding *Legionella* in the water system	4	8	32	High
Swimming pool Showers	Inadequate disinfection method	4	8	32	High
	Low chlorine residual in distribution systems	4	8	32	High
	Event of finding *Legionella* in the water system	2	4	8	Low
Spa Showers	Inadequate disinfection method	1	4	4	Low
	Low chlorine residual in distribution systems	1	4	4	Low
Garden Soil	Event of finding *Legionella* in the water system	1	4	4	Low

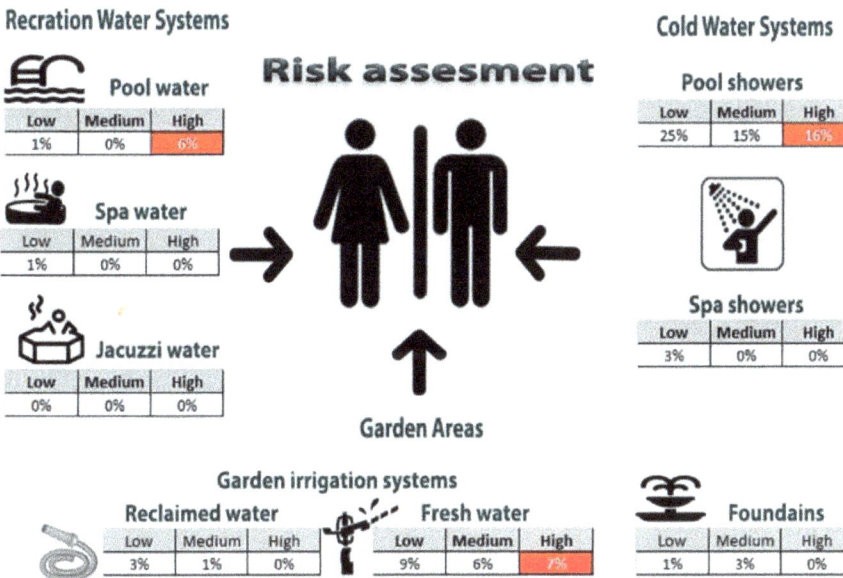

Figure 1. Risk assessment for *Legionella* contamination based on the CFU/L detected in each site tested.

3.4. Evaluation of the Implementation of WSPs

Data from the use of the checklist were collected from 51 hotels. The major recordings had to do with water storage tank protection, clean showers, presence of the proper concentration of residual chlorine, and water temperatures. All findings are summarized into Table 6.

Of the 51 hotels for which the questionnaire for the correct implementation of a WSP was filled in, 24 (36.4%) received a score B (relatively satisfactory) while 37 (63.7%) got a score C (unsatisfactory).

A higher colonization was recorded in the absence of a WSP (R.R. 3.04; *p* value <0.0001; CL 95% 1.73 to 5.34; z-statistic 3.87; NNT (Harm) 8.06) and in hotels where wrong implementation of WSP was recorded (R.R. 3.78; *p* value 0.0077; CL 95% 1.42 to 10.08; z-statistic 2.66; NNT (Harm) 7.33).

Table 6. Findings from the completion of the checklists at the 51 hotels. Only the items, for which a deviation from the normal value was recorded and are presented herein.

Scoring Items	%
No water storage tanks protection	100
* The showers are NOT clean and free of salts	81.2
* The residual chlorine <0.2 mg/L	72.8
The hot water temperature is <50 °C. after 1 min of flowing	63.6
The cold-water temperature in taps is >25 °C. after 2 min of flushing	54.5
Water store and circulation temp <60 °C	54.5
The water exiting the heating unit <60 °C and returning <50 °C	54.5
The amount of stored water is >1 day	45.5
There is NO control book	45.5
* The outgoing temperature (cold) water from the tank is >25 °C	36.3
There are leaks in the network	27.2
* NO random checks of water at least every 6 months	27.2
There is no thermal stratification of the water inside the heaters and storage water	27.2
The water distribution system cannot provide adequate water supply at peak times	18.2
There is a change (increase or decrease) in the consumption of the water	18.2
* Detected *Legionella* the last six months (at a concentration of more than 10^3 CFU/L)	18.2
The filters are NOT in good condition	9
* The network is NOT cleaned and disinfected when remained out of service >1 month	9
* The network and the tanks NOT cleaned with appropriate disinfectants at least annually	9
The water supply is interrupted for a long time	9
* The difference in temperature between 2 successive measurements of hot water is >10 °C/1 min	9
There is a taste and odor problem	9

*: designates a critical item.

4. Discussion

Legionella is a naturally occurring microorganism found in freshwater environments and surface waters where it exploits free-living amoeba cells for survival and multiplication, and, in that context, it is not hard to be introduced in building water systems through the main community water supply network. In fact, it has been stated that in the USA a percentage of 87.5% of Legionellosis outbreaks has been related to community water systems [26]. Even though the colonization of a water system by *Legionella* occurs frequently, this alone is not enough to pose a high risk to humans, unless the bacteria population reaches high numbers and becomes dispersed through appropriate aerosolization. For such conditions to take place, a series of variables must co-occur, such as the increased temperature of cold water or decreased temperature of hot water (optimally 35–46 °C), absence of water disinfectants or under-treated water, out of range pH values (5.5–9.2), presence of substances like iron salts and L-cysteine, as well as, co-existing and supporting microbial flora. Furthermore, other factors such as the complexity of the architecture of the pipe system (high surface to volume ratio), presence of blunt-end pipes, infrequently used pipe terminals, pipelines exposed to the sun heat, close proximity of hot and cold-water pipelines, insufficient maintenance and end-points creating aerosols, have all been evaluated to significantly affect the rate and extent of *Legionella* colonization in water systems [27]. All these factors may well be associated with the formation of biofilms, which can provide a means for the survival and dissemination of the pathogen and undermine the efforts to eradicate bacteria from water systems [28].

The presence of 1559 hotels and accommodation units in Crete with 85,407 rooms and 161,578 beds (data drawn from the Hellenic National Service of Tourism for 2015), could not exclude the island from the presence of TALDs [29]. The current research was focused mostly on the significance of sampling from recreation areas and spas and in particular from pools, spas, jacuzzis, showers next to swimming pools, shower heads and spa showers. The calculated relative risk of *Legionella* colonization was less in swimming pools and in spas, due to the increased surveillance and implementation of proper chlorination procedures, as opposed to the colonization in showers of swimming pools. The analyzed data showed that the high chlorination, the mixed type of contamination and the lower temperatures in the pool are potential factors that may contribute to the prevention of any *Legionella* from reproducing and reaching levels that would represent a health risk for bathers. The pool samples from which *Legionella* were isolated, had significantly lower concentrations of residual free chlorine, in fact less than the 0.4 mg/L required by the current regulations in Greece (0.4–0.7 mg/L). On the other hand, no significant correlation between *Legionella* colonization and pH values was calculated in the current study, agreeing with the study by Fragou et al., where the colonization of *Legionella* in 116 samples collected from hotels and hospitals was evaluated against pH values [30]. In general, such conditions support the growth of *Legionella*, while the frequent vigorous agitation that can occur in spas, pools and whirlpool baths can form aerosols that could create airborne bacteria and transfer them to the lungs of unsuspected individuals [31,32], even if the actual establishments are not actively used by these humans [33]. This is, also, supported by the detection of *Legionella* even in more isolated water facilities such as in spa and pools located on cruise ships that are actually one of the most common sources of *Legionella* infection [32]. It seems that such aerosols-creating settings, along with the close proximity of susceptible individuals, create a potential *Legionella* infectious environment. Such conditions are recorded in showers, especially the ones that have their pipes or at least part of them exposed to the sun heat. Similar results have been described from researches in Italy [4] a country that, like Greece, is a major tourist destination and retains a Mediterranean climate. In fact it has been shown that the risk for travelers is high in southeastern countries (including Greece) compared to countries with moderate climates [19]. Hotel fountains creating aerosols certainly mimic the conditions met in showers and in most cases they use recirculating water that is under a minimal degree of disinfection supervision, if any at all. Therefore, they have already been linked to Legionellosis outbreaks since the bacterium finds it easy to thrive in such conditions and disperse through the formed aerosols to the surrounding environment, or at a much larger distance if favoring conditions exist (for example the presence of wind) [34].

In our study, positive samples were recorded in 43/119 (36.13%) hotels, a result comparable to a similar study in Turkey, where of the 52 hotels included in the study, negative samples for *Legionella* were retrieved in 16 (30.8%) hotels [35]. According to the results of the current study, the seasonal operation of hotels and their presence in municipalities with low population seems to play a role in the increased risk of *Legionella* colonization; this finding has already been supported in a previous study carried out in hotels in Greece [36].

Another point of interest was the high number of *Legionella* species isolated, indicating a widespread dispersion of these microorganisms in the environment. In addition to the isolation of *L. pneumophila* (serogroups 1, 2, 3, 6, 7, 8, 13, 14, 15, and 2–15), other potentially pathogenic environmental species were also isolated, such as *L. anisa*, *L. erythra*, *L. taurinensis*, *L. birminghamensis*, and *L. rubrilucens*, the agent responsible for Pittsburg pneumonia [37] which is similar to Pontiac fever [38]. The presence of non-pneumophila species should not be underestimated since human cases of infection by *Legionella* species other than *L. pneumophila* or even the second most common, *L. anisa*, have been described worldwide, including the Island of Crete [39].

Legionella pneumophila serogroup 1 was detected in swimming pools and swimming pool showers however the low number of samples collected did not allow us to make any correlation among the positive samples, the detected serogroups and the sampling sites. The highest CFU/L was detected for the *L. pneumophila* serogroup 14 (10^5 CFU/L) and for *non-pneumophila* species (200,000 CFU/L). Nevertheless, a larger number of positive samples is required before coming to concrete conclusions on a possible relationship between site of collection and number of bacteria. The prevalence of *Legionella* species at certain environments has, also, been investigated by Litwin and colleagues [26] in which, they isolated *L. pneumophila* serogroup 1 and 6, *L. anisa*, *L. feeleii*, and *L. quateriensis* in the water reservoirs of recreational vehicles. As far as seasonality is concerned, in a similar research it was claimed that the concentrations of *Legionella* recovered from swimming pools, like *L. micdadei* and *L. bozemanii*, did not show any seasonal trend [4].

As regards the use of reclaimed water, ingestion of enteric pathogens causing gastrointestinal disease poses the greatest risk from exposure to wastewater however, inhalation of aerosols or dermal contact can, also, lead to disease. Except from *Vibrio cholerae*, the rest of the enteric pathogens that may cause gastrointestinal illnesses do not grow or survive for ever in water. On the other hand, free-living pathogens, such as *Legionella*, can grow under favorable conditions in treated wastewater and associated biofilms and, under certain circumstances, can survive within amoeba in water distribution systems [40]. That is why, samples from garden drip irrigation systems should be collected and tested in cases where reclaimed water is used and above all, it must be made clear that this type of water should not be used for irrigation through spraying [41].

Concerning WSPs, they already exist in various contexts worldwide. For instance, WSP networks are located in Africa, the Asia-Pacific region and in Latin America. WSPs have been designed in order to monitor water utility and to ensure that its quality standard is consistently kept within accepted limits [42]. In another study carried out in Germany, a decreased number of transgressions was observed following implementation of WSP in all parts of a hospital, supporting its efficacy [43]. In a different study carried out in Iceland, the impacts of WSPs on drinking water quality and health were evaluated and positive conclusions were drawn since implementation of WSPs resulted in better compliance in drinking water, reduced Heterotrophic Plate Count (HPC) numbers in water and decreased incidence of diarrhea in communities served by utilities implementing WSP [44]. It should be noticed however, that it turns out that it not just the presence of a WSP that will ensure the diminishing of the danger for a human infection by water-borne pathogens (including *Legionella*); its proper implementation is sometimes a more crucial factor [45]. In fact, it is possible that the improper implementation or the complete absence of a WSP (leading sometimes to temperature and pH values out of range) may provide the ideal stress conditions for the *Legionella* bacteria to develop a decreased sensitivity to antibiotics [46]. Of course, this is a huge aspect that needs further investigation.

Summing up, there is a need for awareness strategies in concordance with the operators of accommodation sites for the prevention of human *Legionella* infections. Stronger evidence on the source of infection can only be supported through enhanced standardization of *Legionella* investigation, reporting and follow-up, together with the use of high discrimination laboratory techniques. These factors could eventually lead to a more effective measure control [17]. Moreover, maintenance, regular controls, interventions on the hydraulic system, and good hygiene practices together with the assessment of risk analysis and establishment of a routine environmental microbiological surveillance schemes should be implemented to minimize exposure to *Legionella* infection [47,48].

5. Conclusions

The presence of *Legionella* is one of the most serious microbiological risks according to the water safety in distribution hotels. Knowing that *Legionella* bacteria can successfully thrive in natural and artificial water environments with warm waters, certainly directs towards the investigation of establishments with such conditions and with high human use or of those which present more complicated constructions such as pools and spas.

Preventing recreational water LD is a multifaceted issue that requires both the development of a WSP and, above all, its correct implementation, together with the participation of a large group of people like hotel staff and national and local public health authorities.

Acknowledgments: We would like to thank all the environmental health inspectors of the Local Public Health Authorities of the Crete Island who collected the environmental samples during all these years.

Author Contributions: Antonios Papadakis did the collection of the majority of the samples, the analysis of the results and contributed on the writing of the article. Dimosthenis Chochlakis did the analysis of the samples and contributed on the writing of the article. Vassilios Sandalakis did the analysis of the samples and contributed on the writing of the article. Maria Keramarou did the analysis of the samples and the analysis of the results. Yiannis Tselentis was in charge of the proper building and process of the study. Anna Psaroulaki was in charge of the proper processing of the study and contributed on the writing of the article.

Conflicts of Interest: The authors have declared no conflicts of interest.

Appendix A

Table A1. Detailed standardized questionnaire (checklist) used to evaluate risk associated with proper or not implementation of a WSP. * Critical Control Point. The checklist has been adapted from the European Guidelines for Prevention and Control of Travel Associated Legionnaires' disease and from the National School of Public Health 2004 Athens Olympic Games Checklist for building water systems.

	Legionella Prevention and Management Checklist			
	Item to Check	Yes	No	Remarks
	A water safety plan is implemented according to the requirements of the European Legislation and the proposals of the World Health Organization			
	Is there at least one named person responsible for *Legionella* control?			
	Responsible Person: (entity name)			
	Is this person properly trained in the control of Legionella and able to understand the system(s), risk factors and control measures?			
	Is there a written *Legionella* control plan in place for each system which could pose a risk?			
	If the hotel is operating on a seasonal level, is the entire domestic water system disinfected with high level (50 mg/L) chlorine for 2–4 h before the property is reopened?			
	Has there been any new pipe work or changes to existing pipe work in the last two years?			
	If yes, has it been checked to ensure that there are no pipes with intermittent or no water flow?			
	Was the system disinfected with high level chlorine or heat (60 °C) following completion of the work?			
	General Testing Sites of the Water Network			
1	The pressure on the meter is 1–12 atmospheres		−1	
2	The filters are in good condition		−2	
3	The sealing is in good condition		−2	
4	Absence of leaks on the network		−2	
5 *	The storage tank is maintained in good condition and no sediments are observed inside it		−3	
6	The water storage tanks have lids and wire mesh in each open air duct		−1	
7	The amount of water stored is no greater than one day's use		−1	
8 *	The network is cleaned and disinfected when it is not under use for more than a month		−3	
9 *	The network and the tanks are cleaned with appropriate disinfectants at least once a year		−3	
10	The water supply is not interrupted for long periods of time		−1	
11	Unused taps are removed from the network		−2	
12	Checking water network diagrams			
	Cold Water Systems			
13	Chillers are maintained in good condition		−1	
14	Chiller filters are maintained in good condition		−1	
	Hot Water Systems			
15	The system responds well at peak hours		−1	
16	There is no change (increase or decrease) in water consumption		−1	
17 *	No standing water in piping for more than one week		−3	
18 *	If No: Is a flushing procedure used?		−3	
19 *	Shower heads and taps are clean and free from scale		−3	
	Water Heating and Storage Appliances			
20	The appliance is dried and checked		−1	
21	The appliance is cleaned if necessary		−2	
22	The hot water extraction duct is dried		−1	
23	The appliance is maintained in accepted sanitary condition		−2	
	Faucets			
24	Operated and maintained in accordance with the manufacturing instructions		−2	
	Fire Protection Water Supply			
25	No backflow of water fire extinguishing system in the water supply network		−2	
	ANNEX I: Database Book			
26	Are there regular records (logbook for example) of the critical monitoring activities kept on site (temperatures, chlorine levels, etc.)?		−2	
27 *	Random checks of water at least every 6 months		−3	
28	In the control book (if any), there are no abnormal results		−2	
29 *	No *Legionella* detected the last six months (at a concentration of more than 1000 CFU/L)		−3	
	ANNEX II: Recordings			
30 *	Cold water is maintained at temperatures below 25 °C		−3	
31	The cold-water temperature in taps is <25 °C after 2 min flushing		−2	
32	The hot water temperature is >50 °C after 1 min flow		−2	
33 *	The difference in temperature between 2 successive measurements of hot water is NOT > 10 °C/1 min		−3	
34	Hot water store and circulation temp <60 °C		−2	

Table A1. *Cont.*

	Legionella Prevention and Management Checklist	
35	There is NO thermal stratification of the water inside the heaters and storage water	−1
36	The water temperature is >60 °C when exiting the heating unit and >50 °C when returning to it	−2
37	Is the pH maintained at 7.2–7.8?	−2
38 *	There is continuous treatment with chlorine at 0.2–0.5 mg/L?	−3
39	There is no taste and odor problem	−1

Inspection results: (A) satisfactory result (0 to 7 points, <10% of the total negative score, no critical violation); (B) relatively satisfactory result (−8 to 14 points, 11–20% of the total negative score, or a critical violation); (C) unsatisfactory result (more than 14 points, >20% of the total negative score).

References

1. *Legionella*. Developing a Water Management Program. Legionnaires. CDC. Available online: https://www.cdc.gov/legionella/maintenance/wmp-toolkit.html (accessed on 6 December 2017).
2. *Legionella* and the Prevention of Legionellosis. Available online: http://apps.who.int/bookorders/anglais/detart1.jsp?sesslan=1&codlan=1&codcol=15&codcch=633 (accessed on 7 December 2017).
3. Legionnaires' Disease—Annual Epidemiological Report for 2015. Available online: http://ecdc.europa.eu/en/publications-data/legionnaires-disease-annual-epidemiological-report-2015 (accessed on 6 December 2017).
4. Leoni, E.; Legnani, P.P.; Bucci Sabattini, M.A.; Righi, F. Prevalence of *Legionella* spp. in swimming pool environment. *Water Res.* **2001**, *35*, 3749–3753. [CrossRef]
5. Prussin, A.J.; Schwake, D.O.; Marr, L.C. Ten questions concerning the aerosolization and transmission of *Legionella* in the built environment. *Build. Environ.* **2017**, *123*, 684–695. [CrossRef] [PubMed]
6. Sikora, A.; Wójtowicz-Bobin, M.; Kozioł-Montewka, M.; Magryś, A.; Gładysz, I. Prevalence of *Legionella pneumophila* in water distribution systems in hospitals and public buildings of the Lublin region of eastern Poland. *Ann. Agric. Environ. Med. AAEM* **2015**, *22*, 195–201. [CrossRef] [PubMed]
7. Joseph, C. Surveillance of Legionnaires' Disease in Europe. In *Legionella*; Marre, R., Abu Kwaik, Y., Bartlett, C., Cianciotto, N., Fields, B., Frosch, M., Hacker, J., Lück, P., Eds.; ASM Press: Washington, DC, USA, 2002; pp. 311–317. [CrossRef]
8. Fields, B.S.; Benson, R.F.; Besser, R.E. Legionella and Legionnaires' disease: 25 years of investigation. *Clin. Microbiol. Rev.* **2002**, *15*, 506–526. [CrossRef] [PubMed]
9. McDade, J.E. *Legionella* and the Prevention of Legionellosis. *Emerg. Infect. Dis.* **2008**, *14*, 1006. [CrossRef]
10. Diederen, B.M.W. *Legionella* spp. and Legionnaires' disease. *J. Infect.* **2008**, *56*, 1–12. [CrossRef] [PubMed]
11. Marrie, T. Legionella: Molecular microbiology. *Emerg. Infect. Dis.* **2009**, *15*, 139. [CrossRef]
12. European Legionnaires' Disease Surveillance Network (ELDSNet). Available online: http://ecdc.europa.eu/en/about-us/partnerships-and-networks/disease-and-laboratory-networks/eldsnet (accessed on 6 December 2017).
13. Seenivasan, M.H.; Yu, V.L.; Muder, R.R. Legionnaires' disease in long-term care facilities: Overview and proposed solutions. *J. Am. Geriatr. Soc.* **2005**, *53*, 875–880. [CrossRef] [PubMed]
14. Darquenne, C.; Prisk, G.K. Aerosol deposition in the human respiratory tract breathing air and 80:20 Heliox. *J. Aerosol Med. Off. J. Int. Soc. Aerosols Med.* **2004**, *17*, 278–285. [CrossRef] [PubMed]
15. Respiratory Infection—Pennsylvania. Available online: https://www.cdc.gov/mmwr/preview/mmwrhtml/lmrk053.htm (accessed on 6 December 2017).
16. Bollin, G.E.; Plouffe, J.F.; Para, M.F.; Hackman, B. Aerosols containing *Legionella pneumophila* generated by shower heads and hot-water faucets. *Appl. Environ. Microbiol.* **1985**, *50*, 1128–1131. [PubMed]
17. Mouchtouri, V.A.; Rudge, J.W. Legionnaires' disease in hotels and passenger ships: A systematic review of evidence, sources, and contributing factors. *J. Travel Med.* **2015**, *22*, 325–337. [CrossRef] [PubMed]
18. Communicable Disease Threats Report, 12–18 November 2017, Week 46. Available online: http://ecdc.europa.eu/en/publications-data/communicable-disease-threats-report-12-18-november-2017-week-46 (accessed on 6 December 2017).
19. Beauté, J.; Zucs, P.; de Jong, B. Risk for travel-associated Legionnaires' disease, Europe, 2009. *Emerg. Infect. Dis.* **2012**, *18*, 1811–1816. [CrossRef] [PubMed]

20. WHO. Guidelines for Drinking-Water Quality, Fourth Edition. Available online: http://www.who.int/water_sanitation_health/publications/2011/dwq_guidelines/en/ (accessed on 7 December 2017).

21. EUR-Lex-31998L0083-EN-EUR-Lex. Available online: http://eur-lex.europa.eu/legal-content/EN/TXT/?uri=CELEX%3A31998L0083 (accessed on 7 December 2017).

22. EUR-Lex-32015L1787-EN-EUR-Lex. Available online: http://eur-lex.europa.eu/legal-content/EN/TXT/?uri=uriserv%3AOJ.L_.2015.260.01.0006.01.ENG (accessed on 7 December 2017).

23. European Technical Guidelines for the Prevention, Control and Investigation of Infections Caused by *Legionella* Species. Available online: http://ecdc.europa.eu/en/publications-data/european-technical-guidelines-prevention-control-and-investigation-infections (accessed on 7 December 2017).

24. EN 15975-2—European Standards. Available online: https://www.en-standard.eu/csn-en-15975-2-security-of-drinking-water-supply-guidelines-for-risk-and-crisis-management-part-2-risk-management/?gclid=EAIaIQobChMI4JCEqby72AIVWV8ZCh3-SgC7EAAYASAAEgLZofD_BwE (accessed on 3 January 2018).

25. WHO. Water Safety Plan Manual (WSP Manual). Available online: http://www.who.int/water_sanitation_health/publications/publication_9789241562638/en/ (accessed on 3 January 2018).

26. Litwin, C.M.; Asebiomo, B.; Wilson, K.; Hafez, M.; Stevens, V.; Fliermans, C.B.; Fields, B.S.; Fisher, J.F. Recreational vehicle water tanks as a possible source for *legionella* infections. *Case Rep. Infect. Dis.* **2013**, *2013*, 286347. [CrossRef] [PubMed]

27. Whiley, H.; Bentham, R.; Brown, M.H. *Legionella* persistence in manufactured water systems: Pasteurization potentially selecting for thermal tolerance. *Front. Microbiol.* **2017**, *8*, 1330. [CrossRef] [PubMed]

28. Murga, R.; Forster, T.S.; Brown, E.; Pruckler, J.M.; Fields, B.S.; Donlan, R.M. Role of biofilms in the survival of *Legionella pneumophila* in a model potable-water system. *Microbiol. Read. Engl.* **2001**, *147*, 3121–3126. [CrossRef] [PubMed]

29. Chochlakis, D.; Sandalakis, V.; Panoulis, C.; Goniotakis, I.; Makridaki, E.; Tselentis, Y.; Psaroulaki, A. Typing of *Legionella* strains isolated from environmental samples in Crete, Greece, during the period 2004–2011. *J. Water Health* **2013**, *11*, 762–771. [CrossRef] [PubMed]

30. Fragou, K.; Kokkinos, P.; Gogos, C.; Alamanos, Y.; Vantarakis, A. Prevalence of *Legionella* spp. in water systems of hospitals and hotels in south western Greece. *Int. J. Environ. Health Res.* **2012**, *22*, 340–354. [CrossRef] [PubMed]

31. Campese, C.; Roche, D.; Clément, C.; Fierobe, F.; Jarraud, S.; de Waelle, P.; Perrin, H.; Che, D. Cluster of Legionnaires' disease associated with a public whirlpool spa, France, April–May 2010. *Euro Surveill.* **2010**, *15*, 19602. [PubMed]

32. Health Protection Surveillance Centre. *National Guidelines for the Control of Legionellosis in Ireland, 2009*; Health Protection Surveillance Centre: Dublin, Ireland, 2009; ISBN 978-0-9551236-4-1.

33. Coetzee, N.; Duggal, H.; Hawker, J.; Ibbotson, S.; Harrison, T.G.; Phin, N.; Laza-Stanca, V.; Johnston, R.; Iqbal, Z.; Rehman, Y.; et al. An outbreak of Legionnaires' disease associated with a display spa pool in retail premises, Stoke-on-Trent, United Kingdom, July 2012. *Euro Surveill.* **2012**, *17*, 20271. [PubMed]

34. McEvoy, M.; Batchelor, N.; Hamilton, G.; MacDonald, A.; Faiers, M.; Sills, A.; Lee, J.; Harrison, T. A cluster of cases of legionnaires' disease associated with exposure to a spa pool on display. *Commun. Dis. Public Health* **2000**, *3*, 43–45. [PubMed]

35. Erdogan, H.; Arslan, H. Colonization of *Legionella* species in hotel water systems in Turkey. *J. Travel Med.* **2007**, *14*, 369–373. [CrossRef] [PubMed]

36. Mouchtouri, V.; Velonakis, E.; Tsakalof, A.; Kapoula, C.; Goutziana, G.; Vatopoulos, A.; Kremastinou, J.; Hadjichristodoulou, C. Risk factors for contamination of hotel water distribution systems by *Legionella* species. *Appl. Environ. Microbiol.* **2007**, *73*, 1489–1492. [CrossRef] [PubMed]

37. Bäck, E.; Schvarcz, R.; Kallings, I. Community-acquired *Legionella micdadei* (Pittsburgh pneumonia agent) infection in Sweden. *Scand. J. Infect. Dis.* **1983**, *15*, 313–315. [CrossRef] [PubMed]

38. Goldberg, D.J.; Wrench, J.G.; Collier, P.W.; Emslie, J.A.; Fallon, R.J.; Forbes, G.I.; McKay, T.M.; Macpherson, A.C.; Markwick, T.A.; Reid, D. Lochgoilhead fever: Outbreak of non-pneumonic legionellosis due to *Legionella micdadei*. *Lancet Lond. Engl.* **1989**, *1*, 316–318. [CrossRef]

39. Pasparaki, E.; Chochlakis, D.; Damianaki, A.; Psaroulaki, A. Severe community acquired pneumonia due to *Legionella maceachernii* infection. *Arch. Bronconeumol.* **2015**, *51*, 97–98. [CrossRef] [PubMed]

40. Marciano-Cabral, F.; Jamerson, M.; Kaneshiro, E.S. Free-living amoebae, *Legionella* and *Mycobacterium* in tap water supplied by a municipal drinking water utility in the USA. *J. Water Health* **2010**, *8*, 71–82. [CrossRef] [PubMed]
41. WHO. Potable Reuse. Available online: http://www.who.int/water_sanitation_health/publications/potable-reuse-guidelines/en/ (accessed on 8 March 2018).
42. Lockhart, G.; Oswald, W.E.; Hubbard, B.; Medlin, E.; Gelting, R.J. Development of indicators for measuring outcomes of water safety plans. *J. Water Sanit. Hyg. Dev.* **2014**, *4*, 171–181. [CrossRef] [PubMed]
43. Dyck, A.; Exner, M.; Kramer, A. Experimental based experiences with the introduction of a water safety plan for a multi-located university clinic and its efficacy according to WHO recommendations. *BMC Public Health* **2007**, *7*, 34. [CrossRef] [PubMed]
44. Gunnarsdottir, M.J.; Gardarsson, S.M.; Elliott, M.; Sigmundsdottir, G.; Bartram, J. Benefits of Water Safety Plans: Microbiology, compliance, and public health. *Environ. Sci. Technol.* **2012**, *46*, 7782–7789. [CrossRef] [PubMed]
45. Hadjichristodoulou, C.; Goutziana, G.; Mouchtouri, V.; Kapoula, C.; Konstantinidis, A.; Velonakis, E.; Vatopoulos, A.; Kremastinou, J. Evaluation of standardized scored inspections for Legionnaires' disease prevention, during the Athens 2004 Olympics. *Epidemiol. Infect.* **2006**, *134*, 1074–1081. [CrossRef] [PubMed]
46. Sandalakis, V.; Chochlakis, D.; Goniotakis, I.; Tselentis, Y.; Psaroulaki, A. Minimum inhibitory concentration distribution in environmental *Legionella* spp. isolates. *J. Water Health* **2014**, *12*, 678–685. [CrossRef] [PubMed]
47. De Filippis, P.; Mozzetti, C.; Amicosante, M.; D'Alò, G.L.; Messina, A.; Varrenti, D.; Giammattei, R.; Di Giorgio, F.; Corradi, S.; D'Auria, A.; et al. Occurrence of *Legionella* in showers at recreational facilities. *J. Water Health* **2017**, *15*, 402–409. [CrossRef] [PubMed]
48. Napoli, C.; Fasano, F.; Iatta, R.; Barbuti, G.; Cuna, T.; Montagna, M.T. *Legionella* spp. and legionellosis in southeastern Italy: Disease epidemiology and environmental surveillance in community and health care facilities. *BMC Public Health* **2010**, *10*, 660. [CrossRef] [PubMed]

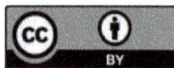

International Journal of
*Environmental Research
and Public Health*

MDPI

Article

Antibiotic Sensitivity Profiling and Virulence Potential of *Campylobacter jejuni* Isolates from Estuarine Water in the Eastern Cape Province, South Africa

Anthony C. Otigbu *, Anna M. Clarke, Justine Fri, Emmanuel O. Akanbi and Henry A. Njom

Microbial Pathogenicity and Molecular Epidemiology Research Group (MPMERG), Department of Biochemistry and Microbiology, Department of Biochemistry & microbiology, University of Fort Hare, Private Bag X1314, Alice 5700, South Africa; aclarke@ufh.ac.za (A.M.C.); jfri@ufh.ac.za (J.F.); femo.emman@gmail.com (O.E.A); Hnjom@ufh.ac.za (H.A.N.)
* Correspondence: aotigbu@gmail.com; Tel.: +2-773-620-7143

Received: 10 April 2018; Accepted: 3 May 2018; Published: 6 May 2018

Abstract: *Campylobacter jejuni (CJ)* is a zoonotic microbe and a major causative organism of diarrheal infection in humans that often has its functional characteristics inactivated in stressed conditions. The current study assessed the correlation between recovered *CJ* and water quality parameters and the drug sensitivity patterns of the pathogen to frontline antibiotics in human and veterinary medicine. Water samples ($n = 244$) from rivers/estuarines were collected from April–September 2016, and physicochemical conditions were recorded on-site. *CJ* was isolated from the samples using standard microbiological methods and subjected to sensitivity testing to 10 antibiotics. Mean *CJ* counts were between 1 and 5 logs (CFU/mL). Ninety-five isolates confirmed as *CJ* by PCR showed varying rates of resistance. Sensitivity testing showed resistance to tetracycline (100%), azithromycin (92%), clindamycin (84.2%), clarithromycin and doxycycline (80%), ciprofloxacin (77.8%), vancomycin (70.5%), erythromycin (70%), metronidazole (36.8%) and nalidixic acid (30.5%). Virulence encoding genes were detected in the majority 80/95, 84.2%) of the confirmed isolates from *cdtB*; 60/95 (63.2%) from *cstII*; 49/95 (51.6%) from *cadF*; 45/95 (47.4%) from *clpP*; 30/95 (31.6%) from *htrB*, and 0/95 (0%) from *csrA*. A multiple resistance *cme*ABC active efflux pump system was present in 69/95 (72.6) isolates. The presence of *CJ* was positively correlated with temperature ($r = 0.17$), pH ($r = 0.02$), dissolved oxygen ($r = 0.31$), and turbidity ($r = 0.23$) but negatively correlated with salinity ($r = -0.39$) and conductivity ($r = -0.28$). The detection of multidrug resistant *CJ* strains from estuarine water and the differential gene expressions they possess indicates a potential hazard to humans. Moreover, the negative correlation between the presence of the pathogen and physicochemical parameters such as salinity indicates possible complementary expression of stress tolerance response mechanisms by wild-type *CJ* strains.

Keywords: *Campylobacter jejuni*; physicochemical; virulence; drug resistance; estuary

---

1. Introduction

Campylobacter spp. are of the epsilonproteobacteria class of microorganism [1]. They are slow growing, Gram-negative, spiral shaped, motile organisms, characterized by their microaerobic nature [2]. They have been reported to be detected in greater quantities in diarrhea infections in humans than any other enteric pathogen and they require less than 100 cells to infect a host [3]. Campylobacteriosis is a chronic enteric infection primarily caused by cytotoxin-producing *Campylobacters* that invade and colonize the gastrointestinal (GI) tract in humans [4]. It is a zoonotic disease mainly transmitted via the consumption of poultry products [2], contact with pets and livestock, ingestion of water contaminated with human faeces originating from sewage, septic tanks, latrines and even animal faeces or from raw milk [5]. In humans, the disease lasts between 4–7 days and is characterized by acute enteritis, fever, vomiting and abdominal pain [4], with the danger of possibly leading to some post-infectious neuropathic diseases, such as bacteraemia, Guillain–Barre syndrome (GBS), reactive arthritis (ReA), and abortion [4,6]. *Campylobacter jejuni* and *C. coli* are the two widely recognized pathogenic species of *Campylobacter* that cause diseases in humans [7]. A large number of recorded campylobacteriosis outbreaks have also been traced to the ingestion of untreated surface water contaminated through human activities or by avian wildlife faeces [8,9]. Recreational and potable water are potential reservoirs of *Campylobacter* infection [5]. Therefore, the role of water in the transmission of *Campylobacter* species is of significant importance.

1.1. Virulence Determinants

Campylobacter jejuni possesses some multiple cell surface expressive virulent factors responsible for its high prevalence and pathogenicity compared to other enteric bacteria [3,10]. The secreted toxin is either enterotoxic or cytotoxic in its mode of action [10]. The target sites of enterotoxins are the cells lining the gastrointestinal (GI) tract of the host where its virulent effect is felt, resulting in either cytotoxin-linked inflammatory diarrhea associated with fever or non-inflammatory diarrhea associated with enterotoxins, characterized by non-leukocyte watery stools [4].

1.1.1. Cytolethal Distending Toxin (CDT)

The Cytolethal Distending Toxin (CDT) is an apoptosis triggering toxin produced by a group of Gram negative bacteria including *Campylobacter jejuni (CJ)* [9]. This toxin plays an important role in the host mucosal inflammatory response for interleukin-8 (IL-8) released by intestinal cells [10]. CDT is suggested to have an AB_2 tripartite structure with *cdtB* as the main effector, while *cdtA* and *cdtC* are makeup units associated with cell membrane binding [11]. The *cdtA* protein has a molecular mass of 27 KDa, *CdtB* has a molecular mass of 29 KDa, and *cdtC* has a molecular mass of 20 KDa [11]. Subunit A is the active unit directly responsible for DNA damage, while subunit B is a binding subunit that helps to bind the toxin to the specific target cells which inhibit cdc2, causing cellular distention and eventually death. The DNase activity of CDT is lethal—causing singular strand breakage with an estimated lethal dose (LD) of 50 pg/mL [11]. The pivotal role played by in cell and DNA degradation not only results in inflammatory diarrhea with faecal leukocytes but can potentially create lesions in fragmented DNA strands that can promote cancer [4,9]. CDT has high cross species sequence similarity and *cdtB* has the highest interspecies similarity [11]. It is, however, believed that some species lack *cdtB* but still have the potential to cause symptoms in children less than 3 years old [11].

1.1.2. Campylobacter Invasion Antigens (*ciaB*)

This is a protein synthesized by *CJ* which facilitates invasion to epithelial cells [10] of the gastrointestinal tract where it inflicts increased damage on the columnar epithelial cells, leading to swelling and rounding of invaded cells as a result of the cytotoxin and enterotoxin activities [8,10]. *Campylobacter* heat labile cytotonic (CTON) and cytotoxin (CTOX) are associated with non-inflammatory and inflammatory diarrhea, respectively [11]. *Cia* proteins are suggested to modify host cell regulatory pathways to promote *CJ* pathogenicity [12].

1.1.3. Fibronectin-Binding Protein (*cadF*)

This outer membrane conserved gene encodes a protein containing 326 amino acids of molar mass 37 kDa and plays a vital role in adherence to intestinal epithelial cells [13]. Internalization of the organism into its host is harnessed by the binding activity of *cadF* to the extracellular fibronectin [14]. However, studies have shown that there may be a reduction in *cadF* functionality when it assumes a defensive viable but non-culturable (VBNC) state [14].

1.1.4. Sialyltransferases (*cstII*)

This is an outer core structure carbohydrate called lipo-oligosaccharide (LOS) expressed by *CJ* that evades detection by mimicry of the human gangliosides [15]. The mechanism of action of this gene is providing the LOS with a protective barrier which facilitates its invasion of the epithelial cells by portraying a resemblance to the human ganglioside in the vertebrate nerve cells, allowing the host's immune system to self-destruct its own ganglioside [15]. It is believed to trigger the development of autoimmune diseases, such as Guillain–Barre Syndrome [16].

1.1.5. Post Transcriptional Regulator (*csrA*)

*csr*A gene is a carbon starvation regulator gene linked to the encoding of protein regulation which plays a vital role in *CJ*'s ability to responsively regulate a stationary phase mechanism to withstand hostile conditions [17]. Other associated virulence expressed by this gene is related to oxidative stress survival, the adherence of intestinal epithelial cells and biofilm formation [18]. Biofilm formation is an adaptive mechanism which complements the fragility of an organism when exposed to stress conditions by triggering a switch into a VBNC state [19].

1.1.6. ATP-Dependent Endopeptidase Protease (*clpP*)

This protease subunit in the bacterial caseinolytic proteases (CLP) contributes to virulence via energy formation through the degradation of virulence regulators [20], while indirectly playing a triggering role in stress tolerance of the organism when subjected to stress conditions [21]. The association of *clpP* with *clp* ATPase subunits enhances the proteolytic activity of the enzyme in the presence of ATP, producing a catalytic action [21]. In many pathogens, *clpP* enhances protein induced growth, under conditions, such as high temperature and oxidative stress [22].

1.1.7. Periplasmic Chaperon (*htrB*)

This is a periplasmic chaperon gene that encodes an acyltransferase for lipid A synthesis [23,24]. Synthesis of this enzyme regulates the organism's response to environmental changes [25]. It is, however, interesting to note that the *Campylobacter* species shows varying diversities of infection outcomes [26] attributable to differences in genetic composition [22].

1.2. Treatment and Drug Resistance

Campylobacter infection is, at times, regarded as self-limiting, but in the case of severe complications, antibiotics are commonly recommended, especially for immunodeficient patients. Antibiotic resistance among *Campylobacter* species has emerged as a global public health burden [4]. There are cases of growing resistance of *Campylobacter* spp. against the front line and alternative treatment therapies, such as macrolides (erythromycin), tetracycline, fluoroquinolones and aminoglycoside (gentamycin) [7,27]. The unregulated use of antimicrobial agents as food additives in livestock in order to prevent and control infections and enhance growth rates [28,29] has contributed to an increased resistance in microbes against multiple antibiotics [9]. The unregulated administration of fluoroquinolones to poultry has contributed to increased resistance of *CJ* to fluoroquinolones in industrialized regions [27].

A survey of the antimicrobial susceptibility of *Campylobacter* species isolated from poultry and pigs was carried out in the Western Cape and Gauteng provinces of South Africa and the results displayed clear traces of resistance to fluoroquinolones, macrolides and tetracycline antibiotics, while some of the isolates displayed multidrug resistance [30]. These characteristic drug resistances were prominent among two specific *Campylobacter* species, *CJ* and *C. coli*, which have very similar epidemiology, but require biochemical tests to distinguish between them [30]. Previous studies have reported variation in *CJ* sensitivity to erythromycin and ciprofloxacin; resistance rates of 79.2% were reported in Nigeria [31], 0% in Djibouti [14] and in Qatar, resistance rates of 63.2% to ciprofloxacin and 8.6% to erythromycin were shown [32]. Resistance to ciprofloxacin, another antimicrobial agent of consideration next to erythromycin, has also been recorded in some other parts of the world [33]. Multidrug resistance in *Campylobacter* is a widely studied area. Previous studies have suggested mutation as a factor responsible for the acquisition of this characteristic [34–36]. *Campylobacters* have an innate resistance trait in combination with externally acquired resistance traits to express virulence [35]. Mutation is believed to play a role in the evolution of the *cme*ABC operon [15,36] in the multidrug efflux system. Drug resistance has, however, been attributed to target modification-mediated enzymatic inactivation and enhanced efflux [37].

2. Materials and Methods

2.1. Study Area

The Swartkops estuary (33°52′ S; 25°38′ E) was selected for this study, and it is one of the most important estuaries in South Africa. It is also an important bird area (IBA) harbouring approximately 4000 migratory birds annually [38]. It is located close to the coastal city of Port Elizabeth in Nelson Mandela Bay Municipality of the Eastern Cape Province. The river is approximately 134 km long, while the estuary is approximately 16.4 km long with a permanent open connection into Algoa Bay in the Indian Ocean [39]. The total catchment area of the Swartkops River (including the tributary) is about 1360 km^2 [39]. Surrounding areas in the catchment of the Swartkops River are used for agriculture, while the lower reaches of the river and the estuary are surrounded by extensive human development, including several industries [40].

2.2. Sampling and Isolation of CJ

Sampling and Isolation

The spot sampling method, as described by the JEEP92 project [41], was used. An Aestuaria Bandi 410 vessel was used for sampling a total distance of 12.775 km of the Swartkops river estuary between the six sample points (Figure 1). Triplicate water samples were collected against water flow from surface level and at a depth below (3 m) using sterile bottles from each sampling point over a 6-month period (April–September 2016) covering three seasons (autumn, winter and spring) of the year and transported at 4 °C to the laboratory and analyzed within 5 h after collection. Physicochemical parameters (temperature, pH, electrical conductivity, salinity and turbidity) of sample stations were recorded in-situ [42] using the YSI 650 MDS multi-parameter reader at two levels (surface and bottom) from each sampling point.

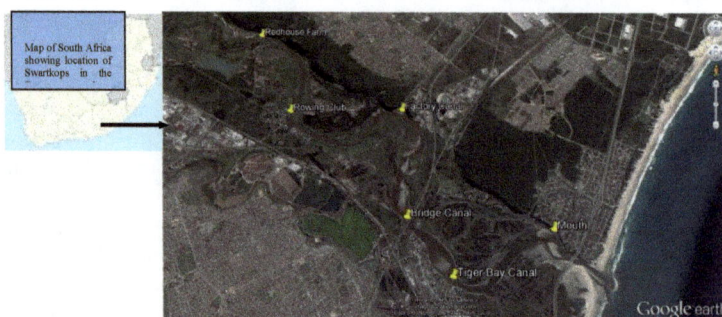

Figure 1. Location and GPS coordinates of the study sites in the Swartkops River estuary, Port Elizabeth. Sampling locations within the estuary; Rowing Club (RC) (33°50′14.60 S; 25°34′14.37 E); Factory Dam (FD) (33°50′12.16 S; 25°35′41.24 E); Redhouse Farm (RF) (33°49′10.56 S; 25°33′37.44 E); Bridge Canal (BC) (33°51′25.99 S; 25°35′49.99 E); Despatch Mouth (DM) (33°51′32.22 S; 25°37′31.33 E); Tiger Bay Canal (TB) (33°52′0.26 S; 25°36′22.32 E) (https://www.google.com.au/maps/).

Bacteria cells were concentrated on a microfilter (0.65 μm pore size cellulose ester Millipore) from raw water (100 mL; 10^{-1}; 10^{-2}) samples. The concentrated filter was aseptically folded and enriched in 20 mL nutrient broth supplemented with Preston *Campylobacter* selective supplement (SR0117-Oxoid) with 5% lysed horse blood and incubated microaerobically at 37 °C for 48 h. One hundred microlitres of enrichment culture was sub-cultured to *Campylobacter* blood-free agar (CCDA; CM739; Oxoid) containing CCDA selective supplement (SR155E; Oxoid) and incubated microaerobically using a campy gas pack (5% O_2, 10% CO_2, 85% N_2, CampyGen Oxoid) at 37 °C for 72 h. All plating was carried out in duplicate. Distinct presumptive colonies on each plate were counted by the surface count method to determine the total viable *Campylobacter* counts (TVCC). Then, 8–10 different colonies per plate were picked and subcultured on the selective medium for purity. A positive control (*Campylobacter jejuni* ATCC 33560 strain) was included with each set of tests. Identification of positive isolates was based on colony morphology, Gram-stain, no-growth in aerobic condition, hippurate hydrolysis and oxidase tests.

2.3. PCR Confirmation of CJ and Detection of Virulence Genes

Genus confirmation was performed using the 23S rRNA gene [43], and species confirmation was done using the *hipO* gene [44]. Screening for the pathogenic virulence genes, *cdtB*, *cadF*, *cstII*, *csrA*, *htrB* and *clpP*, was performed on the *CJ* confirmed isolates. Genomic isolation from the confirmed isolates was carried out using a commercial genomic DNA isolation kit (Qiagen Kit, Invitrogen, Thermo Fisher Scientific, USA) according to the manufacturer's instructions. Table 1 shows the primer sequences (Inqaba biotech, South Africa), amplicon sizes and cycling conditions of the various genes used in this study. The final concentration of the 25 μL PCR reaction consisted of 12.5 μL of the 2X master mix (Sybrselect, USA) 0.5 μL forward and reverse primers, 6.5 μL molecular grade water and 5 μL template DNA. The cycling conditions were as follows: initial denaturation was at 94 °C for 5 min, and then 94 °C for 30 s, with modifications in annealing temperatures specific to the primer pair (as given in Table 1) for 5 min and extension at 72 °C for 50 s. All PCR products were analyzed by electrophoresis on 1.5% agarose gels (CSL-AG100, Cleaver Scientific Ltd. Warwickshire, UK) except for *htrB* and *clpP* genes which were analyzed on 2% agarose gels. The gels were stained with ethidium bromide and visualized with a UV transilluminator and photographed (Alliance 4.7).

Table 1. PCR primer sizes and annealing temperatures.

Name of Gene	Sequence (5'-3')	Product (bp)	Annealing Temperature (°C)	References
Campy 23S	F-AATTGATGGGGTTAGCATTAGC R-CAACAATGGCTCATATACAACTGG	316	55	[43]
hipO	F-AGAGTTTGATCCTGGCTCAG R-ACGGCTACCTTGTTACGACTT	344	58	[44]
cdtB	F-CAC GGT TAA AAT CCC CTG CT R-GCA CTT GGA ATT TGC AAG GC	495	52	[18]
htrB	F-CGC ACC CAA TTT GAC ATA GAA R-TTT TTA GAG CGC TTA GCA TTT GTC T	70	52	[45]
clpP	F-TCG GAG CAT TTT TGC TTA GTT G R-CTC CAC CTA AAG GTT GAT GAA TCA T	90	52	[46]
csrA	F-CAC AGT CAG TGA AGG TGC TT R-ACT CGC ACA ATC GCT ACT TC	878	52	[47]
cstII	F-CAG CTT TCT ATT GCC CTT GC R-ACA CAT ATA GAC CCC TGA GG	570	52	[18]
cadF	F-TTGAAGGTAATTTAGATATG R-CTAATACCTAAAGTTGAAAC	400	42	[10]

2.4. Antimicrobial Sensitivity Testing

Confirmed *CJ* isolates were subjected to antimicrobial sensitivity testing with 10 antimicrobial agents. The Kirby–Bauer disk diffusion method on Mueller–Hinton agar supplemented with 5% horse blood, in accordance with Clinical and Laboratory Standards Institute guidelines [38] was used to perform the antimicrobial profiling. An inoculum of each bacterial isolate was emulsified in 3 mL of sterile normal saline (0.9%) in test tubes and the density was adjusted to 0.5 McFarland standard (0.5 mL of 1% *w/v* $BaCl_2$ and 99.5 mL of 1% *v/v* H_2SO_4), equivalent to 1.0×10^8 cfu/mL. The bacterial suspension was evenly spread on the Mueller–Hinton agar plates using sterile swab sticks and allowed to dry. Antibiotic discs (Mast Diagnostics Ltd., UK) with the following drug concentrations were selected for the assay: nalidixic acid (30 µg), ciprofloxacin (5 µg), azithromycin (15 µg), doxycycline (30 µg), erythromycin (15 µg), clarithromycin (15 µg), vancomycin (15 µg), tetracycline (30 µg), clindamycin (2 µg) and metronidazole (15 µg). Plates were incubated at 37 °C under microaerophilic conditions (5% O_2, 10% CO_2, 85% N_2) with gas generator envelopes (CampyGen; 2.5 L Thermo Scientific, UK) for 48 h, and the diameter zones of inhibition were measured, and the results were interpreted in accordance with the CLSI unit [48].

Detection of Multidrug Resistance Genes (*cmeA*, *cmeB* and *cmeC*)

Detection of the *cmeA*, *cmeB* and *cmeC* genes was determined by PCR, as described by [49], with slight modifications. Table 2 shows the primer sequences (Inqaba biotech, South Africa). The final concentration of the 25 µL PCR reaction consisted of 12.5 µL of the 2X master mix (Sybrselect, USA) 0.5 µL forward and reverse primers, 6.5 µL molecular grade water and 5 µL template DNA. The cycling conditions were as follows: initial denaturation at 94 °C for 7 min, followed by 94 °C for 1 min, annealing temperatures (see Table 2) for 1.5 min, extension at 72 °C for 3 min and then, final extension at 72 °C for 5 min for 30 cycles. All PCR products were analyzed by electrophoresis on 1% agarose gel (CSL-AG100, Cleaver Scientific Ltd. Warwickshire, UK). The gels were stained with ethidium bromide and visualized with a UV transilluminator and photographed (Alliance 4.7). *Campylobacter jejuni* ATCC 33560 strains were used as the positive control.

Table 2. Primers used in the study.

Target Genes	Primer Sequences 5′-3′	Annealing Temp (°C)	Amplicon Size (bp)
CmeA	F-TAGCGGCGTAATAGTAAATAAAC R-ATAAAGAAATCTGCGTAAATAGGA	50	435
CmeB	F-AGGCGGTTTTGAAATGTATGTT R-TGTGCCGCTGGGAAAAG	50	444
CmeC	F-CAAGTTGGCGCTGTAGGTGAA R-CCCCAATGAAAAATAGGCAGAGTA	52	431

3. Results

3.1. Physicochemical Analyses

The mean water temperature in the Swartkops river estuary for the sampled months was between 14.7 °C and 15.6 °C with the Despatch Mouth (DM) recording the highest mean temperature, while the Rowing Club station (RC) had the lowest mean temperature. No clear-cut difference in pH values was recorded for the sample stations, as the mean pH for all the stations ranged between 8.27 and 8.33. However, a high level of variation in the salinity level was recorded at all stations, with the mean salinity ranging between 13.92 practical salinity units (psu) and 32.77 psu. Station E, which is the dispatch point of Swartkops River to Algoa Bay recorded the highest salinity out of all the sampled months, while the Rowing Club (RC) station recorded the lowest salinity. The average dissolved oxygen (DO) concentrations were 53.83 mg/L and 62.9 mg/L, respectively. Station RC also recorded the lowest DO reading, while the Tiger Bay (TB) station recorded the highest overall reading. In terms of turbidity, the Swartkops water was very turbid during the sampled seasons, ranging, on average, between 4.2 Nephelometric Turbidity Units (NTU) and 66.9 NTU. The Factory Dam (FD) station recorded the highest average turbidity (66.9 NTU), especially in July and August, while DM presented more pristine water for all sample periods. The conductivity was between 20.9 ms/cm and 30 ms/cm on average. A low coefficient of variability was observed for all sampled sites (Table 3).

Table 3. Physicochemical parameters of water at different sample stations.

Sample Stations	Parameters	Temp (°C)	pH	Salinity (psu)	DO (mg/L)	Turbidity (NTU)	Conductivity (ms/cm)
RC	M	14.7	8.32	13.9	53.8	37.2	20.9
	Cv	0.16	0.02	0.52	0.68	0.85	0.49
FD	M	14.8	8.33	19.2	60.5	66.9	25.7
	Cv	0.16	0.01	0.4	0.67	0.74	0.43
RF	M	14.9	8.27	14.9	55.3	48.4	22
	Cv	0.17	0.01	0.15	0.7	0.78	0.13
BC	M	14.9	8.31	21.4	56.9	31.9	26.3
	Cv	0.15	0.02	0.5	0.69	0.4	0.55
DM	M	15.6	8.29	32.8	58.9	4.2	26.3
	Cv	0.13	0.01	0.19	0.69	0.7	0.23
TB	M	14.9	8.36	25.4	62.9	24.2	30
	Cv	0.15	0.01	0.38	0.68	1.5	0.44

M = mean; Cv = coefficient of variability; DO = dissolved oxygen.

3.2. PCR Confirmation of CJ and Detection of Virulence Genes

One hundred and twenty isolates were phenotypically confirmed as Campylobacteracea (Figure 2). Further screening at the species level confirmed 95 isolates as *C. jejuni* (Figure 3) and the other 25 identified as *C. coli* (18) and *C. upselensis* (7). Determination of the occurrence of virulence genes in the confirmed *CJ* isolates revealed the *cdtB* gene in 80/95 (84.2%) of the isolates, an indication that the toxin production gene (*cdtB*) was the most prevalent virulence determinant. Forty-nine (52%) of the isolates were identified as having adherence virulence genes (*cadF*), while 60/95 (63.2%) isolates tested positive for the intestinal epithelial invasive virulence gene (*cstII*). This gene is also linked to the risk of Gullian–Barre Syndrome (GBS) development. Thirty (31.6%) of the isolates were positive for the lipid A synthesis gene (*htrB*) responsible for the adjustment of organisms to stressful external environmental changes, while 45/95 (47.4%) of the isolates were identified as having the ATP dependent protease gene (*clpP*), which is responsible for the degradation of damaged proteins due to unfavourable conditions. The carbon starvation regulator gene (*csrA*), which is linked to cell division and the formation of biofilm, was absent in all isolates. Isolates recovered from the Redhouse Farm (RF) and Bridge Canal (BC) sampling sites were confirmed as housing all but the *csrA* gene which was absent in all isolates. Table 4 shows the number of genes detected in confirmed *CJ* isolates.

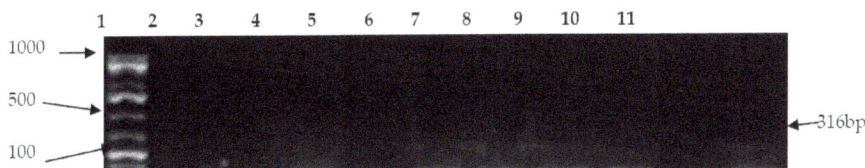

Figure 2. PCR detection of *23S rRNA* gene (316 bp). Lane 1 is themarker, Lanes 2–9 are test isolates, Lane 10 is the negative control, and Lane 11 is the positive control.

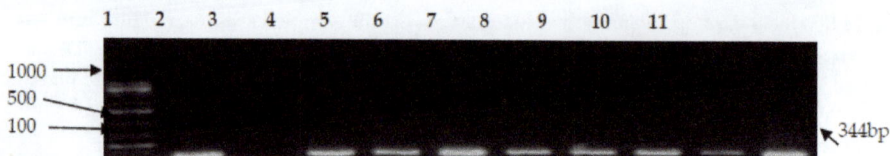

Figure 3. PCR detection of *hipO* gene (344 bp) for *CJ* confirmation. Lane 1 is the marker, Lane 2 is the positive control, Lane 3 is the negative control, and Lanes 4–11 are the test isolates.

Table 4. Detection of pathogenic genes in confirmed *C. jejuni* (*CJ*) isolates.

Sample Source	No. of Samples	No. of Isolates Confirmed as *Campylobacter* Genus for Samples (%)	No. of Isolates Confirmed as *CJ* (%)	Genes Detected in *CJ* Isolates (% Positive)						
Estuarine water	244	23S rRNA	*HipO*	*cdtB*	*cadF*	*cstII*	*csrA*	*htrB*	*ClpP*
		120 (49.2)	95 (79.2)	80 (84.2)	49 (51.6)	60 (63.2)	0 (0)	30 (31.6)	45 (47.4)

3.3. Frequency of CJ Isolation

The frequency of bacterial isolation frequency at all sample sites for the sampling period was recorded (Figure 4). The Despatch Mouth (DM) was the least *Campylobacter*-contaminated site, and the most pristine with an isolation frequency of 33%. No *Campylobacter* count was recorded at DM for April, May, June or July (autumn and winter), but *Campylobacter* were recorded in August and September (spring). The Tiger Bay (TB) site appeared to be the most *Campylobacter*-contaminated site in the Swartkops estuary with an isolation frequency of 100% during the sampled seasons. *Campylobacter* counts were recorded for all sampling months, with higher readings in July, August and September. However, the overall highest average *Campylobacter* counts were recorded at the Factory Dam (FD) and Bridge Canal (BC) sites for the month of August. Consequently, very low counts were recorded in April, May, and June (winter) for all sites.

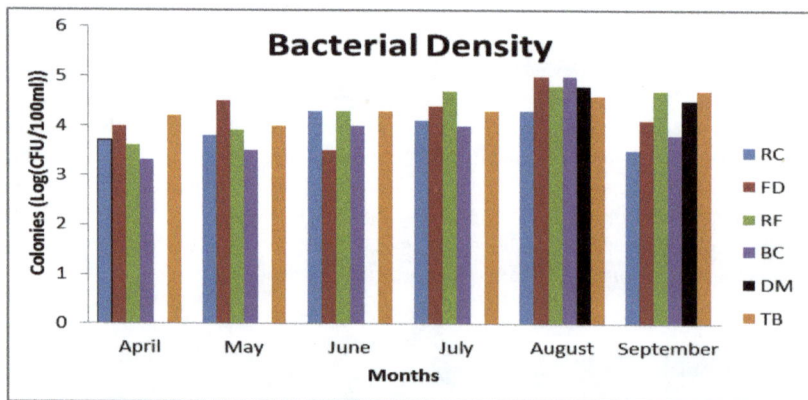

Figure 4. Bacterial density at all sampling sites. * Mean values are expressed in log (cfu per 100 mL).

3.4. Physicochemical Parameters and Occurrence of C. jejuni

No significant positive correlation was observed between the population density of *CJ* and temperature ($r = 0.17$), pH ($r = 0.02$), dissolved oxygen ($r = 0.31$), and turbidity ($r = 0.23$). A negative correlation was observed with salinity ($r = -0.39$) and conductivity ($r = -0.28$). The correlation values were not statistically different for temperature, dissolved oxygen, salinity, turbidity and conductivity, while they were statistically different for pH (Table 5).

Table 5. Correlation (Bravais Pearson) matrix between temperature, bacterial contamination, pH, salinity, turbidity, dissolved oxygen and conductivity.

	Temp	PH	Salinity	DO	Turbidity	Conductivity	CJ
Temp	1						
pH	−0.30	1					
Salinity	−0.60	0.46	1				
DO	0.19	0.07	−0.31	1			
Turbidity	−0.08	−0.03	−0.12	−0.43	1		
Conductivity	−0.53	0.48	0.87	−0.32	0.08	1	
CJ	0.17	0.02	−0.39	0.21	0.23	−0.28	1

3.5. Antimicrobial Sensitivity Testing and Prevalence of Multidrug Resistance (MDR) Efflux Pump Genes

The antibiotic sensitivity of 95 *CJ* isolates was profiled and revealed a higher degree of resistance to tested antimicrobial agents. The highest resistance level, 95/95 (100%), was recorded for tetracycline, followed by azithromycin (87/95, 92%), clindamycin (80/95, 84.2%), clarithromycin and doxycycline (76/95, 80%), ciprofloxacin (78/95, 77.8%), vancomycin (67/95, 70.5%), and erythromycin (67/95, 70%), with the lowest resistance levels recorded for metronidazole (35/95, 36.8%) and nalidixic acid (29/95, 30.5%). Nalidixic acid was the most effective antibiotic with a susceptibility of 57/95 (59%) (Figure 5). The percentage incidences of multidrug resistance (MDR) efflux pump genes of *C. jejuni* are shown in Table 6. A high (69/95, 72.6%) number of *CJs* expressed MDR efflux pump genes with only 6/95 (6.3%) not expressing them. Twenty isolates showed a disruption in the expression of all tripartite efflux systems, which could trigger a malfunction of the *cme*ABC system.

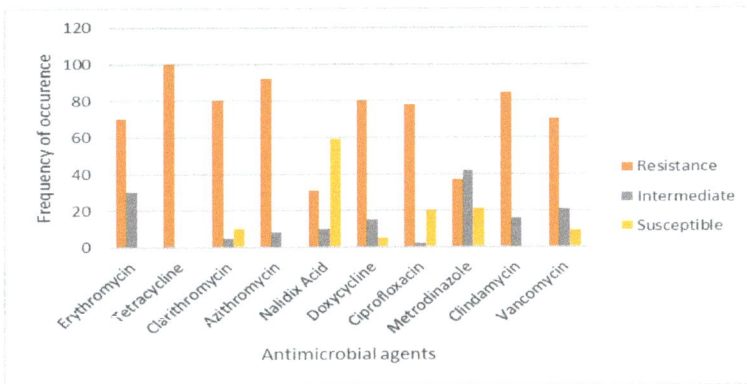

Figure 5. Antimicrobial sensitivity Profile.

Table 6. Incidences of *Campylobacter* multidrug resistance (MDR) efflux pump genes.

Genes	No. of Isolates (n = 95)	
	a (%)	b (%)
*cme*A	11/20 (55)	9/20 (45)
*cme*B	18/20 (90)	2/20 (20)
*cme*C	14/20 (70)	7/20 (30)
*cme*ABC	69/95 (72.6)	6/95 (6.3)

a = positive isolates; b = negative isolates.

4. Discussion

4.1. Survival of Organism

Estuaries are confluent ecosystems where a mixture of salty sea waters and rivers meet with freshwater [42]. They are transition points from land to sea and freshwater to salt water and are rich in organic contents [5]. The dynamic physicochemical nature of the ecosystem is peculiarly detrimental to the survival of fastidious microbes such as *Campylobacter* [14]. However, *Campylobacter* spp. display complex survival mechanisms by transiting to a stationary viable, but non-culturable, form (VBNC) for survival [11]. The recovered strains in this study displayed differential gene expression, which could be peculiarto wild-type *CJ* strains, and morphological evidence showed 66/95 (69%) without flagella. This could be due to the expression of the flagella gene being switched off in a process known as phase variation [49]. The carbon starvation regulator gene (*csrA*) which is linked to the encoding of protein regulation was not detected in the study. The absence of *csrA* could have been complimented by the presence of *htrB* and *clpP* genes. Other associated virulence expressed by this gene is related to oxidative stress survival, adherence of intestinal epithelial cells and in biofilm formation [18,45]. Although the pathogenic potential of wild-type strains is debatable due to the adverse stress conditions which can reduce their colonization and invasive abilities, their ability to live asymptomatically in their hosts may not be fully ruled out, especially as this concerns externally acquired genes from surrounding environs. This is indicated by the presence of the *cstII* gene in some of the strains (Figure 6). Some of the test isolates lacked *cdtB*, and *cadF* genes and could, therefore, be considered non-pathogenic. Most of the isolates lacked motility potential at the point of analysis, inferring the inactivation of the *racR* gene [11]. The results as shown in Figure 7 strongly correlate with the inference drawn in a past study suggesting that *CJ* could still retain its *cadF* adhesion functionality under stressed conditions [14].

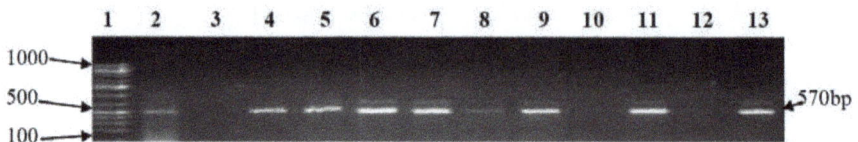

Figure 6. PCR detection of *cstII* gene (570 bp) of *CJ*. Lane 1 is the marker, Lane 2 is the positive control, Lane 3 is the negative control, and Lanes 4–13 are test isolates.

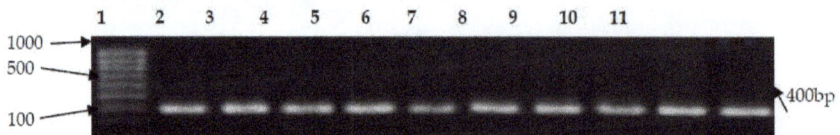

Figure 7. PCR detection of *cadF* gene (400 bp) of *CJ*: Lane 1 is the marker, Lane 2 is the positive control, and Lanes 3–11 are test isolates.

The prevalence of the cytotoxin production gene (*cdtB*) in the confirmed isolates (Figure 8) shows that the organism is capable of retaining its toxin production ability even in a starved state. The presence of *htrB* and *clpP* genes (Figure 9) provides an extra boost in the organism's aero-tolerance survival in environmental waters. However, the survival of microorganisms in oxidative stress environments has been attributed to their ability to develop specialized defensive mechanisms [11]. The existence of *CJ* in the Swartkops could be as a result of oceanic effects rather than continental effects. The FD sample site was the most polluted site in the Swartkops due to effluent discharges from the factory directly to the river. Between FD and BC is the shallowest area; this may be due to high land surface run-off into the river. This area has the highest population of migratory birds and fishing activities with the highest *CJ* density which strongly indicates that avian species are major reservoirs of the organism. Seasonality, on the other hand, could also play a pivotal role in the survival and existence of the organism, as larger population densities of the organism were recorded during spring and the lowest population densities were recorded during winter [2,9]. The Swartkops river estuary has a strong nutrient zonation, which is typified by the variation in salinity distribution in the estuary as a result of upstream shift of salt and fresh waters, which may be responsible for the abundance and distribution of species. Hence, this was the major reason for choosing to investigate the effect of the physicochemical parameters on the survival of the organism. The salinity reading at DM was the highest total average reading of all seasons, but barely affected the survival of the organism.

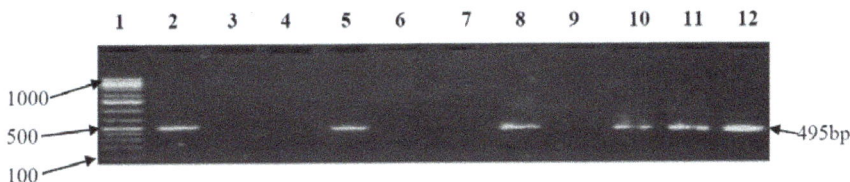

Figure 8. PCR detection of *cdtB* gene (495 bp) of *CJ*. Lane 1 is the marker, Lane 2 is the positive control, Lane 3 is the negative control, and Lanes 4–12 are test isolates.

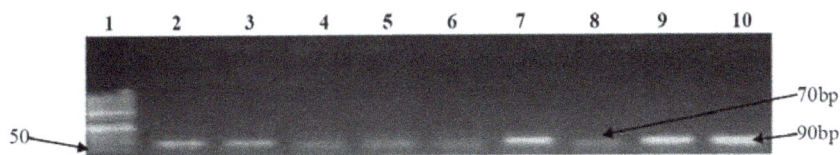

Figure 9. PCR detection of *htrB* (70bp) and *clpP* genes (90bp) of *C. jejuni*. Lane 1 is the marker, Lane 2 is the positive control, Lanes 3, 7, 9 and 10 are *clpP* positive isolates, and Lanes 4, 5, 6 and 8 are *htrB* positive isolates.

4.2. Drug Resistance

Multiple resistances have been reported globally in both *CJ* and *C. coli* in human and animal isolates. The resistance pattern was observed notably in tetracyclines, macrolides and fluoroquinolones [1,7]. In South Africa, antimicrobials with broad-spectrum activity such as tetracyclines are used in both the poultry and pig industries, as they are affordable and easy to administer in food and water [30]. In a recent study, a high level of resistance to tetracyclines was also revealed in *Campylobacter* spp. isolated from broilers and hens [1]. In this study, multidrug resistance was observed in more than 70% of the isolates (Figure 10). The isolates harbored the *Campylobacter* multidrug efflux pump (*cme*ABC) genes responsible for multidrug resistance [7]. Previous studies have shown variation in the resistance pattern of *CJ* in South Africa [7,30]. Some studies revealed a high resistance of the organism to fluoroquinolones, macrolides and tetracyclines [30], while some showed high susceptibility to fluoroquinolones [1]. Resistance to fluoroquinolone is believed to develop more rapidly in *Campylobacter* spp, than in other Gram-negative bacteria, mainly attributed to single-step point mutations in *gyrA* [2]. However, these studies were carried out on *CJ* isolated from avians, porcines and bovines. In this study, multidrug resistance was shown for fluoroquinolones, macrolides and tetracyclines. A high resistance to tetracycline (100%) was observed and the highest susceptibility (59%) was shown to nalidixic acid. Previous studies have suggested that aquatic environments (surface and groundwater bodies) are perfect for horizontal gene exchange of mobile genetic elements (MGEs) which results in antibiotic resistance [2].

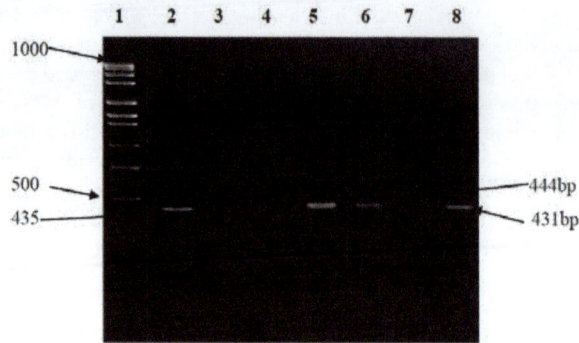

Figure 10. PCR detection of *cme*ABC in isolates. Lane 1 is the marker, Lane 2 is the positive control, Lane 8 is the *CmeA* positive isolate (435 base pair, Lane 4 is the negative control, Lanes 5 and 6 are *cmeB* positive isolates (444 bp), and Lane 3 is the *cmeC* positive isolate (431 bp).

5. Conclusions

This is the first study to report the occurrence of differential gene expressions in wild-type *CJ* isolated from the Swartkops in the Eastern Cape Province. The results showed that the estuarine water could potentially harbour multiple resistant *CJ* strains of public health concern among estuarine users. Although the extent of their pathogenicity is not fully ascertained, it could be assumed that pathogens with similar traits are likely to be found in other similar ecosystems.

6. Future Direction of Study

This study focused on the detection of active virulence-inducing genes and antimicrobial sensitivity profiling of environmentally recovered *CJ* strains. More elaborate future studies should include a comparative genomic analysis using whole genome sequencing (WGS) for other related water sources of high importance around the Eastern Cape Province to fully understand the pathophysiological mechanisms of recovered wild-type *Campylobacter* strains. Moreover, a comparative study of the antimicrobial profile and analysis of expressed virulence of wild-type isolates and clinical strains should be investigated. Other important virulence determinants which were not investigated in this study such as *racR* and *flaA* genes associated with motility and *cosR*, *rrpA* or *rrpB* associated with the oxidative stress response should be studied in wild-type isolates. It is also necessary to conduct the same study on other closely-related organisms, such as *Arcobacter* species, to document their pathogenicity.

Author Contributions: A.C.O. carried out the project experimental design, sample collection, performed the experiments, analysed data, and drafted the manuscript, H.A.N. and J.F. contributed to data analysis, study design and proof reading of manuscript, O.E.A. assisted in sample collection and proof reading of manuscript, A.M.C. contributed to the study design and organisation of sampling.

Acknowledgments: This work was supported by the National Research Foundation (NRF) and the South African Institute for Aquatic Biodiversity (SAIAB) under the NRF/SAIAB innovative scholarship.

Conflicts of Interest: The authors declare no conflict of interest.

References

1. Bester, L.; Essack, S. Prevalence of antibiotic resistance in *Campylobacter* isolates from commercial poultry suppliers in KwaZulu-Natal, South Africa. *J. Antimicrob. Chemother.* **2008**, *62*, 1298–1300. [CrossRef] [PubMed]

2. Nichols, G.; Richardson, J.; Sheppard, S.; Lane, K.; Sarran, C. *Campylobacter* epidemiology: A descriptive study reviewing 1 million cases in England and Wales between 1989 and 2011. *BMJ* **2012**, *2*, e001179. [CrossRef] [PubMed]

3. Croinin, O.; Backert, S. Host epithelial cell invasion by *Campylobacter jejuni*: Trigger of zipper mechanism? *Research Advances in the study of Campylobacter, Helicobacter and related organisms. Front. Cell. Infect. Microbiol.* **2012**, *2*, 25. [CrossRef] [PubMed]

4. World Health Organization. *The Increasing Incidence of Human Campylobacteriosis Report and Proceedings of a WHO Consultation of Experts, Copenhagen, Denmark 21–25 November 2000*; World Health Organization: Copenhagen, Denmark; pp. 21–25.

5. EFSA (European Food Safety Authority); ECDC (European Centre for Disease Prevention and Control). The European Union summary report on trends and sources of zoonoses, zoonotic agents and food-borne outbreaks in 2012. *EFSA J.* **2014**, *12*, 3547. [CrossRef]

6. Skirrow, M.; Blaser, M. Clinical aspects of *Campylobacter* infection. In *Campylobacter*, 2nd ed.; Nachamkin, I., Blaser, M.J., Eds.; ASM Press: Washington, DC, USA, 2000; pp. 69–88.

7. Engberg, J.; Aarestrup, F.; Taylor, D.; Gerner-Smidt, P.; Nachamkin, I. Quinolone and macrolide resistance in *Campylobacter jejuni* and *C. coli*: Resistance mechanisms and trends in human isolates. *Emerg. Infect. Dis.* **2001**, *7*, 24–34. [CrossRef] [PubMed]

8. Sopwith, W.; Birtles, A.; Matthews, M.; Fox, A.; Gee, S.; Painter, M. *Campylobacter jejuni* multilocus sequence types in humans, northwest England, 2003–2004. *Emerg. Infect. Dis.* **2006**, *12*, 1500–1507. [CrossRef] [PubMed]

9. DefFraites, F.; Sanchez, L.; Brandt, A.; Kadlec, P.; Haberberger, L.; Lin, J.; Taylor, N. An outbreak of *Campylobacter* enteritis associated with a community water supply on a US military installation. *MSMR* **2014**, *21*, 10–15.

10. Perera, V.; Nachamkin, I.; Ung, H.; Patterson, J.; McConville, M. Molecular mimicry in *Campylobacter jejuni*: Role of the lipo-oligosaccharide core oligosaccharide in inducing anti-ganglioside antibodies. *FEMS Immunol. Med. Microbiol.* **2007**, *50*, 27–36. [CrossRef] [PubMed]

11. Samosornsuk, W.; Asakura, M.; Yoshida, E.; Taguchi, T.; Eampokalap, B.; Chaicumpa, W.; Yamasaki, S. Isolation and characterization of *Campylobacter* strains from diarrheal patients in Bangkok and its suburb in Thailand. *Jpn. J. Infect. Dis.* **2015**, *68*, 209–215. [CrossRef] [PubMed]

12. Saouaf, J.; Li, B.; Zhang, G.; Shen, Y.; Furuuchi, N.; Hancock, W.; Greene, I. Deacetylase inhibition increases regulatory T cell function and decreases incidence and severity of collagen-induced arthritis. *Exp. Mol. Pathol.* **2009**, *87*, 99–104. [CrossRef] [PubMed]

13. Sails, A.; Bolton, F.; Fox, A.; Wareing, D.; Greenway, D. Detection of *Campylobacter jejuni* and *Campylobacter coli* in environmental waters by PCR enzyme- linked immunosorbent assay. *Appl. Environ. Microbiol.* **2002**, *68*, 1319–1324. [CrossRef] [PubMed]

14. Patrone, V.; Campana, R.; Vallorani, L.; Dominici, S.; Federici, S.; Casadei, L.; Gioacchini, A.M.; Stocchi, V.; Baffone, W. CadF expression in *Campylobacter jejuni* strains incubated under low-temperature water microcosm conditions which induce the viable but non-culturable (VBNC) state. *Antonie Van Leeuwenhoek* **2013**, *103*, 979–988. [CrossRef] [PubMed]

15. Pérez-Boto, D.; López-Portolés, J.; Simón, C.; Valdezate, S.; Echeita, M. Study of the molecular mechanisms involved in high-level macrolide resistance of Spanish *Campylobacter jejuni* and *Campylobacter coli* strains. *J. Antimicrob. Chemother.* **2010**, *65*, 2083–2088.

16. Bach, J. Infections and autoimmune diseases. *J. Autoimmun.* **2005**, *25*, 74–80. [CrossRef] [PubMed]

17. Fields, J.; Thompson, S. *Campylobacter jejuni* CsrA mediates oxidative stress responses, biofilm formation, and host cell invasion. *J. Bacteriol.* **2008**, *190*, 3411–3416. [CrossRef] [PubMed]

18. González-Hein, G.; Huaracán, B.; García, P.; Figueroa, G. Prevalence of virulence genes in strains of *Campylobacter jejuni* isolated from human, bovine and broiler. *Braz. J. Microbiol.* **2013**, *44*, 1223–1229.

19. Thakur, S.; Zhao, S.; McDermott, P.; Harbottle, H.; Abbott, J.; Gebreyes, W.; White, D. Antimicrobial resistance, virulence, and genotypic profile comparison of *Campylobacter jejuni* and *Campylobacter coli* isolated from humans and retail meats. *Foodborne Pathog. Dis.* **2010**, *7*, 835–844. [CrossRef] [PubMed]

20. Hlaváček, O.; Vachova, L. ATP- dependent proteinases in bacteria. *Folia Microbiol.* **2002**, *47*, 203–212. [CrossRef]

21. Frees, D.; Brøndsted, L.; Ingmer, H. Bacterial proteases and virulence. In *Regulated Proteolysis in Microorg*; Springer Science: Dordrecht, The Netherlands, 2013; pp. 161–192.
22. Hughes, R.; Cornblath, D. Guillain-Barre´ syndrome. *Lancet* **2005**, *366*, 1653–1666. [CrossRef]
23. Parkhill, J.; Wren, B.W.; Mungall, K.; Ketley, J.M.; Churcher, C.; Basham, D.; Chillingworth, T.; Davies, R.M.; Feltwell, T.; Holroyd, S.; et al. The genome sequence of the food-borne pathogen *Campylobacter jejuni* reveals hypervariable sequences. *Nature* **2000**, *403*, 665–668. [CrossRef] [PubMed]
24. Hausdorf, L.; Neumann, M.; Bergmann, I.; Sobiella, K.; Mundt, K.; Fröhling, A.; Schlüter, O.; Klocke, M. Occurrence and genetic diversity of *Arcobacter* spp. in a spinach processing plant and evaluation of two *Arcobacter*-specific quantitative PCR assays. *Syst. Appl. Microbiol.* **2013**, *36*, 235–243. [CrossRef] [PubMed]
25. Mihaljevic, R.; Sikic, M.; Klancnik, A.; Brumini, G.; Mozina, S.; Abram, M. Environmental stress factors affecting survival and virulence of *Campylobacter jejuni*. *Microb. Pathog.* **2007**, *43*, 120–125. [CrossRef] [PubMed]
26. Sheppard, S.; Dallas, J.; Strachan, N.; MacRae, M.; McCarthy, N.; Wilson, D.; Gormley, F.J.; Falush, D.; Ogden, I.; Maiden, M.; et al. *Campylobacter* genotyping to determine the source of human infection. *Clin. Infect. Dis.* **2009**, *48*, 1072–1078. [CrossRef] [PubMed]
27. Koolman, L.; Whyte, P.; Burgess, C.; Bolton, D. Distribution of virulence- associated genes in a selection of *Campylobacter* isolates. *Foodborne Pathol. Dis.* **2016**, *12*, 424–432. [CrossRef] [PubMed]
28. Igimi, S.; Okada, Y.; Ishiwa, A.; Yamasaki, M.; Morisaki, N.; Kubo, Y.; Asakura, H.; Yamamoto, S. Antimicrobial resistance of *Campylobacter*: Prevalence and trends in Japan. *Food Addit. Contam.* **2008**, *25*, 1080–1083. [CrossRef]
29. Rożynek, E.; Dzierżanowska-Fangrat, K.; Szczepańska, B.; Wardak, S.; Szych, J.; Konieczny, P.; Albrecht, P.; Dzierżanowska, D. Trends in antimicrobial susceptibility of *Campylobacter* isolates in Poland (2000–2007). *Polskie Tow. Mikrobiol. Pol. Soc. Microbiol.* **2009**, *58*, 111–115.
30. Jonker, A.; Picard, J. Antimicrobial susceptibility in thermophilic *Campylobacter* spp. isolated from pigs and chickens in South Africa. *J. S. Afr. Vet. Assoc.* **2010**, *81*, 228–236. [CrossRef] [PubMed]
31. Coker, O.; Adefeso, O. The changing patterns of *Campylobacter jejuni/coli* in Lagos, Nigeria after ten years. *East African Med. J.* **1994**, *71*, 437–440.
32. Ghunaim, H.; Behnke, J.; Aigha, I.; Sharma, A.; Doiphode, S.; Deshmukh, A.; Abu-Madi, M. Analysis of Resistance to Antimicrobials and Presence of Virulence/Stress Response Genes in *Campylobacter* Isolates from Patients with Severe Diarrhoea. *PLoS ONE* **2015**, *10*, e0119268. [CrossRef] [PubMed]
33. Nachamkin, I.; Mishu-Allos, B.; Ho, T. *Campylobacter* species and Guillain-Barre´ Syndrome. *J. Clin. Microbiol.* **1998**, *11*, 555–567.
34. Vacher, S.; Menard, A.; Bernard, E.; Santos, A.; Megraud, F. Detection of mutation associated with macrolide resistance in thermophilic *Campylobacter* spp. By real-time PCR. *Microb. Drug Resist.* **2005**, *11*, 40–47. [CrossRef] [PubMed]
35. Qin, S.; Wang, Y.; Zhang, Q.; Chen, X.; Shen, Z.; Deng, F. Identification of a novel genomic island conferring resistance to multiple amino glycoside antibiotics in *Campylobacter coli*. *Antimicrob. Agents Chemother.* **2012**, *56*, 5332–5339. [CrossRef] [PubMed]
36. Iovine, N. Resistance mechanisms in *Campylobacter jejuni*. *Virulence* **2013**, *4*, 230–240. [CrossRef] [PubMed]
37. Gibreel, A.; Taylor, D.E. Macrolide resistance in *Campylobacter jejuni* and *Campylobacter coli*. *J. Antimicrob. Chemother.* **2006**, *58*, 243–255. [CrossRef] [PubMed]
38. Department of Water Affairs. *Revision of general authorizations in terms of Section 39 of the National Water Act, 1998 (At No. 36 of 1998)*; Published under Government Notice 665 in Government Gazette 36820 No. 665; Department of Water Affairs: Cape Town, South Africa, 2013.
39. Scharler, M.; Baird, D. A comparison of selected ecosystem attributes of three South African estuaries with different freshwater inflow regimes using network analysis. *J. Mar. Syst.* **2005**, *56*, 283–308. [CrossRef]
40. Baird, D.; Marais, J.; Martin, P. *The Swartkops Estuary: Proceedings of a Symposium at the University of Port Elizabeth*; Foundation for Research Development: Pretoria, South Africa, 2007; p. 8.
41. Heip, C.; Herman, P. Major biological processes in European tidal estuaries: A synthesis of the JEEP-92 Project. *Hydrobiologia* **1995**, *311*, 1–7. [CrossRef]
42. EPA. *Guidelines for Water Reuse*; EPA/625/R-04/108; Environmental Protection Agency, Municipal Support Division Office of Wastewater Management Office of Water: Washington, DC, USA; Agency for International Development: Washington, DC, USA, 2012.

43. Vacher, S.; Menard, A.; Bernard, E.; Mégraud, F. PCR-Restriction Fragment Polymorphism analysis for detection of point mutations associated with macrolide resistance in *Campylobacter* spp. *Antimicrob. Agents Chemother.* **2003**, *47*, 1125–1128. [CrossRef] [PubMed]

44. Persson, S.; Olsen, K.E. Multiplex PCR for identification of *Campylobacter coli* and *Campylobacter jejuni* from pure cultures and directly on stool samples. *J. Med. Microbiol.* **2005**, *54*, 1043–1047. [CrossRef] [PubMed]

45. Phongsisay, V. *Campylobacter jejuni* and the Guillain-Barré Syndrome. Ph.D. Thesis, RMIT University, Melbourne, Australia, 2006.

46. Cohn, M.; Ingmer, H.; Mulholland, F.; Jørgensen, K.; Wells, J.; Brøndsted, L. Contribution of conserved ATP-dependent proteases of *Campylobacter jejuni* to stress tolerance and virulence. *Appl. Environ. Microbiol.* **2007**, *73*, 7803–7813. [CrossRef] [PubMed]

47. Lin, J.; Overbye Michel, L.; Zhang, Q. CmeABC functions as a multidrug efflux system in *Campylobacter jejuni*. *Antimicrob. Agents Chemother.* **2002**, *46*, 2124–2131. [CrossRef] [PubMed]

48. CLSI. *Methods for Antimicrobial Dilution and Disk Susceptibility Testing of infrequently Isolated or Fastidious Bacteria*, Approved Guidelines-2nd ed.; CLSI: Wayne, PA, USA, 2012.

49. De Vries, S.P.; Gupta, S.; Baig, A.; L'Heureux, J.; Pont, E.; Wolanska, D.P.; Maskell, D.J.; Grant, A.J. Motility defects in *Campylobacter jejuni* defined gene deletion mutants caused by second-site mutations. *Microbiology* **2015**, *161*, 2316–2327. [CrossRef] [PubMed]

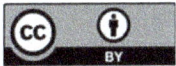

International Journal of
Environmental Research and Public Health

MDPI

Article

Occurrence of Antibiotic-Resistant Bacteria in Therapy Pools and Surrounding Surfaces

Daniela E. Koeck [1,*], Stefanie Huber [1], Nadera Hanifi [1], Manfred Köster [2], Martina B. Schierling [1] and Christiane Höller [1]

[1] Bavarian Health and Food Safety Authority, Veterinärstraße 2, 85764 Oberschleißheim, Germany; stefanie.huber@lgl.bayern.de (S.H.); Nadera.hanifi@lgl.bayern.de (N.H.); Martina.Schierling@lgl.bayern.de (M.B.S.); christiane.hoeller@lgl.bayern.de (C.H.)
[2] Bavarian Health and Food Safety Authority, 91058 Erlangen, Germany; Manfred.koester@lgl.bayern.de
[*] Correspondence: daniela.koeck@lgl.bayern.de; Tel.: +49-(0)9131-6808-5215

Received: 4 October 2018; Accepted: 21 November 2018; Published: 27 November 2018

Abstract: The number of patients colonized with antibiotic-resistant bacteria is increasing in health care facilities. Because transmission of antibiotic-resistant bacteria is feared, there exist reports that the affected patients are frequently excluded from hydrotherapy, which is a non-invasive and beneficial treatment used for patients with different diseases. Data from the literature suggest that deficient water disinfection measures exist, which are not always sufficient to kill all released bacteria. If the pool water is not disinfected properly, it may also infect the bathers. Immunocompromised patients are particularly susceptible to be infected with (antibiotic-resistant) bacteria. In order to determine the distribution of antibiotic-resistant bacteria in the pool water treatment system and the pool environment and to estimate the associated transmission risk we analyzed samples from eleven health care facilities. Antibiotic-resistant bacteria were found in the water and surface samples collected. One hundred and two antibiotic-resistant isolates from water samples and 307 isolates from surrounding surfaces were obtained, respectively. The majority of the isolates belonged to non-fermenting Gram-negative rods, like *Pseudomonas* spp. Some isolates were resistant to a wide range of the tested antibiotics. The results indicate a relation between the number of isolates in water samples and the number of patients using the pools in combination with deficiencies in water treatment. In the pool environment the highest number of isolates was obtained from barefoot areas and floor cleaning equipment.

Keywords: antibiotic resistance; hydrotherapy; pool; water; treatment; transfer

1. Introduction

Emerging and increasing antibiotic microbial resistance (AMR) represents one major threat to human health in Europe and worldwide. Resistance to antibiotics is widely distributed among Gram-positive and Gram-negative bacteria that may cause serious infections in humans, and AMR is increasing in the EU, especially among Gram-negative bacteria. The major drivers behind the occurrence and spread of AMR are the use of antimicrobial agents and the transmission of antibiotic-resistant microorganisms between humans; between animals; and between humans, animals, and the environment [1].

Bacteria that are resistant to three or more classes of antibiotics are called multidrug-resistant. Infections with these bacteria are associated with increased morbidity, mortality, length of hospitalization, and financial costs [2]. For a long time, methicillin-resistant *Staphylococcus aureus* (MRSA) have been the main point of concern in public health, but during the last couple of years extended-spectrum-ß-lactamase (ESBL)–producing bacteria have become a much more severe problem. While MRSA are predominantly acquired in connection with medical treatments, the picture concerning multidrug-resistant Gram-negative bacteria is much less clear and differs from species to species [3]. The production of ESBL is the most frequent resistance mechanism among Gram-negative bacteria. The corresponding gene sequences of the ESBLs are mostly on mobile DNA elements and can be transmitted horizontally, which contributes to the spread of these resistance genes [4]. Due to the resistance of the microorganisms to β-lactam antibiotics and other classes of antibiotics such as the fluoroquinolones (e.g., ciprofloxacin and levofloxacin), the therapeutic spectrum is strongly restricted in the case of infection with ESBL-producing bacteria [5]. Options for treatment of patients who are infected with multidrug-resistant bacteria are limited to only a few remaining last-line antibiotics, such as carbapenems (e.g., imipenem, ertapenem, meropenem). However, the increasing carbapenem-resistance limits options for the treatment of infected patients [6,7]. For the KRINKO (German Commission on Hospital Hygiene and Infection Prevention) definition of multidrug-resistant Gram-negative rods (MRGN), only resistance to antibiotics which are used as primary therapeutics for severe infections (acylaminopenicillins, third and fourth generation cephalosporins, carbapenems, and fluoroquinolones) has been included: 3MRGN (with resistance to three of the four antibiotic groups) and 4MRGN (with resistance to four of the four antibiotic groups). Aminoglycosides, like amikacin, gentamicin, and tobramycin, were not included in the KRINKO classification of multidrug-resistant Gram-negative rods, as they are generally not used as monotherapeutics [8].

Hydrotherapy is a non-invasive and beneficial treatment for many patients, like patients with chronic diseases, disabilities, or trauma. Very often those patients have a long history of medical treatments, including antibiotic treatments. Thus, the probability that they have a disturbed microflora with an increased rate of carriage of AMR and also a reduced colonization resistance against AMR is relatively high [9]. Although pool water is usually disinfected, infections are known to occur either due to deficiencies in water treatment or due to colonization of swimming pool equipment [10–13]. Therapies performed in a swimming pool cause a large release of bacteria. Bathers transfer approximately 10^5–10^6 CFU per person in 15 min to the surrounding water body [14]. Bacteria should be inactivated by disinfectants in the pool water; however, this is not always the case, because they can be attached to particles or be protected by an EPS (extrapolymeric substance) and thus not be exposed to the disinfectant. Bacteria can form biofilms on pool surfaces, especially in areas of the pool where the concentration of disinfectant is low [15–17]. Additionally, they can be attached to swimming aids, which are made from plastics, often foams, which provide a large surface. They can also be found on tools for cleaning, where they are exposed occasionally but not permanently to disinfectants. *Pseudomonas aeruginosa*, a species very often involved in biofilm formation, has been commonly isolated from the pool environment [18,19].

Immunocompromised patients are particularly susceptible to infections with pathogens (including antibiotic-resistant bacteria) via the mucous membranes and via penetration of bathing water into auditory canals and the nasopharynx. Although some literature exists on antibiotic-resistant bacteria in swimming pools [16,17,20], little is known about the prevalence of AMR. To this day, to our knowledge, no information exists about the public health impact of therapy pools in the dissemination of antibiotic-resistant bacteria. In order to assess the extent of contamination with antibiotic-resistant bacteria, their distribution, and the associated transmission risk in clinical therapy pools, we performed a study on this topic. The main objective of the project was to investigate the occurrence of antibiotic-resistant bacteria in water of therapy pools, in filters, balance tanks, and on surrounding surfaces. Factors contributing to their occurrence will be discussed with regard to details in pool water treatment and disinfection, number of patients entering the pools, and usage of the pools for other purposes. Finally, we derive recommendations for the management of patients colonized with antibiotic-resistant bacteria in hydrotherapy pools.

2. Materials and Methods

2.1. Sampling

Eleven pre-selected therapy pools located in different hospitals in Bavaria were sampled in accordance with the requirements of DIN EN ISO 19458 [21]. Bottles with capacities of 250 and 1000 mL, prepared with sufficient (100 mg/L) sodium thiosulfate ($Na_2S_2O_3$, sodium thiosulfate pentahydrate, Merck, Darmstadt, Germany) for dechlorination, were used. Pool water and balance tank water samples were collected from a depth of 30 cm, at a point about 40 cm away from the basin edge, filtrate was taken from a sampling tap, and filter backwash water was taken directly before the drain. The samples were transferred to the laboratory within 1–2 h from collection, using appropriate insulated coolers, and they were processed immediately after arrival at the laboratory. In addition to the water samples, samples from the surrounding surfaces (especially sanitary areas and pool equipment) were taken with sterile, wet swabs, moistened with 0.9% NaCl (w/v). All sampling sites are summarized in Table 1. The swabs were transported to the laboratory immediately after the collection. In order to isolate microorganisms, the tips of the swabs were cut off and placed in tubes containing 10 mL of sterile CASO-broth (BD BBL™ Trypticase™ Soy Broth, Becton Dickinson GmbH, Heidelberg, Germany). The tubes were vortexed (for 2 min) to remove microbial cells from the swab material and incubated for 24 h +/− 2 h at 37 °C. Four samples of each sampling point (water and surfaces) were collected over the course of one year (one sampling per quarter).

Table 1. Sampling sites of water samples (left column) and surrounding surfaces (right column).

Water Samples	No.	Volume	Sampling Points in the Pool Surroundings	No.
pool water	1	1000 mL	swimming aid	1
filtrate	2	100 mL	seats	2
balance tank water	3	100 mL	spillway	3
filter backwash water	4	100 mL	hand rail	4
			toilet	5
			shower rooms	6
			barefoot areas	7
			cleaning trolley	8
			cleaning equipment	9

2.2. Determination of Water Quality Parameters According to DIN 19643-1

Typical water quality parameters (chemical and microbial) were determined from all water samples according to DIN 19643-1 [21]. The parameter limits and all references for the methods used are listed in Table 2.

For the measurement of chlorates and chlorites by LC-MS, a hypercarb column (100 × 2.1 mm, 5 μm, Thermo Scientific, Waltham, MA, USA) was used. The eluents used were deionate/methanol 95/5 with 1% (w/v) formic acid (A) and methanol with 1% (w/v) formic acid (B). The flow rate was 0.3 mL/min with an injection rate of 10 μL. For subsequent mass spectrometry with the API 5500 device (SCIEX, Darmstadt, Germany), the software package Analyst 1.6.2 (SCIEX, Darmstadt, Germany) was used. For the measurement, a three-point calibration with bracketing was performed. The concentrations of the standards were 10, 50, and 100 μg/L. The samples were diluted according to the calibration line. The internal standard used was $^{18}O_3$-chlorate.

Table 2. Parameter limits are according to DIN 19643-1 [21]. Limits are only valid for pool water and filtrate (not for balance tank water and filter backwash water).

Microbial Parameter	Method	Parameter Limits	Chemical Parameter	Method	Parameter Limits
Total heterotrophic counts at 36 °C	TrinkwV, appendix 5	<100 CFU/mL	THM (mg/L)	DIN EN ISO 10301:1997	<0.02
Escherichia coli	DIN EN ISO 9308-2	<1 CFU/100 mL	Bromate (mg/L)	DIN EN ISO 15061	<2.0
Pseudomonas aeruginosa	DIN EN ISO 16266	<1 CFU/100 mL	Chlorate and chlorite (mg/L)	LC-MS	<30
			Al (mg/L)	DIN EN ISO 11885	<0.05
			Fe (mg/L)	DIN EN ISO 11885	<0.02
			pH	DIN EN ISO 10523	6.5–7.5
			$K_{S4.3}$ (mmol/L)	DIN 38409-1	>0.7
1			Nitrate (mg/L)	EN ISO 10304:1995	<20
			Ox. (mg/L)	DIN EN ISO 8467	<0.75
			Redox (mV)	DIN 38404-6	>750
			Free chlorine (mg/L)	DIN EN ISO 7393-1	0.3–0.6
			Bound chlorine (mg/L)	DIN EN ISO 7393-1	<0.2

THM: Trihalogenmethane; LC-MS: Liquid chromatography–mass spectrometry.

To determine the acid capacity (K$_{S4.3}$), the samples were titrated with 0.1 mol/L hydrochloric acid until a pH of 4.3 was reached (DIN 38409-1). The necessary amount of acid was documented and the acid capacity was calculated as follows:

$$Ks = \frac{a \times 1000 \times 0.1 \times f}{W} \tag{1}$$

where Ks refers to acid capacity, *a* refers to the titrated volume in mL of 0.1 mol/L HCl, *W* refers to the sample volume (100 mL), and *f* refers to the titer of 0.1 m HCl (=1.000).

The oxidation–reduction potential was recorded on site using the continuously operating measuring systems the pools applied to control the necessary addition of chemicals. The measurement was performed with platinum or gold electrodes against a silver/silver chloride reference electrode and the measured voltage was converted to the standard hydrogen electrode.

2.3. Determination of the Total Number of CFU (Colony Forming Units) from the Pool Surroundings

Contact plates (ICRplus (Isolators and Clean Rooms) TSA (Tryptic Soy Agar) contact plates with LTHThio neutralizers, Millipore, Darmstadt, Germany) were used to determine the total number of CFU from the surrounding surfaces. All sampling sites are summarized in Table 1. The agar plates were incubated for 24 h +/− 2 h at 37 °C. It is important to ensure that sampling is carried out at representative and similar sites to ensure comparability between the therapy pools. Based on the DGfdB (German Society for Bathing) guideline 94.04 [22], it can be determined whether or not the surface cleaning and disinfection was performed adequately.

2.4. Isolation of Antibiotic-Resistant Bacteria

The abovementioned water samples (1000 mL or 100 mL, respectively; Table 1) were filtrated through sterile 0.45 μm membrane filters (Millipore, Darmstadt, Germany). Filters were subsequently placed on MacConkey agar (Oxoid, Wesel, Germany) supplemented with cefotaxime (1 mg/L), Brilliance carbapenem-resistant *Enterobacteriaceae* (CRE) Agar (Oxoid), ChromID™ VRE Agar (bioMérieux, Nurtingen, Germany), and ChromID$_{TM}$ MRSA SMART Agar (bioMérieux, Nurtingen, Germany), and incubated for 24 h +/− 2 h at 37 °C under aerobic conditions. Next, 200 μL from the liquid enrichments of the culture swabs were plated on the same selective media and incubated for 24 h +/− 2 h at 37 °C. One colony of each phenotype was picked from the selective plates, subcultured on 10% defibrinated sheep blood agar (Oxoid), and incubated at 37 °C for 24 h. Identification to the species or genus level was performed using BD Phoenix™ 100 (Becton Dickinson Diagnostic systems, Heidelberg, Germany) and MALDI-TOF-MS Microflex LT (Bruker, Bremen, Germany). The MALDI Biotyper Real Time Classification System (Bruker) and the BD EpiCenter™ Software (Becton Dickinson, Heidelberg, Germany) were used for the identification and taxonomical classification of bacteria.

2.5. Antimicrobial Susceptibility Testing

Antimicrobial susceptibility testing was performed by Phoenix™ Panels NMIC 448794 (Becton Dickinson Diagnostic systems, Heidelberg, Germany) for Gram-negative bacteria, with 21 antimicrobial substances (ampicillin, piperacillin, piperacillin-tazobactam, cefuroxime, cefotaxime, ceftazidime, cefepime, imipenem, meropenem, aztreonam, gentamicin, tobramycin, amikacin, ciprofloxacin, levofloxacin, trimethoprim-sulfamethoxazole, amoxicillin-clavulanic acid, ertapenem, fosfomycin+G6P, tigecycline) and Panel NMIC 448796 for Gram-positive bacteria, with 23 antimicrobial substances (penicillin G, ampicillin, oxacillin, cefoxitin, imipenem, clindamycin, erythromycin, vancomycin, teicoplanin, linezolid, fusidic acid, rifampicin, nitrofurantoin, gentamicin, tobramycin, ciprofloxacin, moxifloxacin, tetracycline, trimethoprim-sulfamethoxazole, daptomycin, fosfomycin, gentamicin-syn, tigecycline) according to the manufacturer's guidelines (Becton Dickinson Diagnostic Systems, Heidelberg, Germany). Results of all antimicrobials tested were interpreted according to the European

Committee on Antimicrobial Susceptibility Testing (EUCAST) breakpoints (http://www.eucast.org/clinical_breakpoints). The calculation of MIC50 (representing the minimal inhibitory concentration (MIC) of 50% of the isolates) and MIC90 (representing the MIC of 90% of the isolates) were calculated using the obtained values from Phoenix™.

2.6. Questionnaire

A standardized questionnaire was developed and given to the facilities operating the therapy pools to document the technical details of the pool, their water treatment, cleaning procedures, and frequency and duration of pool usage (Supplementary Materials S1).

2.7. Statistical Analysis

Pearson's χ^2 test was used to test whether observed differences in contamination of water samples and surface samples between the sampling locations were statistically significant. An interactive calculation tool for chi-square tests (available from http://quantpsy.org) was employed for all statistical analyses and the significance level was set at 95% ($p \leq 0.05$) for all analyses.

3. Results

3.1. Water Quality Parameters According to DIN 19643-1

The number of bathers/patients using the pool clearly differed between the sampled facilities (ranging from <50 patients per year to 35,000 patients per year). None of the pools exceeded the maximal bathing load per hour (according to DIN 19643-1 [21]). The chemistry of the pool water samples is shown in Table 3. Location six and eight were only sampled twice and location ten only three times, because the bathing facilities were closed down during the study. The results of the filtrate, balance tank water, and filter backwash water samples are not shown, since there are no standard requirements specified in DIN 19643-1 [21]. The filtrate should only be investigated in case of problems with the pool water. Most of the chemical parameters of the pool water met the requirements. Only the acid capacity was often (59%) too low, which is an indicator for a low puffer capacity and may hinder a proper flocculation. The aluminum concentration was above the limit value in 64% of the sampled basins, which is an indication of a flocculation failure due to too much flocculant or an inadequate flocculation (e.g., due to insufficient mixing). Furthermore, a relationship was observed between the high number of visitors (indicated in grey) in pool number two and eight and a distinctly higher concentration of bound and free chlorine.

The microbiological quality of the investigated pools was considered acceptable/unacceptable according to the German standards DIN 19643 [21]. The limits are valid for pool water and filtrate (not for balance tank water and filter backwash water). All pool water samples examined met the microbiological standards specified in Table 2. We detected three exceedances in the filtrate: >12,600/mL CFU total heterotrophic counts (36 °C) and >200 CFU/100 mL *P. aeruginosa* in one sample and again 108/mL CFU total heterotrophic counts (36 °C) in another sample. Both samples came from facility number ten. *E. coli* was not detected in any of the samples analyzed.

Table 3. Chemistry in pool water samples (according to DIN 19643-1) and number of visitors per year (date from the questionnaire).

Hospital Number	1	2	3	4	5	6	7	8	9	10	11
Visitors/per year	2500	7200	4500	4500	10,800	1680	1450	35,000	3000	<50	300
THM (mg/L)	0.0	0.007	0.006	0.000	0.005	0.000	0.001	0.008	0.000	0.002	0.000
Bromate (mg/L)	0.055	<LOD	<LOQ	0.009	0.011	0.054	0.003	0.005	0.005	0.004	0.005
Chlorate and chlorite (mg/L)	18.0	2.0	0.8	3.2	2.1	33.5 [a]	9.0	4.7	5.4	16.1	9.2
Al (mg/L)	0.06 [a]	0.07 [a]	<LOQ	0.07 [a]	<LOQ	0.07 [a]	<LOQ	0.08 [a]	<LOQ	0.1 [a]	0.08 [a]
Fe (mg/L)	<LOQ	<LOQ	<LOQ	<LOQ	<LOQ	<LOQ	<LOQ	<LOQ	<LOQ	0.0	<LOQ
pH	6.7	7.0	7.0	7.2	7.3	6.7	7.1	7.2	6.7	7.2	7.5
$K_{S4.3}$ (mmol/L)	0.3 [b]	0.9	0.6 [b]	0.9	0.71	0.2 [b]	0.4 [b]	1.0	0.2 [b]	0.5 [b]	1.3
Nitrate (mg/L)	10.8	7.5	28.8 [a]	26.8 [a]	14.3	30.0 [a]	<NG	3.5	13.3	30.7 [a]	14.3
Ox (mg/L)	0.7	0.5	0.7	0.5	1.4	<LOD	0.4	0.9 [a]	0.3	0.3	1.0 [a]
Redox (mV)	780.80	821.50	806.00	738.30 [b]	819.30	767.00	675.00 [b]	716.30 [b]	823.00	803.30	919.00
Free chlorine (mg/L)	0.51	0.72 [a]	0.40	0.27 [b]	0.50	0.33	0.54	0.77 [a]	0.46	0.49	0.59
Bound chlorine (mg/L)	0.11	0.15	0.06	0.06	0.06	0.01	0.03	0.25 [a]	0.04	0.02	0.02

<LOD = below limit of detection; <LOQ = below limit of quantification; [a] above requirements acc. DIN 19643-1; [b] below requirements acc. DIN 19643-1 [21].

3.2. Determination of Total Heterotrophic Counts from the Pool Surroundings

An analysis of the samples revealed that 78% of the total plate count samples (370) showed bacterial growth, i.e., were counted as positive (Table 4). One hundred and seventeen samples (32%) exceeded the action value (800 CFU/100 cm^2) from the DGfdB guideline 94.04 [22]. However, as our samples were taken when bathers were present, these results should be interpreted with caution, because the guideline values refer to areas after cleaning and/or disinfection in order to determine if the surface cleaning and disinfection has been performed adequately.

Table 4. Number of positive samples from contact agar plates and percentage of positive samples ($n = 370$).

Hospital Number	1	2	3	4	5	6	7	8	9	10	11	% Positive Samples
swimming aid	4	2	2	4	4	1	2	1	3	3	3	66
seats	4	4	0	4	4	2	4	2	4	3	3	77
spillway	1	3	4	1	4	1	1	1	1	2	1	45
hand rail	4	4	2	4	4	2	4	2	4	2	3	80
toilet	3	3	1	4	3	2	3	2	4	3	3	70
shower rooms	2	2	1	4	4	2	4	2	3	3	3	68
barefoot areas	4	3	3	4	3	2	4	1	4	3	3	77
cleaning trolley	3	3	4	3	2	1	3	1	3	2	ND	57
cleaning equipment	1	4	3	4	3	2	4	2	4	4	ND	70
% positive samples	72	78	56	89	86	83	81	78	83	69	70	

ND = not determined.

3.3. Bacterial Isolates

A total of 307 isolates from 23% positive samples (growth on selective media) were obtained from all surface samples ($n = 371$). A significant difference between the surface samples across the sampled pools was observed ($X^2 = 200.138$, p-value = 0). Most isolates were obtained from hospital number eight, which was only sampled twice (Figure 1). Hospital number two and five, which have the second and third highest number of pool visitors per year, also yielded a high number of isolates. A relationship was observed between the high number of visitors (Table 3) and the number of isolates. The highest number of isolates was obtained from barefoot areas (78) and floor cleaning equipment (49).

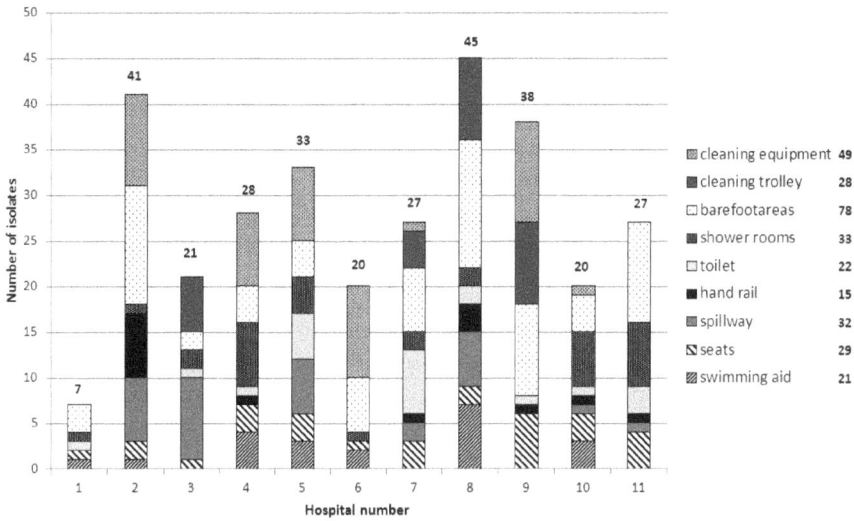

Figure 1. Number of antibiotic-resistant isolates (growth on selective media) from the surrounding surface samples (*n* = 371).

A total of 102 isolates from 32% positive samples (growth on selective media) were obtained from all water samples (*n* = 155) (Figure 2). A significant difference between the water samples across the sampled pools was observed (X^2 = 52.778, *p*-value = 0.002). The two therapy pools with the highest number of isolates (number five and number eight) also had the highest number of visitors, even if pool number eight was only sampled twice. Most of the positive water samples were from the balance water and filtrate; the pool water itself was contaminated less frequently. Isolates could be obtained directly from the pool water in only pool number two, six, eight, nine, and ten.

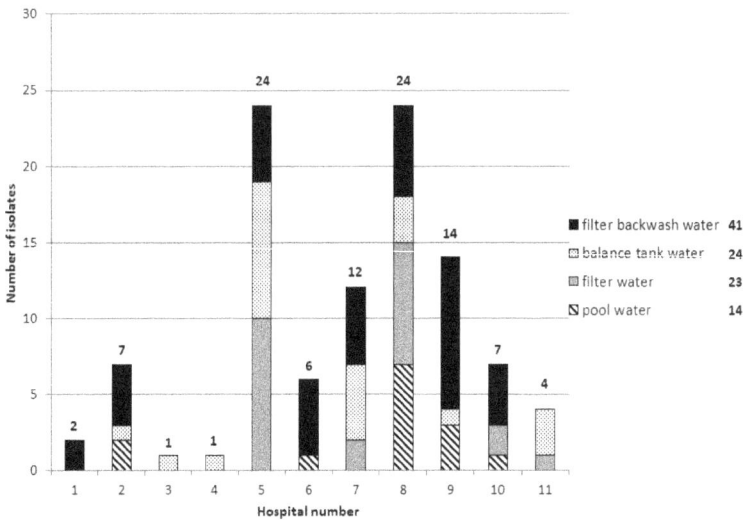

Figure 2. Number of antibiotic-resistant isolates (growth on selective media) from the water samples (*n* = 155).

Not all isolates could be classified up to species level (Figure 3). For genetically closely related species the applied identification methods (BD Phoenix™ and MALDI-TOF-MS) only allowed assignment to the genus level. The majority of the isolates belonged to the taxonomically heterogeneous group of non-fermenting Gram-negative bacteria. Typical genera like Burkholderia spp., *Moraxella* spp., *Pseudomonas* spp., *Stenotrophomonas* spp., and *Sphingomonas* spp. were found. Some of them are typical water borne bacteria, like *Pseudomonas* spp. *E. coli* was not isolated and other coliform bacteria were very rare. *Acinetobacter* spp. were also not isolated. The abundant Gram-positive genera are mostly inhabitants of the natural skin flora (like *Staphylococcus epidermidis*) or environmental bacteria (like *Bacillus subtilis*). There was only one *S. aureus* isolate from a handrail, which was oxacillin sensitive. Some genera appeared in high abundances only in water samples (like *Sphingomonas* and *Sphingobacterium*) and some were mainly found in environmental samples (like *Stenotrophomonas*, *Bacillus*, *Achromobacter*, *Ochrobactrum*). *Pseudomonas* spp. is one of the most abundant genera in both kinds of samples. Isolates from the pool water (*n* = 14) were mostly *Pseudomonas* spp. (*n* = 3), *Sphingobacterium* spp. (*n* = 4), and *Staphylococcus* spp. (*n* = 4).

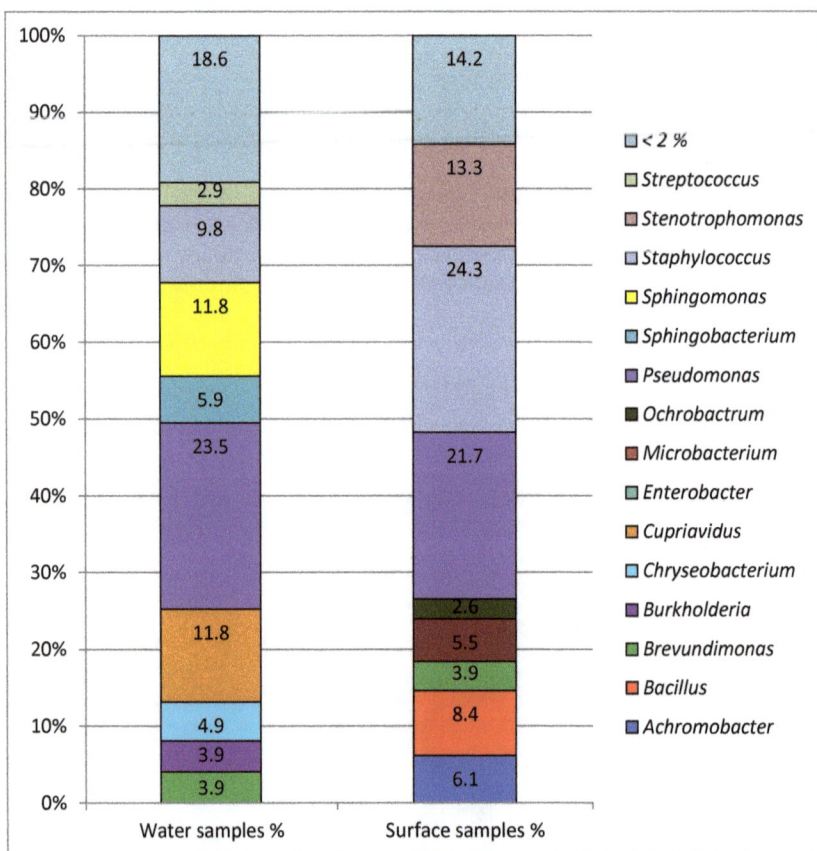

Figure 3. Taxonomic profile up to genus level for all antibiotic-resistant isolates. Left column: percentage of water isolates (*n* = 102); right column: percentage of isolates from surfaces (*n* = 307). Other genera present in <2%. Identification to the species or genus level was performed using BD Phoenix™ and MALDI-TOF-MS.

3.4. Antimicrobial Susceptibility

The isolated Gram-positive genera have no or very rare clinical relevance, therefore the antibiotic resistance patterns (antibiograms) of Gram-positive isolates were not further analyzed. There were abundant Gram-negative genera, like *Pseudomonas*, *Stenotrophomonas*, and *Sphingomonas*, which can cause infections especially in immunocompromised patients; their antibiograms are shown in Table 5. *Sphingobacterium* and *Achromobacter* are the two other abundant Gram-negative genera. These are rarely involved in human infections; their resistance patterns are shown in Table 6. For these five bacteria genera, the MIC50 (minimal inhibitory concentration (MIC) for 50% of the isolates) and the MIC90 (MIC for 90% of the isolates) were calculated using the obtained values from the Phoenix^{TM} experiments (Tables 7 and 8).

The antibiograms of other *Pseudomonas* species (e.g., *P. putida*) isolates ($n = 136$), are not shown, as they are seldom associated with infections in humans. The total abundance of all *Pseudomonas aeruginosa* isolates was 5%. Among these isolates five were resistant to ciprofloxacin (MIC50: 0.25 μg/mL; MIC90: 2 μg/mL) and levofloxacin (MIC50: 1 μg/mL; MIC90: 4 μg/mL). Three *P. aeruginosa* isolates were simultaneously resistant to imipenem (MIC50: 2 μg/mL; MIC90: 8 μg/mL), ertapenem (MIC50: 2 μg/mL; MIC90: 2 μg/mL) and all tested fluoroquinolones. But all *P. aeruginosa* isolates were susceptible against piperacillin, ceftazidime and cefepime. The 39 *Stenotrophomonas maltophilia* isolates were resistant to almost all tested antibiotic substances. All isolates were susceptible against trimethoprim-sulfamethoxazole. The susceptibility against polymyxins was not investigated. Among the 14 *Sphingomonas paucimobilis* isolates there existed a high diversity between the resistance patterns. One isolate was susceptible to at least one antibiotic substance of all classes of antibiotics. The majority of the isolates was resistant to all tested carbapenems and sensitive to other classes. But there was also one isolate, which was resistant to 4 of 4 antibiotic groups from the KRINKO classification for MRGN.

The isolates from the genus *Achromobacter* could not be resolved up to species level, as the databases lack appropriate reference spectra. All *Sphingobacterium* spp. isolates belong either to the species *S. spiritivorum* or *S. multivorum*. Some isolates were resistant to a wide range of the tested antibiotics.

Table 5. Antibiotic resistance patterns of all *Pseudomonas aeruginosa*, *Stenotrophomonas maltophilia*, and *Sphingomonas paucimobilis* isolates from water and surface samples.

Class of Antibiotics	Antibiotic																	
Penicillins	ampicillin	r	r	r	r	r	r	s	r	r	r	s	r	r	s	s	s	s
	piperacillin	s	s	s	s	s	s	s	s	s	r	s	s	r	s	s	r	s
	piperacillin-tazobactam	s	s	s	s	s	s	s	s	s	r	s	s	r	s	r	r	s
Penicillins/ Beta-lactamase inhibitor	amoxicillin-clavulanic acid	r	r	r	r	r	r	r	r	r	r	r	r	r	s	r	r	r
Cephalosporins (2nd)	cefuroxime	r	r	r	r	r	r	r	r	r	r	r	r	r	s	r	r	r
Cephalosporins (3rd)	cefotaxime	r	r	r	r	r	r	r	r	r	r	r	r	r	s	r	r	r
Cephalosporins (3rd)	ceftazidime	s	s	s	s	s	s	s	s	r	r	s	s	r	s	s	s	s
Cephalosporins (4th)	cefepime	s	s	s	s	s	s	r	r	r	r	s	s	r	s	r	s	s
Carbapenems	imipenem	s	s	s	s	s	s	r	r	r	r	r	r	r	s	s	s	s
	ertapenem	r	r	r	r	r	r	r	r	r	r	r	r	r	r	r	r	r
Aminoglycosides	gentamicin	s	s	s	s	s	s	r	r	r	r	s	s	r	s	s	s	s
	tobramycin	s	s	s	s	s	s	r	r	r	r	s	s	r	s	s	s	r
	amikacin	s	s	s	s	s	s	r	r	r	r	s	s	r	s	r	s	s
Fluoroquinolones	ciprofloxacin	s	s	s	r	r	r	s	s	s	r	s	s	s	r	r	s	s
	levofloxacin	s	r	s	r	r	r	s	s	s	r	s	s	s	r	r	s	s
Sulfonamide antibiotic	trimethoprim-sulfam.	r	r	r	r	r	r	s	s	s	r	r	r	r	s	s	s	s
Fosfomycin	fosfomycin	ND	ND	ND	ND	ND	ND	s	s	r	r	r	s	s	s	r	r	r
Glycylcycline	tigecycline	r	r	r	r	r	r	r	r	r	r	ND	ND	ND	ND	ND	ND	ND
Number of Isolates		16	3	2	2	2	13	24	6	2	1	1	1	1	1	1	1	1
Species		*Pseudomonas aeruginosa* (26)					*Stenotrophomonas maltophilia* (39)			*Sphingomonas paucimobilis* (14)							

Susceptibility (s) and resistance (r) were automatically determined with the BD Phoenix™ System; ND = Not determined.

Table 6. Antibiotic resistance patterns of all *Achromobacter* spp. and *Sphingobacterium* spp. isolates from water and surface samples.

Class of Antibiotics	Antibiotic												
Penicillins	ampicillin	r	r	ND	r	r	r	r	r	r	r	r	s
	piperacillin	s	s	s	s	s	s	s	s	s	s	r	s
	piperacillin-tazobactam	s	s	s	s	s	r	s	s	s	s	s	s
Penicillins/Beta-lactamase inhibitor	amoxicillin-clavulanic acid	r	r	r	r	r	r	r	r	r	r	r	r
Cephalosporins (2nd)	cefuroxime	r	r	r	r	r	r	r	r	r	r	r	r
Cephalosporins (3rd)	cefotaxime	r	r	r	r	r	r	r	r	r	r	r	r
Cephalosporins (3rd)	ceftazidime	s	s	s	s	s	r	s	s	s	r	r	s
Cephalosporins (4th)	cefepime	s	s	s	s	s	r	r	s	s	s	s	s
Carbapenems	imipenem	ND	ND	ND	ND	s	r	ND	r	s	r	r	s
	ertapenem	ND	ND	ND	ND	s	r	ND	r	r	r	r	r
Aminoglycosides	gentamicin	s	s	r	r	r	r	s	s	s	r	r	s
	tobramycin	s	s	r	r	r	r	r	s	s	r	r	r
	amikacin	s	s	s	r	r	r	s	s	s	r	r	s
Fluoroquinolones	ciprofloxacin	s	r	r	r	r	r	s	s	s	s	s	s
	levofloxacin	s	r	s	r	s	r	s	s	s	s	s	s
Sulfonamide antibiotic	trimethoprim-sulfam.	s	s	s	s	s	s	s	s	s	s	s	s
Fosfomycin	fosfomycin	r	r	r	r	r	r	r	r	r	r	r	r
Glycylcycline	tigecycline	ND	ND	ND	r	ND	ND	ND	r	ND	r	ND	ND
Number of Isolates		1	2	1	10	3	1	1	4	1	3	2	1
Species		*Achromobacter* spp. (19)							*Sphingobacterium* spp. (11)				

Susceptibility (s) and resistance (r) was automatically determined with the BD Phoenix™ System; ND = Not determined.

Table 7. MIC50 and MIC90 values of *Pseudomonas aeruginosa*, *Stenotrophomonas maltophilia*, and *Sphingomonas paucimobilis* isolates from water and surface areas.

Class of Antibiotics	Antibiotic	Pseudomonas aeruginosa		Stenotrophomonas maltophilia		Sphingomonas paucimobilis	
		MIC50	MIC90	MIC50	MIC90	MIC50	MIC90
Penicillins	ampicillin	16	16	16	16	8	16
	piperacillin	4	8	32	32	4	32
	piperacillin-tazobactam	4/4	8/4	32/4	32/4	4/4	29.2/4
Penicillins/beta-lactamase inhibitor	amoxicillin-clavulanic acid	64/2	64/2	64/2	64/2	32/2	60.8/2
Cephalosporins (2nd)	cefuroxime	16	16	16	16	16	16
Cephalosporins (3rd)	cefotaxime	8	8	8	8	8	8
Cephalosporins (3rd)	ceftazidime	2	4	8	16	4	8
Cephalosporins (4th)	cefepime	4	4	16	16	1	2
Carbapenems	imipenem	2	8	16	16	16	16
	ertapenem	2	2	2	2	2	2
Aminoglycosides	gentamicin	1	2	8	8	8	8
	tobramycin	1	1	8	8	8	8
	amikacin	4	4	32	32	32	32
Fluoroquinolones	ciprofloxacin	0.25	2	2	2	0.5	0.9
	levofloxacin	1	4	1	4	0.5	0.5
Sulfonamide antibiotic	trimethroprim-sulfam.	4/76	8/76	1/19	1/19	4/76	7.6/76
Fosfomycin	fosfomycin	ND	ND	>64	>64	32	64
Glycylcycline	tigecycline	4	4	1	2	ND	ND

The MIC values used for calculation of the MIC50 and MIC90 were determined with the BD Phoenix™ System; ND = not determined.

Table 8. MIC50 and MIC90 values of *Achromobacter* spp. and *Sphingobacterium* spp. isolates from water and surface areas.

Class of Antibiotics	Antibiotic	*Achromobacter* spp.		*Sphingobacterium* spp.	
		MIC50	MIC90	MIC50	MIC90
Penicillins	ampicillin	16	16	16	16
	piperacillin	4	5.2	16	32
	piperacillin–tazobactam	4/4	4/4	8/4	32/4
Penicillins/Beta-lactamase inhibitor	amoxicillin–clavulanic acid	16/2	64/2	4/2	4.4/2
Cephalosporins (2nd)	cefuroxime	16	16	16	16
Cephalosporins (3rd)	cefotaxime	8	8	8	8
Cephalosporins (3rd)	ceftazidime	8	16	4	16
Cephalosporins (4th)	cefepime	16	16	1	16
Carbapenems	imipenem	ND	ND	4	8
	ertapenem	ND	ND	2	2
Aminoglycosides	gentamicin	8	8	8	8
	tobramycin	8	8	8	8
	amikacin	32	32	32	32
Fluoroquinolones	ciprofloxacin	2	2	0.25	0.5
	levofloxacin	2	4	0.5	0.5
Sulfonamide antibiotic	trimethoprim-sulfam.	1/19	1/19	1/19	1/19
Fosfomycin	fosfomycin	>64	>64	>64	>64
Glycylcycline	tigecycline	2	2	1*	1*

The MIC values used for calculation of the MIC50 and MIC90 were determined with the BD Phoenix™ System; ND = not determined. * calculated from three values.

4. Discussion

The therapy pool with the highest number of isolates obtained directly from the pool water and from the sampled surfaces had not only the highest number of visitors but also seemed to have problems with the water treatment (high bound chlorine levels). The cleaning intervals of the pool areas were the same between the different health care facilities (once per day, according to the evaluation of the questionnaire); hence there is no detectable correlation between the number of isolates and the cleaning interval. These results indicate a correlation of the incidence of antibiotic-resistant bacterial isolates with the number of patients in combination with deficiencies in water treatment. The isolation of potential human pathogens, particularly *P. aeruginosa*, *S. maltophilia*, and *S. paucimobilis* strains, indicates that these inhabitants of the nosocomial environment may have been released by bathers, with contact to surfaces in the surrounding of the pool and the hospital environment, after entering the pool. *P. aeruginosa* can potentially cause disease in healthy humans, but more often it colonizes immunocompromised patients, like those with cystic fibrosis or cancer [23]. *P. aeruginosa* is intrinsically resistant to the majority of antimicrobial agents due to the low permeability of its outer membrane and the constitutive expression of various efflux pumps. Any additional acquired resistance severely limits the therapeutic options for treating serious infections. The antimicrobial groups that remain active against the susceptible *P. aeruginosa* phenotype include some fluoroquinolones (e.g., ciprofloxacin and levofloxacin), aminoglycosides (e.g., gentamicin, tobramycin, and amikacin), some beta-lactams (piperacillin- tazobactam, ceftazidime, cefepime, imipenem, doripenem, and meropenem), and polymyxins (polymyxin B and colistin). Resistance of *P. aeruginosa* to these agents can be acquired through one or more of several mechanisms, like the acquisition of plasmid-mediated resistance genes coding for various β-lactamases and aminoglycoside-modifying enzymes [24,25]. Some strains that have been isolated exhibited resistance to essentially antipseudomonal antibiotics, like fluoroquinolones and carbapenems.

Another problematic nosocomial pathogen is *S. maltophilia*, which is also naturally resistant to many broad-spectrum antibiotics (including all carbapenems). *S. maltophilia* is the third most common nosocomial pathogen with multi-drug-resistance [26]. *S. maltophilia* is often associated with pulmonary infections, urinary tract infections, bloodstream infections, and colonization of individuals with cystic fibrosis, especially in immunocompromised patients. The treatment of infected patients is very difficult [27,28]. It can be considered positive that all *S. maltophilia* isolates were susceptible against trimethoprim-sulfamethoxazole, as trimethoprim-sulfamethoxazole is still the treatment of choice for suspected or culture-proven *S. maltophilia* infections [29]. If a patient is infected with one of these strains, polymyxins may also be effective treatment options, though not without frequent adverse effects.

Sphingomonas paucimobilis has been implicated in various types of clinical infection. Although infections by *S. paucimobilis* are rarely serious and could be effectively treated with antibiotics, *S. paucimobilis* is capable of causing active infections in humans [30,31]. However, 93% of the isolates in this study were resistant to aminoglycosides, and one isolate was resistant to ceftazidime. Another study describes carbapenems, against which all isolates were resistant, as the most effective therapy for infections with *S. paucimobilis* [32]. *Achromobacter* spp. have been identified as opportunistic human pathogens in people with certain immunosuppressive conditions, such as cystic fibrosis, cancer, and kidney failure [33]. Notably, 80% of the isolates originated from barefoot areas or the floor cleaning equipment, which indicates a transmission due to insufficient management of floor cleaning equipment.

Like *Achromobacter* spp., *Sphingobacterium spiritivorum/multivorum* is rarely involved in human infection. Sphingobacterium species are intrinsically resistant to many commonly used antibiotics and can grow in antiseptics and disinfectants [34]. S. multivorum can produce an extended-spectrum β-lactamase and a metallo-β-lactamase, conferring resistance to third-generation cephalosporins and carbapenems, respectively [35]. Two isolates were both resistant to carbapenems and third-generation cephalosporins.

In addition to these quite important human pathogens, some uncommon antibiotic-resistant Gram-negative bacterial species, like *Chryseobacterium indologenes* and *Ochrobactrum anthropi*, were isolated. The isolation of *Chryseobacterium indologenes* and *Ochrobactrum anthropi* from swimming pool water was described previously by Papadopoulou et al. [17]. In this study, *Ochrobactrum anthropi* could only be isolated from the surface samples in the pool surroundings and not from the water samples. For both species, rare clinical significance and resistance to a wide variety of antimicrobial agents has been reported [36,37].

However, whether such resistant strains can contaminate bathers and cause infection strongly depends on the immune status of the patient. The study has revealed deficiencies in the operation of the pools, although the extent to which immunocompetent patients may be at risk from multidrug resistant bacteria in the pool water could not be determined. The question of whether patients who are proven carriers of multidrug resistant bacteria may use therapy pools has to be clarified in individual cases, taking the respective bacterial species into account. In the case of unsafe operation or outdated technology and patients colonized with 4MRGN, a ban on use should be considered.

5. Conclusions

Despite the reduction of antibiotic-resistant bacteria due to water treatment and disinfection, some antibiotic-resistant bacteria are still present in the water of therapy pools and on surrounding surfaces. There they can potentially persist and infect other patients and staff alike. Adequate pool water treatment and management of cleaning and cleaning equipment can prevent the transmission of these bacteria. The capacity of the water treatment defines the maximum bathers load. This maximum number of visitors should not be exceeded to ensure good water quality.

Supplementary Materials: The following are available online at http://www.mdpi.com/1660-4601/15/12/2666/s1, S1: questionnaire for the study "resistant pathogens in hospital swimming pools", S2: raw data.

Author Contributions: All authors made substantial contributions to study conception and the interpretation of data. The analyses were carried out by N.H., M.K., M.B.S., and D.E.K. and the drafting of the manuscript was carried out by D.E.K. All authors read and approved the final version of the manuscript.

Funding: This study was not supported by any external funding.

Acknowledgments: The authors wish to thank Laura Perez Alleres, Marijana Duilo-Bening, Christiane Christian, Sylvia Kühnel, Angelika Mahr, and Christiane Strauss for their excellent technical assistance.

Conflicts of Interest: The authors declare no conflict of interest.

References

1. European Centre for Disease Prevention and Control, European Food Safety Authority, European Medicines Agency. ECDC/EFSA/EMA first joint report on the integrated analysis of the consumption of antimicrobial agents and occurrence of antimicrobial resistance in bacteria from humans and foodproducing animals. *EFSA J.* **2015**, *13*, 114. [CrossRef]
2. Cerceo, E.; Deitelzweig, S.B.; Sherman, B.M.; Amin, A.N. Multidrug-resistant gram-negative bacterial infections in the hospital setting: Overview, implications for clinical practice, and emerging treatment options. *Microb. Drug Resist.* **2016**, *22*, 412–431. [CrossRef] [PubMed]
3. Valenza, G.; Nickel, S.; Pfeifer, Y.; Eller, C.; Krupa, E.; Lehner-Reindl, V.; Holler, C. Extended-spectrum-beta-lactamase-producing *Escherichia coli* as intestinal colonizers in the German community. *Antimicrob. Agents Chemother.* **2014**, *58*, 1228–1230. [CrossRef] [PubMed]
4. Munita, J.M.; Arias, C.A. Mechanisms of antibiotic resistance. *Microbiol. Spectr.* **2016**, *4*. [CrossRef]
5. Ramphal, R.; Ambrose, P.G. Extended-spectrum beta-lactamases and clinical outcomes: Current data. *Clin. Infect. Dis.* **2006**, *42* (Suppl. 4), S164–S172. [CrossRef]
6. European Centre for Disease Prevention and Control. ECDC publishes a directory of online resources for prevention and control of antimicrobial resistance and healthcare-associated infections. *Eur. Surveill.* **2014**, *19*. [CrossRef]

7.   World Health Organization. *Critically Important Antimicrobials for Human Medicine, 5th Revision*; World Health Organization: Geneva, Switzerland, 2017.

8.   Empfehlung der Kommission für Kranken- haushygiene und Infektionsprävention (KRINKO) beim Robert Koch-Institut (RKI). Hygienemaßnahmen bei Infektionen oder Besiedlung mit multiresistenten gramnegativen Stäbchen. *Bundesgesundheitsbl* **2012**, *55*, 1311–1354. [CrossRef] [PubMed]

9.   Sassone-Corsi, M.; Raffatellu, M. No vacancy: How beneficial microbes cooperate with immunity to provide colonization resistance to pathogens. *J. Immunol.* **2015**, *194*, 4081–4087. [CrossRef] [PubMed]

10. Hollyoak, V.; Allison, D.; Summers, J. *Pseudomonas aeruginosa* wound infection associated with a nursing home's whirlpool bath. *Commun. Dis. Rep. CDR Rev.* **1995**, *5*, R100–R102. [PubMed]

11. Rice, S.A.; van den Akker, B.; Pomati, F.; Roser, D. A risk assessment of *Pseudomonas aeruginosa* in swimming pools: A review. *J. Water Health* **2012**, *10*, 181–196. [CrossRef] [PubMed]

12. Schlech, W.F., III; Simonsen, N.; Sumarah, R.; Martin, R.S. Nosocomial outbreak of *Pseudomonas aeruginosa* folliculitis associated with a physiotherapy pool. *CMAJ* **1986**, *134*, 909–913. [PubMed]

13. Tate, D.; Mawer, S.; Newton, A. Outbreak of *Pseudomonas aeruginosa* folliculitis associated with a swimming pool inflatable. *Epidemiol. Infect.* **2003**, *130*, 187–192. [CrossRef] [PubMed]

14. Elmir, S.M.; Wright, M.E.; Abdelzaher, A.; Solo-Gabriele, H.M.; Fleming, L.E.; Miller, G.; Rybolowik, M.; Peter Shih, M.T.; Pillai, S.P.; Cooper, J.A.; et al. Quantitative evaluation of bacteria released by bathers in a marine water. *Water Res.* **2007**, *41*, 3–10. [CrossRef] [PubMed]

15. Friedman, M.S.; Roels, T.; Koehler, J.E.; Feldman, L.; Bibb, W.F.; Blake, P. *Escherichia coli* O157:H7 outbreak associated with an improperly chlorinated swimming pool. *Clin. Infect. Dis.* **1999**, *29*, 298–303. [CrossRef] [PubMed]

16. Kahanov, L.; Kim, Y.K.; Eberman, L.; Dannelly, K.; Kaur, H.; Ramalinga, A. *Staphylococcus aureus* and community-associated methicillin-resistant *Staphylococcus aureus* (CA-MRSA) in and around therapeutic whirlpools in college athletic training rooms. *J. Athletic Train.* **2015**, *50*, 432–437. [CrossRef] [PubMed]

17. Papadopoulou, C.; Economou, V.; Sakkas, H.; Gousia, P.; Giannakopoulos, X.; Dontorou, C.; Filioussis, G.; Gessouli, H.; Karanis, P.; Leveidiotou, S. Microbiological quality of indoor and outdoor swimming pools in Greece: Investigation of the antibiotic resistance of the bacterial isolates. *Int. J. Hyg. Environ. Health* **2008**, *211*, 385–397. [CrossRef] [PubMed]

18. Pereira, S.G.; Paixao, J.; Leitao, R.; Cardoso, O. *Pseudomonas aeruginosa* in a hydropathic facility: Diversity, susceptibility and imipenem resistance mutation. *Lett. Appl. Microbiol.* **2011**, *53*, 518–524. [CrossRef] [PubMed]

19. Schets, F.M.; van den Berg, H.H.; Baan, R.; Lynch, G.; de Roda Husman, A.M. *Pseudomonas aeruginosa* on vinyl-canvas inflatables and foam teaching aids in swimming pools. *J. Water Health* **2014**, *12*, 772–781. [CrossRef] [PubMed]

20. Tolba, O.; Loughrey, A.; Goldsmith, C.E.; Millar, B.C.; Rooney, P.J.; Moore, J.E. Survival of epidemic strains of healthcare (HA-MRSA) and community-associated (CA-MRSA) meticillin-resistant *Staphylococcus aureus* (MRSA) in river-, sea- and swimming pool water. *Int. J. Hyg. Environ. Health* **2008**, *211*, 398–402. [CrossRef] [PubMed]

21. DIN 19643:2012-11, Aufbereitung von Schwimm- und Badebeckenwasser—Teil 1: Allgemeine Anforderungen. Available online: https://www.beuth.de/de/norm/din-19643-1/164174095 (accessed on 27 November 2018).

22. DGfdB Guideline R 94.04:2013-12, Reinigung, Desinfektion und Hygiene in Bädern. Available online: http://www.drnuesken.de/uploads/media/94.04_Reinigung__Desinfektion_und_Hygiene_in_Baedern_Blaudruck_2013.pdf (accessed on 27 November 2018).

23. Botzenhardt, K.; Döring, G. *Ecology and Epidemiology of Pseudomonas aeruginosa*; Campa, M., Bendinelli, M., Friedman, H., Eds.; Springer: Boston, MA, USA, 1993.

24. Eurosurveillance editorial team. ECDC publishes 2014 surveillance data on antimicrobial resistance and antimicrobial consumption in Europe. *Eur. Surveill.* **2015**, *20*. [CrossRef]

25. Strateva, T.; Yordanov, D. *Pseudomonas aeruginosa*—A phenomenon of bacterial resistance. *J. Med. Microbiol.* **2009**, *58*, 1133–1148. [CrossRef] [PubMed]

26. Denton, M.; Kerr, K.G. Microbiological and clinical aspects of infection associated with *Stenotrophomonas maltophilia*. *Clin. Microbiol. Rev.* **1998**, *11*, 57–80. [CrossRef] [PubMed]

27. McGowan, J.E., Jr. Resistance in nonfermenting gram-negative bacteria: Multidrug resistance to the maximum. *Am. J. Infect. Control* **2006**, *34*, S29–S37. [CrossRef] [PubMed]

28. Waters, V.G.M.; Soong, G.; Amin, S.; Ernst, R.; Prince, A. Immunostimulatory properties of the emerging pathogen *Stenotrophomonas maltophilia*. *Infect. Immun.* **2007**, *75*, 1698–1703. [CrossRef] [PubMed]

29. Abbott, I.J.; Slavin, M.A.; Turnidge, J.D.; Thursky, K.A.; Worth, L.J. *Stenotrophomonas maltophilia*: Emerging disease patterns and challenges for treatment. *Expert Rev. Anti-Infect. Ther.* **2011**, *9*, 471–488. [CrossRef] [PubMed]

30. Lin, J.N.; Lai, C.H.; Chen, Y.H.; Lin, H.L.; Huang, C.K.; Chen, W.F.; Wang, J.L.; Chung, H.C.; Liang, S.H.; Lin, H.H. *Sphingomonas paucimobilis* bacteremia in humans: 16 case reports and a literature review. *J. Microbiol. Immunol. Infect.* **2010**, *43*, 35–42. [CrossRef]

31. Ryan, M.P.; Adley, C.C. *Sphingomonas paucimobilis*: A persistent Gram-negative nosocomial infectious organism. *J. Hosp. Infect.* **2010**, *75*, 153–157. [CrossRef] [PubMed]

32. Bayram, N.; Devrim, I.; Apa, H.; Gulfidan, G.; Turkyilmaz, H.N.; Gunay, I. *Sphingomonas paucimobilis* infections in children: 24 case reports. *Mediterr. J. Hematol. Infect. Dis.* **2013**, *5*, e2013040. [CrossRef] [PubMed]

33. Liu, L.; Coenye, T.; Burns, J.L.; Whitby, P.W.; Stull, T.L.; LiPuma, J.J. Ribosomal DNA-directed PCR for identification of *Achromobacter (Alcaligenes) xylosoxidans* recovered from sputum samples from cystic fibrosis patients. *J. Clin. Microbiol.* **2002**, *40*, 1210–1213. [CrossRef] [PubMed]

34. Fass, R.J.; Barnishan, J. In vitro susceptibilities of nonfermentative Gram-negative bacilli other than *Pseudomonas aeruginosa* to 32 antimicrobial agents. *Rev. Infect. Dis.* **1980**, *2*, 841–853. [CrossRef] [PubMed]

35. Blahova, J.; Kralikova, K.; Krcmery, V., Sr.; Kubonova, K. Hydrolysis of imipenem, meropenem, ceftazidime, and cefepime by multiresistant nosocomial strains of *Sphingobacterium multivorum*. *Eur. J. Clin. Microbiol. Infect. Dis.* **1997**, *16*, 178–180. [CrossRef] [PubMed]

36. Holmes, B.P.M.; Kiredjian, M.; Kersters, K. *Ochrobactrum anthropi* gen. nov., sp. nov. from Human Clinical Specimens and Previously Known as Group Vd. *Int. J. Syst. Bacteriol.* **1998**, *38*, 406–416. [CrossRef]

37. Sudharani, A. *Chryseobacterium indologenes* bacteremia in a preterm baby. *Indian J. Med. Microbiol.* **2011**, *29*, 196–198. [CrossRef] [PubMed]

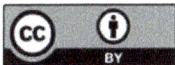

International Journal of
Environmental Research and Public Health

MDPI

Article

Salmonella enterica Serovar Typhimurium and Escherichia coli Survival in Estuarine Bank Sediments

Mahbubul H. Siddiqee [1,2], Rebekah Henry [1], Rebecca Coulthard [1], Christelle Schang [1], Richard Williamson [1], Rhys Coleman [3], Graham Rooney [3], Ana Deletic [1] and David McCarthy [1,*]

[1] Environmental and Public Health Microbiology Laboratory (EPHM LAB), Department of Civil Engineering, Monash University, Melbourne, VIC-3168, Australia; mhsiddiqee@gmail.com (M.H.S.); Rebekah.Henry@monash.edu (R.H.); Rebecca.Coulthard@wsp.com (R.C.); Christelle.Schang@monash.edu (C.S.); Richard.Williamson@monash.edu (R.W.); a.deletic@unsw.edu.au (A.D.)

[2] Molecular and Environmental Microbiology Laboratory (MEM LAB), Department of Mathematics and Natural Sciences, BRAC University, Dhaka 1212, Bangladesh

[3] Melbourne Water Corporation, Docklands, VIC-3008, Australia; Rhys.Coleman@melbournewater.com.au (R.C.); grahamrrooney@gmail.com (G.R.)

* Correspondence: David.McCarthy@monash.edu; Tel.: +61-3-9905-5068

Received: 2 October 2018; Accepted: 14 November 2018; Published: 21 November 2018

Abstract: Estuarine bank sediments have the potential to support the survival and growth of fecal indicator organisms, including *Escherichia coli*. However, survival of fecal pathogens in estuarine sediments is not well researched and therefore remains a significant knowledge gap regarding public health risks in estuaries. In this study, simultaneous survival of *Escherichia coli* and a fecal pathogen, *Salmonella enterica* serovar Typhimurium, was studied for 21 days in estuarine bank sediment microcosms. Observed growth patterns for both organisms were comparable under four simulated scenarios; for continuous-desiccation, extended-desiccation, periodic-inundation, and continuous-inundation systems, logarithmic decay coefficients were 1.54/day, 1.51/day, 0.14/day, and 0.20/day, respectively, for *E. coli*, and 1.72/day, 1.64/day, 0.21/day, and 0.24/day for *S.* Typhimurium. Re-wetting of continuous-desiccated systems resulted in potential re-growth, suggesting survival under moisture-limited conditions. Key findings from this study include: (i) Bank sediments can potentially support human pathogens (*S.* Typhimurium), (ii) inundation levels influence the survival of fecal bacteria in estuarine bank sediments, and (iii) comparable survival rates of *S.* Typhimurium and *E. coli* implies the latter could be a reliable fecal indicator in urban estuaries. The results from this study will help select suitable monitoring and management strategies for safer recreational activities in urban estuaries.

Keywords: fecal indicator; fecal pathogen; waterborne pathogens; recreational risks; QMRA

1. Introduction

Urban estuaries deliver multiple benefits to communities, including access to aquatic recreation, amenity, transport, and supporting cultural traditions. As a result, 22 of the largest cities in the world are located adjacent to estuaries [1]. However, community benefits from estuaries are under increasing threat from pollution due to progressive urbanization and population growth [2]. Fecal contamination is one of the leading threats to public health in these systems, via exposure to harmful organisms during aquatic recreation [3–5].

Monitoring of public health risks in estuaries has historically relied on fecal indicator organisms, such as *Escherichia coli* and *Enterococcus* spp.—principally due to the practical limitations and costs associated with measuring pathogens. In many cases, significant correlations have been observed between health outcomes (i.e., illness rates) and indicator organism concentrations in marine waters and some freshwater systems [6,7]. However, there is a paucity of epidemiological studies for estuarine environments [8], meaning that the link between indicator organisms and human health outcomes in these systems is more uncertain.

There are an increasing number of studies that show that fecal indicators can survive and grow in estuarine systems, especially in their sediments where they are protected from competition and predation and have a rich nutrient supply [9]. For example, Solo-Gabriele et al. (2000) and Desmarais et al. (2002) found that coastal bank sediments are a suitable habitat for the survival and growth of E. coli. Further, Solo-Gabriele et al. (2000) found that that growth of E. coli was a function of soil moisture content and hence, different soil moisture scenarios (as a result of tidal fluctuation) could potentially exert various degrees of stress, leading to differential survival of fecal organisms. At the same time, the survival potential of pathogens in these sediments may indeed be different to that of the indicator organism, E. coli. Moreover, the survival of fecal organisms in the bank sediments of estuaries in temperate climates is not well understood.

There are only a handful of studies that have explored the survival of pathogens in estuarine systems, and even fewer which have focused on estuarine sediments. Indeed, there are only two reported studies which have explored pathogen survival within the sediments of estuaries [9,10]. This lack of pathogen-survival studies in these types of systems is especially important considering the salient features of estuarine bank sediment as opposed to other soils in terms of its particle size distribution, organic content, composition of minerals, and organic matters [11]. With others having demonstrated extended survival and resuspension [12,13] of fecal indicator organisms from the bank sediments, this paucity in pathogen-survival data leaves a critical knowledge gap regarding the reliability of these indicators for predicting public health risk in these systems.

This study aims to determine: (a) Whether different sections of tidally-influenced estuarine bank sediments (fully inundated, periodically inundated, occasionally inundated, and fully desiccated) can support the extended survival of a human pathogen (*Salmonella enterica* serovar Typhimurium), and (b) whether the survival of a commonly used fecal contamination indicator (*E. coli*) is comparable to *Salmonella* Typhimurium. *Salmonella* Typhimurium is recommended by the US EPA as a suitable pathogen for water-based monitoring [14] and it is also responsible for the majority of *Salmonella*-related infections (nearly 80% in Australia) [15].

2. Materials and Methods

2.1. Bacterial Strains and Inoculum Development

In this study, *Escherichia coli* K1 was used as a model indicator organism and S. Typhimurium NVSL 6993 as the model enteric pathogen. *E. coli* and S. Typhimurium were subcultured from glycerol stock (maintained at −80 °C) onto Eosine-Methylene-Blue (EMB) (Oxoid, UK) agar and Xylose-Lysine-Deoxcolate (XLD) (Oxoid, UK) agar, respectively. Plate cultures were incubated overnight at 37 °C. Single colonies were isolated and transferred to 150 mL LB broth and incubated for 12 h at 37 °C with shaking (60 rpm). The cultures were pelleted at $4000 \times g$ for 15 min (at 10 °C). Supernatants were discarded, and the pellets resuspended in 5 mL Phosphate Buffered Saline (PBS) (1×; pH 7.4). Pelleting was repeated, the supernatant discarded, and the final pellet resuspended in 5 mL PBS (1×; pH 7.4).

2.2. Collection and Processing of Bank Sediment

The top 8 cm layer of bank sediments (20 kg) were collected at low tide from the Yarra River estuary at South Yarra (Victoria, Australia). The sediment was mixed to ensure homogeneity followed by sterilization by autoclaving before cooling it to room temperature. Since the main focus of this study was to test the influence of inundation scenarios, autoclaving of the bank sediment before inoculation with the two test microorganisms was done. This sterilization was essential to ensure that the survival rates of E. coli and S. Typhimurium were not influenced by predation, competition, or parasitism by native microorganisms present in natural sediments, which are known to have differential effects on these two organisms in different scenarios [16–18]. The influence of autoclaving on the nutritional properties of the sediment was tested prior to experimentation; no significant change in concentrations of total phosphorus (TP) and total dissolved nitrogen (TN) was observed when measured according to the Australian Laboratory Handbook of Soil and Water Chemical Methods, 1992 (see Figure A1 and Table A1). Changes in particle size distribution were also investigated using the electro-resistance counting method [19] and no detectable change was observed between autoclaved and non-autoclaved sediments.

The sterilized sediment was inoculated with both bacterial strains to reach a final concentration of 10^7 g^{-1} (wet sediment) cells. After mixing, the inoculated sediment was distributed into sterilized plastic containers by sub-sampling 10×100 g aliquots into 14 open plastic containers, using a randomization approach [20], to achieve a 3 cm thick layer consisting of 1 kg of sediment.

2.3. Experimental Matrix

Four experimental configurations were investigated in triplicate to represent four typical exposed tidally influenced bank sediment areas (Table 1): (i) continuous desiccation (CD), which received no inundation and represented bank sediment above the high tide mark, which does not receive any moisture from inundation; (ii) extended desiccation (ED), no inundation for the first seven days followed by periodic inundation after this period and represented the section of bank sediment that is only inundated during extreme conditions (including high flow periods and/environmental flow releases); (iii) periodically inundated (PI), representing tidally influenced sediment between high and low tide marks, which received the normal tidal of the condition of the Yarra estuary with a 12.4 h inundation cycle; and (iv) continuously inundated (CI) systems, which were permanently inundated with water and represent bank sediments just below the low tide mark. A non-inoculated control (NI) was used to monitor for environmental contamination that may occur during the experiment as a result of the open system design. Sediment containers were faced toward the sun with a slope of 7° (same as observed in the bank at the South Yarra site from where the sediment was collected).

Table 1. Experimental configurations tested for survival of E. coli and S. Typhimurium and their properties.

Configuration	No. of Replicates	Inoculation with E. coli and S. Typhimurium	Extent of Inundation
Continuous desiccation (CD)	3	Yes	Never
Extended desiccation (ED)	3	Yes	Starts on Day 7; periodic (cycles of 12.4 h)
Periodic inundation (PI)	3	Yes	Periodic (cycles of 12.4 h)
Continuous inundation (CI)	3	Yes	Continuous
Non-inoculated (NI)	2	No	Periodic (cycles of 12.4 h)

2.4. Experimental Procedure

All configurations were placed outdoor (Figure 1) under a Perspex sheet to protect the configurations from rain and direct fecal deposition by local wildlife. ED configurations were placed on a high platform to ensure shorter exposure to inundations compared to the PI configurations. The remaining configurations were placed on the low platforms in a randomized manner to account for differences related to spatial distribution. ED, PI, and NI containers were connected with silicon hoses to sterile plastic bottles (autoclaved) containing 1 L (each) of sterile semi-synthetic river water; representing water quality parameters of the Yarra River during a similar dry weather period at the same location. Data from a previous project (data not shown) was used to calculate target TP, TN, and total suspended solid (TSS) concentrations (0.09 mgL^{-1}, 0.91 mgL^{-1}, and 23 mgL^{-1}, respectively). The stock semi-synthetic water was made using autoclaved bed sediment (collected from the river at South Yarra) to produce a final TSS concentration of 23 mgL^{-1}. As sediment alone was unable to reproduce the target TN and TP concentrations, inorganic salts (KH$_2$PO$_4$ for TP and a mixture of KNO$_3$, NH$_4$Cl, and C$_6$H$_5$O$_2$N for TN) were added as outlined by Bratieres et al. (2008) to achieve the target concentrations [21]. The stock water was stored in room temperature and periodically tested to ensure sterility throughout experimentation. The water containers (all containing 1 L each) were kept on a platform, which had a periodic vertical movement mimicking the tidal fluctuations of the Yarra River (12.4 h cycle) covering the intended sediment configurations. The inundating water was replaced every week.

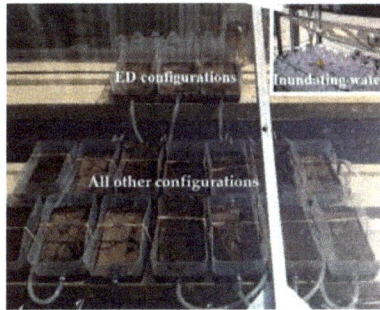

Figure 1. Outdoor experimental set up for the bank sediment survival study, which is covered by a transparent Perspex sheet; ED configurations placed on a higher platform and all the others on the lower platforms. Bottles containing water for inundating sediments (see upper right corner) were located on a vertically moving platform.

The survival experiment was conducted over 21 days. The first three days of the experiment coincided with a heat wave experienced in Melbourne; on each day, the maximum atmospheric temperature exceeded 40 °C. The average daily maximum temperature during this experiment was 29.4 °C and the average solar radiation was 25.6 MJ/m^2 (BOM, Australia, 2014).

2.5. Collection and Processing of Samples

A total of 6 g of top layer sediment was sampled (in four sub-samples) from each configuration on Days 0, 2, 7, 14, and 21. Further samples were collected from PI and ED on Day 1. The four sub-samples were homogeneously mixed to make a uniform mixture. Moisture content measurements were conducted on ~1.5 g of sediment following Standards Australia, (2005) [22]. For culture-based assays, ~1.5 g of sediment was dissolved in 25 mL sterile de-ionized water and mixed for 1 min at 120 shakes min^{-1} to dislodge particle-bound bacteria. The homogenized mix was pelleted at $400 \times g$ for 5 min. From the supernatant, a single 5 mL aliquot was diluted in 5 mL PBS (1×; pH 7.4) and vortexed for 3 s. The diluted supernatants were then further diluted to a final concentration of 10^{-4} in PBS (1×; pH 7.4).

2.6. Enumeration of E. coli and S. Typhimurium and Calculation of Die-Off Rates

A volume of 100 µL was plated, in triplicate, from the 10^{-3} and 10^{-4} dilutions on EMB agar for *E. coli*, and on XLD agar for *S.* Typhimurium for culturable counts as two differential media are needed to monitor two different organisms in the same system [23,24]. Plate counts were converted to cfu/g (dry weight) based on the relevant dilution factor and corresponding moisture content. Colony counts were then log-transformed and used to construct a line of best fit and the gradient of this line was used to estimate the die-off rate [25]. In cases where no colony was observed in any of the triplicate plates, data points were replaced with half of the detectable limit (i.e., 0.5 cfu/plate [26]). Data points that fluctuated around the lowest detectable limit were not used to estimate die-off rates. Colony counts of below 30 cfu/plate were considered for calculation of die-off rates, with possible uncertainties taken into consideration during data analysis and interpretation. The overall die-off rates were calculated as the logarithmic difference of initial and final numbers divided by the number of days elapsed.

3. Results and Discussion

3.1. The Impact of Experimental Design

Preliminary investigations demonstrated the insignificant impact that autoclaving had on particle size distributions and nutrient contents. Furthermore, other analyses (Appendices A and B) demonstrated that the process of autoclaving did not significantly impact microbial survival through the re-release of nutrients from dead microorganisms. However, since the experiment was conducted in an outdoor environment, it was influenced by the prevailing atmospheric conditions.

The initial phase of the experiment coincided with high atmospheric temperatures (>40 °C) and solar radiation, both known to reduce survival of *E. coli* and *S.* Typhimurium [11,26,27]. During this initial period, a sharp decrease in moisture level was observed in configurations without inundation (CD and ED). In fact, on Day 2, there was almost no moisture remaining in these systems (Figure 2). Overall, the moisture content readings of different configurations were reduced significantly (from 41% to as low as 10%) in all configurations, except for the CI system.

Another by-product of the heat wave was an increase in TP and TN concentration in the sediment and inundating water (Tables A1 and A2). However, since the water was replaced weekly, exposure to the increased nutrient levels was not persistent. Furthermore, the concentration of TN and TP within the sediment (0.21 and 0.81 mg/g, respectively, at the beginning) showed very little change (up to 0.4 mg/g for TP and up to 1.4 mg/g for TN) across the experimental period. Thus, it can be assumed that the alteration in water column concentrations did not have a significant effect on sediment survival rates.

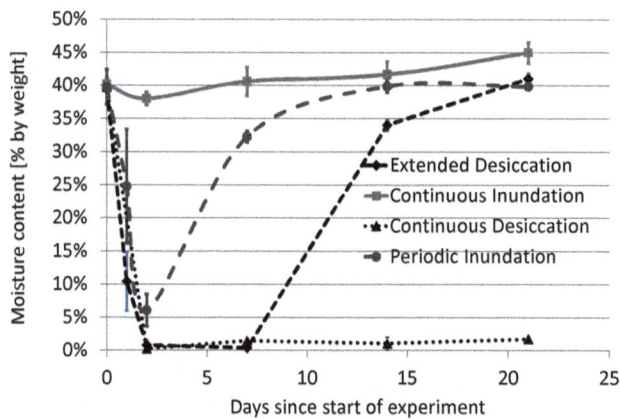

Figure 2. Levels of moisture content in four test sediment configurations during the experiment (error bars represent standard deviations around the mean values for each of the configurations).

3.2. Survival of E. coli and S. Typhimurium

The results of the survival study indicate that both *E. coli* and *S.* Typhimurium are able to survive for up to 21 days in all three configurations that received moisture (ED, PI, and CI). Both microorganisms withstood the first 24 h of the experiment after sediment inoculation, which was evident from the culture counts of the two tested configurations (PI and ED; Figure 3). Notably, even though the atmospheric temperature reached 43 °C within a few hours of inoculation, *E. coli* counts increased marginally, and *S*. Typhimurium counts increased nearly 10 times of the initial number. This initial growth could reflect the fact that fecal microorganisms are adapted to animal gut environments (37 °C for mammals and 42 °C for birds). Sediment properties that are widely known to influence bacterial survival include available nutrients [28], organic matter [29], particle size [30], and clay content [31]. Among these, estuarine bank sediment is generally known to have finer particles [32,33], as well as higher organic matter content [34], which can offer several advantages, such as protection from UV light [35,36] and nutritional support. Therefore, it is perhaps not surprising to see extended survival of fecal microorganisms, including the potential pathogen, in estuarine banks even in unfavorable weather conditions. This, in turn, suggests that in the absence of other stressors, *S*. Typhimurium can probably grow in estuarine bank sediments in high-temperature conditions when moisture is available and potentially serve as a source of this pathogen to the water column if re-suspended.

The initial phase of growth in the first 24 h was followed by a sharp die-off, consistent across organisms and configurations (Figure 3). The CD system had the highest die-off rates for both types of bacteria during the experiment; 1.54/day for *E. coli* and 1.72/day for *S*. Typhimurium. Since significant losses in soil moisture took place during the early phase of the experiment (moisture content decreased from 40% to <1%), these very fast die-off rates were consistent with the literature [11,37]. In addition, high die-off rates might have been facilitated by very high air temperatures [38] coupled with high radiation levels [39].

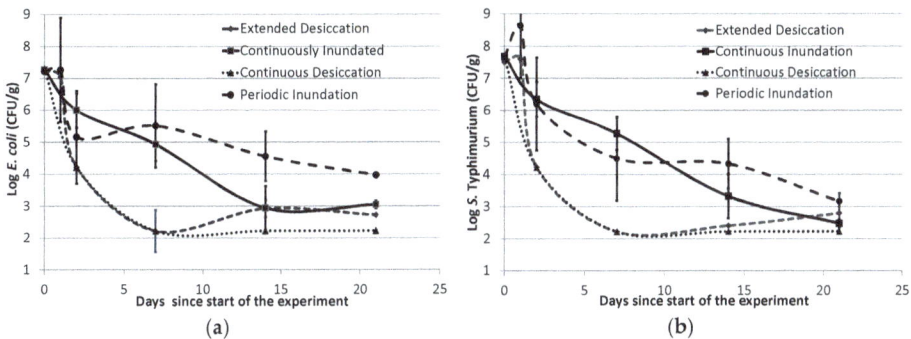

Figure 3. Survival of the test organisms; (**a**) *E. coli* K1 densities (cfu/g dw) and (**b**) *S*. Typhimurium NVSL 6993 densities (cfu/g dw) in the four experimental configurations (error bars represent standard deviations around the mean values of the replicates tested).

The two test organisms in the ED systems behaved similarly to the CD systems in the first week of the experiment (Figure 3). The die-off rate for *E. coli* was calculated to be 1.51/day and for *S*. Typhimurium it was 1.64/day. Interestingly, when inundation was restored to these systems after Day 7 (although the ED system received a shorter duration of inundation compared to PI counterparts), an increase in moisture content coincided with the detection of *E. coli* colonies on both Days 14 and 21 (in two of the three replicates on both days). *S*. Typhimurium was also detected on Day 21 in one of the replicate boxes while the NI controls remained negative. An increase in moisture level due to inundation restoration might have influenced this regrowth/recurrence of both test organisms.

The detection of culturable bacteria after a period of drying indicates that both bacteria may survive either in dormant form or at least survive in very low densities. It is important to note that although above the limit of detection, the colony counts were below 30 cfu/plate, and therefore may have higher associated uncertainties. However, colonies were reproducibly isolated within the replicate, suggesting a level of survival was possible. Dormancy and subsequent regrowth of *S*. Typhimurium upon increasing moisture has previously been reported [40]. Also, desiccation has been shown for both *E. coli* and *S*. Typhimurium to significantly enhance resistance towards environmental stressors, including high temperature [41,42]. This could perhaps partly explain the recurrence of these two organisms in the ED systems. Therefore, it is possible that bank sediments, which only receive moisture very intermittently (i.e., bank sediments above the usual high-tide mark, which are inundated only during king tides or high flows) could support the growth of viable fecal pathogens that, if washed, could get resuspended back into the water column [43]. Resuspension could also occur due to other natural and anthropogenic activities, like storms, floods, recreational activities, and commercial dredging, which have all been known to cause resuspension of sediment borne bacteria and causing elevated levels of fecal organisms [44,45]. Therefore, extended survival of potential fecal pathogens, like *S.* Typhimurium, in estuarine bank sediment could comprise a potential human health risk.

PI systems had higher levels of survival for both *E. coli* and *S.* Typhimurium compared to the desiccated CD and ED systems (Figure 3). For PI, the decay rate of *E. coli* was 0.14/day, while a slightly higher decay rate was observed for *S.* Typhimurium (0.21/day). The decrease in cell counts after Day 1 may be associated with very high air temperatures and solar radiation, which also resulted in a very low moisture content (close to 5%; Figure 2). It has previously been reported that Gram-negative bacteria require a moisture content of 93% or more for optimal growth [46]. However, despite some variation among the three biological replicates for the PI configurations, it was evident that the scenario still supported the survival of both test organisms for up to three weeks. Therefore, under more favorable conditions (lower atmospheric temperature, lower solar radiation, and higher moisture), it is likely that survival of these fecal organisms (including potential pathogens) would be higher.

Survival rates of *E. coli* and *S.* Typhimurium in the PI configuration were found to be comparable. This contradicts the notion that fecal pathogens cannot survive in estuarine sediments, and suggests that *E. coli* could be a reliable indicator of this pathogen in this scenario. Furthermore, the extended survival of a potential fecal pathogen in the tidally influenced zone of an estuarine bank could have human health implications. This is especially the case for bank sediments, where natural and anthropogenic activities (including tide, storm, flood, recreation, dredging, etc.) can readily cause resuspension into the water column [10,45,47].

The CI systems showed slightly higher die-off rates when compared to PI (0.20/day for *E. coli* and 0.24/day for *S.* Typhimurium). It was interesting to see higher die-off rates compared to those of PI, especially since the organisms in the CI systems were exposed to higher moisture levels and reduced solar irradiation. However, the water used for inundating the experimental containers was stagnant in the CI configurations, which led to some interference due to the formation of algae after the first week, and this may have resulted in a faster die-off. The algal growth resulted in lower TP and TN concentrations in the inundating water in the CI systems compared to the other configurations (Table A2).

In the estuarine context, better survival of *E. coli* in areas of coastal bank sediment with intermittent drying effect compared to continuously moist sediment has previously been reported by Solo-Gabriele et al. (2000). They argued that this better survival was due to having a better competitive advantage over the predators existing in natural sediment. Although our study attempted to exclude the biotic factors by sterilizing the soil beforehand, the CI systems with algal interference supports the idea that algal bloom (which could occur in estuarine systems) could potentially reduce the survival of fecal organisms in estuarine bank sediments. In this scenario, even under these algae-influenced conditions, the survival rates of both organisms were again comparable, reinforcing the ability of *E. coli* to represent *S.* Typhimurium in complex systems, including those with algae blooms. It is also important to note that apart from the CI systems, no other configurations showed any sign of algal interference.

This study was conducted under open atmospheric conditions, which led to some challenges, including changing TP and TN concentrations. However, other studies have demonstrated that increases in TP does not necessarily impact the survival of fecal organisms, like *E. coli* [48,49]. Likewise, increased levels of organic or inorganic nitrogen do not necessarily impact the survival of fecal bacteria in ambient waters [48]. Therefore, it can be assumed that the changes in TP and TN concentrations did not significantly influence the die-off rates of the test organisms. In fact, conducting the study in an ambient environment allowed a unique opportunity to explore the comparative survival of these organisms under highly unfavorable conditions.

In combination, the survival data suggests, for the first time, that both *E. coli* and *S.* Typhimurium were able to withstand severe environmental conditions in estuarine bank sediments. Overall, the die-off rates observed in this study ranged from 0.14/day to 1.54/day for *E. coli* and 0.21/day to 1.72/day for *S.* Typhimurium. In three of the four configurations (i.e., CD, PI, CI), die-off rates for the two organisms were similar. A wide range of die-off rates has been reported in soil sediment systems for these organisms [27,40,50,51], and differences have been attributed to both biotic and abiotic factors [11,38,49,52–54] that are also encountered in bank sediments.

This study investigated the influence of different bank sediment scenarios on the survival of two fecal microorganisms in potentially extreme weather conditions with respect to temperature, radiation, and desiccation. Our underlying hypothesis is that if the test organisms survive in this study's extreme climatic conditions, then they can also survive in the less extreme conditions that exist in many systems year-round. With an absence of previous studies focusing on bank sediments under similar experimental conditions, the results of this study significantly enhance our knowledge of the survival of fecal organisms in estuarine bank sediments. Further, this study demonstrates that, without studying fecal pathogen survival in all environments (estuarine bank sediment in this case), perhaps it could be premature to conclude that *E. coli* is not a good indicator organism.

4. Conclusions

This study presented data on the survival of the faecal indicator organism, *E. coli*, and the human fecal pathogen, *S.* Typhimurium, in estuarine bank sediments. Different degrees of tidal inundation were observed to influence the survival for both test organisms, with periodic inundation, mimicking natural tidal cycles, being the most conducive to persistence. While the simultaneous survival rates for these two organisms were found to be comparable, for the first time, this experiment presents evidence that *S.* Typhimurium may survive for over three weeks in estuarine bank sediments, which could be of critical importance. This, in turn, highlights the potential of bank sediments as a source of viable pathogens to the water column, especially when natural processes and anthropogenic activities cause resuspension. Considering the comparable survival patterns of *E. coli* and *S.* Typhimurium in the contrasting experimental conditions, *E. coli* cannot be excluded from being a reliable indicator of public health risks associated with *S.* Typhimurium in estuarine bank sediments.

Author Contributions: Conceptualization: M.H.S., R.H., R.C. (Rebecca Coulthard), C.S. and D.M.; Methodology: M.H.S., R.H., R.C. (Rebecca Coulthard), C.S. and D.M.; Validation: M.H.S., R.C. (Rebecca Coulthard), C.S., R.W.; Formal analysis: M.H.S., R.C. (Rebecca Coulthard), C.S., D.M.; Writing—original draft preparation: M.H.S., D.M.; Writing—review and editing: M.H.S., R.H., R.C. (Rhys Coleman), A.D. and D.M.; Supervision: R.H., A.D. and D.M.; Funding acquisition: D.M., R.C. (Rhys Coleman) and G.R.

Funding: This research was funded by [Melbourne Water] and the [Australian Research Council], grant number [LP120100718].

Acknowledgments: We gratefully acknowledge the timely help we received from Peter Kolotelo, Dusan Jovanovic, Gayani Chandrasena, and Scott Coutts during various stages of the study.

Conflicts of Interest: The authors declare no conflict of interest.

Appendix A

Effect of Autoclaving

Autoclaving was done in this experiment to exclude the interference from predation and competition by native organisms present in natural sediments. However, a combination of very high temperature and pressure kills the naturally occurring microbes in the sediment and releases nutrients into the sediment. Also, some other reports suggest that autoclaving can change sediment's own nutritional properties [42–44]. Therefore, it was essential to check if autoclaving was introducing any bias towards higher or lower survival. Therefore, along with the experimental configurations (Table 1), another set (triplicate) of sediments was augmented with a mixture of *E. coli* and *S.* Typhimurium culture (each at a concentration of 10^9 g^{-1} wet sediment and hereby named as Nutritionally Augmented) before autoclaving. These sediments were eventually inoculated with both test organisms and were tested along the test configurations as mentioned above (Figure A1).

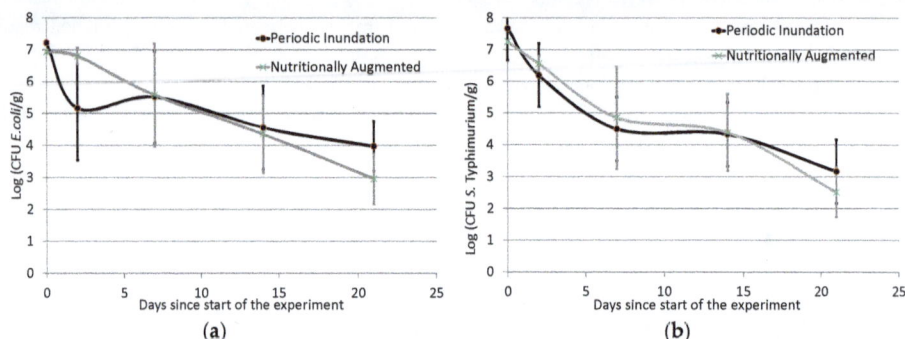

(a) (b)

Figure A1. Influence of augmented nutrition on survival of (**a**) *E. coli* K1 and (**b**) *S.* Typhimurium NVSL 6993 (error bars represent standard deviations around the mean values for each of the configurations).

It was observed in this study that there was no obvious impact of nutritional augmentation on *E. coli* or *S.* Typhimurium survival where additional microorganisms were added to the sediment before autoclaving. This could suggest that the extra nutrition (if at all) available to *E. coli* and *S.* Typhimurium through the autoclaving process did not cause significant bias in the observed die-off rates.

Appendix B

Changes in Sediments

Table A1. Mean (and relative standard deviations in %) of total phosphorus (TP) and total nitrogen (TN) concentrations of sediment samples.

Time during Experiment	*E. coli* (cfu/g dw)	*S.* Typhimurium (cfu/g dw)	TP (mg/g dw)	TN (mg/g dw)
	Original bank conditions—not inoculated, not autoclaved			
Day = 0	540	Nil	0.21 *	0.77 *
	Autoclaved, not inoculated			
Day = 0	Nil	Nil	0.18 *	0.78 *
Day = 21 (PI)	Nil	Nil	0.4 (12)	1.4 (5)
	Autoclaved, spiked with *E. coli*, *S.* Typhimurim and mixed culture			
Day = 0	**	**	0.20 *	0.77 *
Day = 21 (PI)	**	**	0.4 (2)	1.3 (1)
	Autoclaved, spiked with *E. coli*, *S.* Typhimurim			
Day = 0	***	***	0.21 *	0.81 *
Day = 21 (ED)	***	***	0.4 (7)	1.4 (3)
Day = 21 (CI)	***	***	0.4 (12)	1.3 (8)
Day = 21 (CD)	***	***	0.4 (4)	1.4 (0)
Day = 21 (PI)	***	***	0.4 (3)	1.4 (3)

* only one sample analysed, ** data presented in Appendix A, *** data presented in Section 3.2.

Table A2. Changes of nutrients in inundating water; means (and relative standard deviations in %) of TP and TN concentration of weekly inflow samples.

Time during Experiment	TP (mg/L)	TN (mg/L)	pH	EC (mS/cm)	Turbidity (NTU)
		Fresh Inflow			
	0.13 (37)	0.9 (4)	6.6 (4)	0 (17)	2.14 *
		Extended Desiccation			
Day = 7			7.4 (2)	0.5 (8)	
Day = 14			5.8 (6)	1.7 (6)	
Day = 21	0.25 (48)	6.4 (48)	5.7 (7)	1 (38)	8.1 (62)
		Non-Inoculated			
Day = 7	0.27 (45)	13 (22)	7.2 (1)	2.5 (20)	
Day = 14	0.17 (42)	4.2 (67)	6.1 (1)	0.3 (6)	
Day = 21			5.8 (10)	2.7 (46)	4.4 (37)
		Continuously Inundated			
Day = 7			7.5 (0)	2.4 (10)	
Day = 14			6.7 (2)	0.7 (1)	
Day = 21	0.37 (25)	3.6 (19)	7.1 (0)	0.4 (4)	12.3 (44)
		Periodically Inundated			
Day = 7	0.27 (19)	10.83 (19)	6.7 (3)	1.9 (23)	
Day = 14	0.2 (12)	5.8 (9)	6 (9)	0.7 (1)	
Day = 21	0.25 (13)	12.2 (43)	5.8 (11)	1.7 (36)	4.4 (30)
		Nutritionally Augmented			
Day = 7	0.25 (43)	10.33 (49)	0.1 (1)	1.8 (46)	
Day = 14	0.23 (11)	7.27 (12)	6.4 (9)	0.9 (23)	
Day = 21			6.3 (14)	1.9 (7)	3.7 (27)

* Only one sample was tested against three for the others.

References

1. Ross, D.A. *Introduction to Oceanography*; Harper Collins College Publishers: New York, NY, USA, 1995; ISBN 978-0-673-46938-0.
2. Mallin, M.A.; Williams, K.E.; Esham, E.C.; Lowe, R.P. Effect of human development on bacteriological water quality in coastal watersheds. *Ecol. Appl.* **2000**, *10*, 1047–1056. [CrossRef]
3. Catalao-Dionisio, L.P.; Joao, M.; Ferreiro, V.S.; Fidalgo, M.L.; Garcia-Rosado, M.E.; Borrego, J.J. Occurrence of *Salmonella* spp. in estuarine and coastal waters of Portugal. *Antonie Van Leeuwenhoek* **2000**, *78*, 99–106. [CrossRef] [PubMed]
4. Samhan, F.A.; Kronlein, M.R.; Fakher, U.; Kronlein, C.; Stedtfeld, R.D.; Hashsham, S.A. Detection and occurrence of indicator organisms and pathogens. *Water Environ. Res.* **2009**, *81*, 959–980. [CrossRef] [PubMed]
5. Henry, R.; Schang, C.; Chandrasena, G.I.; Deletic, A.; Edmunds, M.; Jovanovic, D.; Kolotelo, P.; Schmidt, J.; Williamson, R.; McCarthy, D. Environmental monitoring of waterborne *Campylobacter*: Evaluation of the Australian standard and a hybrid extraction-free MPN-PCR method. *Front. Microbiol.* **2015**, *6*, 74. [CrossRef] [PubMed]
6. Edberg, S.C.; Allen, M.J.; Smith, D.B.; Kriz, N.J. Enumeration of total coliforms and *Escherichia coli* from source water by the defined substrate technology. *Appl. Environ. Microbiol.* **1990**, *56*, 366–369. [PubMed]
7. Odonkor, S.T.; Ampofo, J.K. *Escherichia coli* as an indicator of bacteriological quality of water: An overview. *Microbiol. Res.* **2013**, *4*, e2. [CrossRef]
8. Australian Government. *Guidelines for Managing Risks in Recreational Water*; NHMRC: Canberra, Australia, 2008.
9. Schang, C.; Lintern, A.; Cook, P.L.M.; Osborne, C.A.; McKinley, A.; Schmidt, J.; Coleman, R.; Rooney, G.; Henry, R.; Deletic, A.; et al. Presence and survival of culturable *Campylobacter* spp. and *Escherichia coli* in temperate urban estuaries. *Sci. Total Environ.* **2016**, *569–570*, 1201–1211. [CrossRef] [PubMed]

10. Hood, M.A.; Ness, G.E. Survival of *Vibrio cholerae* and *Escherichia coli* in estuarine waters and sediments. *Appl. Environ. Microbiol.* **1982**, *43*, 578–584. [PubMed]

11. Venkatramanan, S.; Ramkumar, T.; Anithamary, I. Distribution of grain size, clay mineralogy and organic matter of surface sediments from Tirumalairajanar Estuary, Tamilnadu, east coast of India. *Arab. J. Geosci.* **2013**, *6*, 1371–1380. [CrossRef]

12. Solo-Gabriele, H.M.; Wolfert, M.A.; Desmarais, T.R.; Palmer, C.J. Sources of *Escherichia coli* in a Coastal Subtropical Environment. *Appl. Environ. Microbiol.* **2000**, *66*, 230–237. [CrossRef] [PubMed]

13. Desmarais, T.R.; Solo-Gabriele, H.M.; Palmer, C.J. Influence of soil on fecal indicator organisms in a tidally influenced subtropical environment. *Appl. Environ. Microbiol.* **2002**, *68*, 1165–1172. [CrossRef] [PubMed]

14. US-EPA. *Fact Sheet: Final Third Drinking Water Contaminant Candidate List (CCL 3)*; Office of Water: Washington, DC, USA, 2009.

15. OzFoodNet Working Group. *Burden and Causes of Foodborne Disease in Australia: Annual Report of the OzFoodNet Network, 2005*; Office of Health Protection, Australian Government Department of Health and Ageing: Canberra, Australia, 2006; Volume 30.

16. Chandran, A.; Mohamed Hatha, A.A. Relative survival of *Escherichia coli* and *Salmonella typhimurium* in a tropical estuary. *Water Res.* **2005**, *39*, 1397–1403. [CrossRef] [PubMed]

17. Feng, F.; Goto, D.; Yan, T. Effects of autochthonous microbial community on the die-off of fecal indicators in tropical beach sand. *FEMS Microbiol. Ecol.* **2010**, *74*, 214–225. [CrossRef] [PubMed]

18. Wanjugi, P.; Harwood, V.J. The influence of predation and competition on the survival of commensal and pathogenic fecal bacteria in aquatic habitats. *Environ. Microbiol.* **2013**, *15*, 517–526. [CrossRef] [PubMed]

19. Vdović, N.; Obhođaš, J.; Pikelj, K. Revisiting the particle-size distribution of soils: Comparison of different methods and sample pre-treatments. *Eur. J. Soil Sci.* **2010**, *61*, 854–864. [CrossRef]

20. McCarthy, D.T. Modelling microorganisms in urban stormwater. Ph.D. Thesis, Department of Civil Engineering, Monash University, Melbourne, Australia, 2008.

21. Bratieres, K.; Fletcher, T.D.; Deletic, A.; Zinger, Y. Nutrient and sediment removal by stormwater biofilters: A large-scale design optimisation study. *Water Res.* **2008**, *42*, 3930–3940. [CrossRef] [PubMed]

22. Australia Standard. *AS 1289.2.1.1: Methods of Testing Soils for Engineering Purposes—Soil Moisture Content Tests—Determination of the Moisture Content of a Soil-Oven Drying Method (Standard Method)*; SAI Global: Sydney, Australia, 2005.

23. Roszak, D.B.; Grimes, D.J.; Colwell, R.R. Viable but nonrecoverable stage of *Salmonella enteritidis* in aquatic systems. *Can. J. Microbiol.* **1984**, *30*, 334–338. [CrossRef] [PubMed]

24. Bogosian, G.; Sammons, L.E.; Morris, P.J.; O'Neil, J.P.; Heitkamp, M.A.; Weber, D.B. Death of the *Escherichia coli* K-12 strain W3110 in soil and water. *Appl. Environ. Microbiol.* **1996**, *62*, 4114–4120. [PubMed]

25. Nguyen, H.T.M.; Le, Q.T.P.; Garnier, J.; Janeau, J.L.; Rochelle-Newall, E. Seasonal variability of faecal indicator bacteria numbers and die-off rates in the Red River basin, North Viet Nam. *Sci. Rep.* **2016**, *6*, 21644. [CrossRef] [PubMed]

26. Whitcomb, B.W.; Schisterman, E.F. Assays with lower detection limits: Implications for epidemiological investigations. *Paediatr. Perinat. Epidemiol.* **2008**, *22*, 597–602. [CrossRef] [PubMed]

27. Mallmann, W.L.; Litsky, W. Survival of Selected Enteric Organisms in Various Types of Soil. *Am. J. Public Health Nations Health* **1951**, *41*, 38–44. [CrossRef] [PubMed]

28. Pommepuy, M.; Guillaud, J.F.; Dupray, E.; Derrien, A.; Le Guyader, F.; Cormier, M. Enteric bacteria survival factors. *Water Sci. Technol.* **1992**, *25*, 93–103. [CrossRef]

29. Pote, J.; Haller, L.; Kottelat, R.; Sastre, V.; Arpagaus, P.; Wildi, W. Persistence and growth of faecal culturable bacterial indicators in water column and sediments of Vidy Bay, Lake Geneva, Switzerland. *J. Environ. Sci.* **2009**, *21*, 62–69. [CrossRef]

30. Garzio-Hadzick, A.; Shelton, D.R.; Hill, R.L.; Pachepsky, Y.A.; Guber, A.K.; Rowland, R. Survival of manure-borne *E. coli* in streambed sediment: Effects of temperature and sediment properties. *Water Res.* **2010**, *44*, 2753–2762. [CrossRef] [PubMed]

31. Burton, G.A.; Gunnison, D.; Lanza, G.R. Survival of pathogenic bacteria in various freshwater sediments. *Appl. Environ. Microbiol.* **1987**, *53*, 633–638. [PubMed]

32. Malham, S.K.; Rajko-Nenow, P.; Howlett, E.; Tuson, K.E.; Perkins, T.L.; Pallett, D.W.; Wang, H.; Jago, C.F.; Jones, D.L.; McDonald, J.E. The interaction of human microbial pathogens, particulate material and nutrients in estuarine environments and their impacts on recreational and shellfish waters. *Environ. Sci. Process. Impacts* **2014**, *16*, 2145–2155. [CrossRef] [PubMed]

33. Perkins, T.L.; Clements, K.; Baas, J.H.; Jago, C.F.; Jones, D.L.; Malham, S.K.; McDonald, J.E. Sediment composition influences spatial variation in the abundance of human pathogen indicator bacteria within an estuarine environment. *PLoS ONE* **2014**, *9*. [CrossRef] [PubMed]

34. Gerba, C.P.; McLeod, J.S. Effects of sediments on the survival of *Escherichia coli* in marine waters. *Appl. Environ. Microbiol.* **1976**, *32*, 114–120. [PubMed]

35. Sinton, L.W.; Davies-Colley, R.J.; Bell, R.G. Inactivation of enterococci and fecal coliforms from sewage and meatworks effluents in seawater chambers. *Appl. Environ. Microbiol.* **1994**, *60*, 2040–2048. [PubMed]

36. Davies-Colley, R.J.; Donnison, A.M.; Speed, D.J.; Ross, C.M.; Nagels, J.W. Inactivation of faecal indicator micro-organisms in waste stabilisation ponds: Interactions of environmental factors with sunlight. *Water Res.* **1999**, *33*, 1220–1230. [CrossRef]

37. Byappanahalli, M.N.; Nevers, M.B.; Korajkic, A.; Staley, Z.R.; Harwood, V.J. Enterococci in the Environment. *Microbiol. Mol. Biol. Rev.* **2012**, *76*, 685–706. [CrossRef] [PubMed]

38. Carlucci, A.F.; Pramer, D. An evaluation of factors affecting the survival of *Escherichia coli* in sea water. II. Salinity, pH, and nutrients. *Appl. Microbiol.* **1960**, *8*, 247–250. [PubMed]

39. Korajkic, A.; McMinn, B.R.; Shanks, O.C.; Sivaganesan, M.; Fout, G.S.; Ashbolt, N.J. Biotic Interactions and Sunlight Affect Persistence of Fecal Indicator Bacteria and Microbial Source Tracking Genetic Markers in the Upper Mississippi River. *Appl. Environ. Microbiol.* **2014**, *80*, 3952–3961. [CrossRef] [PubMed]

40. Marsh, P.; Morris, N.Z.; Wellington, E.M.H. Quantitative molecular detection of *Salmonella typhimurium* in soil and demonstration of persistence of an active but non-culturable population. *FEMS Microbiol. Ecol.* **1998**, *27*, 351–363. [CrossRef]

41. Chen, Z.; Diao, J.; Dharmasena, M.; Ionita, C.; Jiang, X.; Rieck, J. Thermal Inactivation of Desiccation-Adapted *Salmonella* spp. in Aged Chicken Litter. *Appl. Environ. Microbiol.* **2013**, *79*, 7013–7020. [CrossRef] [PubMed]

42. Begley, M.; Hill, C. Stress adaptation in foodborne pathogens. *Annu. Rev. Food Sci. Technol.* **2015**, *6*, 191–210. [CrossRef] [PubMed]

43. Frey, S.K.; Gottschall, N.; Wilkes, G.; Grégoire, D.S.; Topp, E.; Pintar, K.D.M.; Sunohara, M.; Marti, R.; Lapen, D.R. Rainfall-induced runoff from exposed streambed sediments: An important source of water pollution. *J. Environ. Qual.* **2015**, *44*, 236–247. [CrossRef] [PubMed]

44. An, Y.J.; Kampbell, D.H.; Breidenbach, G.P. *Escherichia coli* and total coliforms in water and sediments at lake marinas. *Environ. Pollut.* **2002**, *120*, 771–778. [CrossRef]

45. Grimes, D.J. Release of Sediment-Bound Fecal Coliforms by Dredging. *Appl. Microbiol.* **1975**, *29*, 109–111. [PubMed]

46. D'Aoust, J.Y.; Maurer, J. *Salmonella* species. In *Food Microbiology: Fundamentals and Frontiers*; Doyle, M.P., Beuchat, L.R., Eds.; ASM Press: Washington, DC, USA, 1997.

47. Stephenson, G.R.; Rychert, R.C. Bottom Sediment: A Reservoir of *Escherichia coli* in Rangeland Streams. *J. Range Manag.* **1982**, *35*, 119–123. [CrossRef]

48. Chudoba, E.A.; Mallin, M.A.; Cahoon, L.B.; Skrabal, S.A. Stimulation of fecal bacteria in ambient waters by experimental inputs of organic and inorganic phosphorus. *Water Res.* **2013**, *47*, 3455–3466. [CrossRef] [PubMed]

49. Ferguson, C.M.; Coote, B.G.; Ashbolt, N.J.; Stevenson, I.M. Relationships between indicators, pathogens and water quality in an estuarine system. *Water Res.* **1996**, *30*, 2045–2054. [CrossRef]

50. Tate, R.L. Cultural and Environmental Factors Affecting the Longevity of *Escherichia coli* in Histosols. *Appl. Environ. Microbiol.* **1978**, *35*, 925–929. [PubMed]

51. Zibilske, L.M.; Weaver, R.W. Effect of Environmental Factors on Survival of *Salmonella typhimurium* in Soil1. *J. Environ. Qual.* **1978**, *7*, 593–597. [CrossRef]

52. Fujioka, R.S.; Hashimoto, H.H.; Siwak, E.B.; Young, R.H. Effect of sunlight on survival of indicator bacteria in seawater. *Appl. Environ. Microbiol.* **1981**, *41*, 690–696. [PubMed]

53. Crane, S.R.; Moore, J.A. Modeling enteric bacterial die-off: A review. *Water Air Soil Pollut.* **1986**, *27*, 411–439. [CrossRef]

54. Semenov, A.V.; van Overbeek, L.; Termorshuizen, A.J.; van Bruggen, A.H. Influence of aerobic and anaerobic conditions on survival of *Escherichia coli* O157:H7 and *Salmonella enterica* serovar Typhimurium in Luria-Bertani broth, farm-yard manure and slurry. *J. Environ. Manag.* **2011**, *92*, 780–787. [CrossRef] [PubMed]

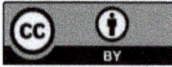

International Journal of
Environmental Research and Public Health

MDPI

Review

Relationships between Microbial Indicators and Pathogens in Recreational Water Settings

Asja Korajkic [1,*], Brian R. McMinn [1] and Valerie J. Harwood [2]

[1] National Exposure Research Laboratory, Office of Research and Development, United States Environmental Protection Agency, 26 West Martin Luther King Drive, Cincinnati, OH 45268, USA; mcminn.brian@epa.gov

[2] Department of Integrative Biology, University of South Florida, 4202 East Fowler Ave, SCA 110, Tampa, FL 33620, USA; vharwood@usf.edu

* Correspondence: korajkic.asja@epa.gov

Received: 16 November 2018; Accepted: 11 December 2018; Published: 13 December 2018

Abstract: Fecal pollution of recreational waters can cause scenic blight and pose a threat to public health, resulting in beach advisories and closures. Fecal indicator bacteria (total and fecal coliforms, *Escherichia coli*, and enterococci), and alternative indicators of fecal pollution (*Clostridium perfringens* and bacteriophages) are routinely used in the assessment of sanitary quality of recreational waters. However, fecal indicator bacteria (FIB), and alternative indicators are found in the gastrointestinal tract of humans, and many other animals and therefore are considered general indicators of fecal pollution. As such, there is room for improvement in terms of their use for informing risk assessment and remediation strategies. Microbial source tracking (MST) genetic markers are closely associated with animal hosts and are used to identify fecal pollution sources. In this review, we examine 73 papers generated over 40 years that reported the relationship between at least one indicator and one pathogen group or species. Nearly half of the reports did not include statistical analysis, while the remainder were almost equally split between those that observed statistically significant relationships and those that did not. Statistical significance was reported less frequently in marine and brackish waters compared to freshwater, and the number of statistically significant relationships was considerably higher in freshwater ($p < 0.0001$). Overall, significant relationships were more commonly reported between FIB and pathogenic bacteria or protozoa, compared to pathogenic viruses (p: 0.0022–0.0005), and this was more pronounced in freshwater compared to marine. Statistically significant relationships were typically noted following wet weather events and at sites known to be impacted by recent fecal pollution. Among the studies that reported frequency of detection, FIB were detected most consistently, followed by alternative indicators. MST markers and the three pathogen groups were detected least frequently. This trend was mirrored by reported concentrations for each group of organisms (FIB > alternative indicators > MST markers > pathogens). Thus, while FIB, alternative indicators, and MST markers continue to be suitable indicators of fecal pollution, their relationship with waterborne pathogens, particularly viruses, is tenuous at best and influenced by many different factors such as frequency of detection, variable shedding rates, differential fate and transport characteristics, as well as a broad range of site-specific factors such as the potential for the presence of a complex mixture of multiple sources of fecal contamination and pathogens.

Keywords: recreational water; fecal indicators; pathogens; relationships

---

1. Introduction

Approximately 39% of the United States (US) population and more than 50% of the global population live near a coastal area [1,2]. Coastal tourism accounts for 85% of all tourism revenue in the US [3], with the average beachgoer spending ~$35 per beach visit [4], resulting in a massive contribution to local economy and national gross domestic product [5,6]. During 2013, approximately 10% of US beach samples (out of total 116,230 samples collected) at 3485 beaches exceeded the US Environmental Protection Agency beach action value (BAV) for fecal indicator bacteria (FIB), indicating unacceptable water quality [5]. Similarly, a more recent report for the European Union (EU) indicated that ~15% of beach samples failed to meet the most stringent "excellent" quality standard at nearly 22,000 coastal beaches and inland sites across EU [7].

Because of a wide array of potential pathogens and typically low concentrations in environmental waters, direct monitoring of waterborne pathogens can be costly, technically challenging, and in some cases not feasible. Therefore, recreational waters are typically monitored for FIB levels instead. Monitoring is intended to ensure that the water body is safe for human recreational contact, and the resulting data are used to determine whether beach advisories or closures are needed. General FIB such as total coliforms, fecal coliforms, *Escherichia coli* and enterococci have been used worldwide for over a century in sanitary assessment of recreational waters [8–12]. The type of FIB measured and values used in recreational water guidelines vary by country [13]. Other general fecal microorganisms, such as *Clostridium perfringens* and various bacteriophages, are considered alternative indicator organisms, and are also frequently measured in various water quality monitoring programs worldwide [13–19]. However, FIB and alternative indicator organisms are common inhabitants of gastrointestinal tracts of mammals and birds [14,20], and their detection in environmental waters provides no information about the source of pollution. Considering that ambient waters can be influenced by multiple point and non-point pollution sources, identification of source is crucial for any remedial efforts and risk assessment determinations since not all fecal sources pose the same risk to human health. For example, human fecal pollution typically presents the greatest risk because of the possible presence of human viral pathogens, while cattle manure may be a close second because of the possible presence of zoonotic pathogens such as *Cryptosporidium* spp. and enteropathogenic *E. coli* [21]. Exposure to gull, chicken, and pig feces carries a known risk, because of possible presence of zoonotic pathogens associated with these animals including hepatitis E virus [22], *Campylobacter* spp., *Brucella* spp., pathogenic *E. coli* and *Salmonella* spp. [23–25]. Microbial source tracking (MST) has emerged in response to a need to identify the source(s) of fecal pollution to better safeguard human health and aid in remediation efforts. The majority of MST genetic markers target the 16S rRNA gene of *Bacteroides* spp., although some amplify other genes and, in some instances, viral targets [13,14]. Earlier technology centered on end-point PCR, which provides a binary, presence/absence result, but more recent studies estimate the concentration of a given MST genetic marker via real-time quantitative PCR (qPCR) [14]. Of note, more rapid technology in lieu of molecular enrichment followed by qPCR is also being developed for monitoring of *Staphylococcus aureus* and *Pseudomonas aeruginosa*, indicator species used to monitor the water quality in swimming pools [26].

The majority of waterborne disease outbreaks associated with recreational use of untreated waters (e.g., lakes and oceans) are caused by pathogenic microorganisms including bacteria, parasites, and viruses, while chemicals (including toxins) accounted for approximately 6% of outbreaks with confirmed etiology [27]. Among the pathogenic bacteria, virulent *Escherichia coli* serotypes (e.g., O157:H7), *Campylobacter* spp., *Legionella* spp., *Shigella* spp., *Salmonella* spp., and *Pseudomonas* spp. were most commonly identified etiologic agents [28–32]. While other protozoan species are occasionally identified as the cause (e.g., *Naegleria* spp.), [27,30], *Cryptosporidium* spp., followed by *Giardia* spp. are etiological agents for the majority of recreational waterborne outbreaks [28,29,31,32]. Regarding viral pathogens, noroviruses and adenoviruses were most frequently identified as causative agents in outbreaks where etiology was confirmed [27,30,32,33]. In treated waters (e.g., swimming pools and spas), *Cryptosporidium* spp. are most often identified as etiological agents [30–32], although noroviruses and adenoviruses are becoming more frequently detected [33]. It is important to note that etiological agents in nearly 30% of outbreaks in the US alone remain unidentified [27], and that sporadic recreational waterborne illnesses not associated with outbreaks are excluded from this report.

Even though the concepts of FIB, alternative indicators, and MST markers were developed to indicate fecal contamination and its sources, the same paradigm is often employed to indicate pathogen presence under the assumption that indicators consistently covary with pathogen presence. The goals of this review are: (1) to examine reported relationships between various indicators and pathogen species to determine the feasibility of indicators as pathogen sentinels in recreational waters; and (2) to identify factors that affect this relationship (or lack thereof). In addition, we also queried epidemiological studies to determine which indicator(s) most commonly correlated with illness in recreational waters. Our search criteria mandated that each study measured at least one indicator (FIB or alternative) or MST marker along with at least one pathogen. We focused on studies conducted in waters intended for primary human contact (e.g., swimming, wading, diving, and surfing) such as beaches and swimming pools, but also included ambient waters used for secondary or non-contact (e.g., boating, fishing) human activities. Our methodology for collecting the manuscripts involved querying "PubMed" (www.ncbi.nlm.nih.gov/pubmed/) and "Google Scholar" (https://scholar.google.com/) databases for following keywords: "recreational water pathogens", "recreational water viral pathogens", "recreational water bacterial pathogens", "recreational water protozoan pathogens", "recreational water fungal pathogens", "swimming pools pathogens", "swimming pools viral pathogens", "swimming pools bacterial pathogens, "swimming pools protozoan pathogens" and "swimming pools fungal pathogens" regardless of the year published. For the purposes of this review, a relationship is identified as a significant correlation (e.g., Pearson Product Momentum Correlation, Wilcoxon signed-rank tests) and/or significant predictive relationship (e.g., binary and other logistic regression modelling). Assumptions made in our analyses included the following: (1) all measurement strategies yielded equivalent results (e.g., various culture-based, molecular and microscopy were equally sensitive); and (2) data were not affected by characteristics of the water samples (e.g., we assumed that the water chemistry did not influence performance of the methods). In total, we collected 73 papers spanning over four decades of research from 25 countries: Argentina, Australia, Bolivia, Brazil, Canada, China, Cyprus, Democratic Republic of Congo, France, Greece, Germany, Hungary, Iceland, Italy, Japan, Luxembourg, Netherlands, New Zealand, Poland, Portugal, South Africa, Taiwan, United Kingdom, US, and Venezuela. The majority of studies were conducted in freshwaters (lakes, rivers and streams), followed by marine/brackish waters and swimming pools (Figure 1). Since some studies were conducted in both fresh and marine/brackish waters, they were included in each water type in Figure 1. This resulted in a total of 126 observations (i.e., report on a relationship between indicator and pathogen) since some studies were conducted in both, marine and freshwater, and/or measured more than one type of indicator or pathogen. The majority of observations ($n = 52$) did not report any relationship between indicator(s) and pathogen(s), while those that did, were split into relationships that were statistically significant ($n = 30$) and those that were not ($n = 44$). Statistically significant relationships (or the lack thereof) and rationale for the observed trends are further examined in the following sections.

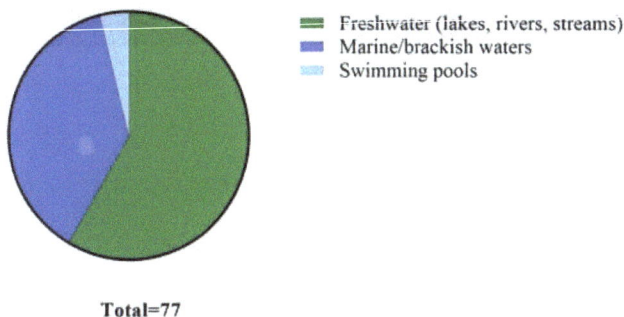

Total=77

Figure 1. Documented relationships between various indicators and pathogens in freshwaters ($n = 45$), marine/brackish waters ($n = 29$) and swimming pools ($n = 3$).

2. Relationships between Indicators and Pathogens in Recreational Waters

We queried studies conducted in marine, brackish, freshwater, and swimming pool waters meeting our search criteria for FIB, alternative indicators, MST markers, and pathogen data. FIB levels were typically reported as colony forming units (CFU), or most probable number (MPN), depending whether studies measured concentrations using membrane filtration on selective-differential media or defined substrate technology (e.g., Enterolert and Colilert), respectively (Tables 1 and 2). However, a few studies quantified general FIB using qPCR and expressed concentrations usually as gene copies per unit volume (Tables 1 and 2). Alternative indicators of fecal pollution such as *C. perfringens* and different bacteriophages [34] were also of interest for inclusion to assess their reliability for estimating pathogen presence compared to general FIB. *C. perfringens* was measured using membrane filtration on selective-differential media with concentrations expressed as CFU per unit volume, while bacteriophage concentrations were usually measured via single or double agar layer (SAL, DAL) techniques, with data expressed as plaque forming units (PFU) per unit volume (Table 3).

Lastly, studies using molecular assays targeting MST markers were gathered to determine any potential relationships with pathogenic organisms. Depending on the detection assay used, MST data was reported as either presence/absence (end-point PCR) or as gene copies (qPCR) per unit volume. Assays for general MST markers included those targeting 16S rRNA gene of *Bacteroidales* spp. (i.e., Bac23F, GenBac3, AllBac), and pepper mild mottle viruses (PMMoV) (Table 4). For human-associated MST markers, most assays targeted 16S rRNA or other functional genes of *Bacteroidales* or *Bacteroidales*-like organisms (e.g., HF183, *gyrB*, *Bfra*, HF134, *B. thetaiotamicron*, BacHum-UCD, *B. dorei*, *B. uniformis*, *B. stericoris*, HumM2, HumM19), as well as 16S rRNA of human -associated *C. coccoides*, *nifH* gene of *Methanobrevibacter smithii*, and *esp* gene of *Enterococcus faecium* (Table 4). Bovine/ruminant-associated MST markers typically target 16S rRNA genes of *Bacteroidales* spp. (e.g., BacCow, CF128, and CF193) or toxin-genes of *E. coli* (e.g., LTIIa), while swine-associated MST markers target *Bacteroidales* spp. (e.g., PF163) or *E. coli* (e.g., STII) (Table 4). Since pets and waterfowl can influence water quality, dog-associated markers have been developed targeting 16S rRNA of *Bacteroidales* spp. (BacCan and DogBac), as well as seagull associated markers targeting 16S rRNA from *Catelicoccus marimammalium* or *Bacteroides* spp. (Gull) (Table 4).

We also gathered data for various bacterial, viral, and protozoan pathogens. For bacterial pathogens, we collected data on 10 genera (*Vibrio*, *Salmonella*, *Shigella*, *Mycobacteria*, *Pseudomonas*, *Escherichia*, *Aeromonas*, *Campylobacter*, *Legionella*, and *Listeria*). Measurement strategies ranged from culture-based (data reported as CFU, MPN or presence/absence) to end-point PCR (presence/absence) and qPCR (gene copies) (Tables 1–4). For viral pathogens, we collected data on eight different species including enteroviruses, adenoviruses, noroviruses, hepatitis A and E, astroviruses, rotaviruses, reoviruses, and sapoviruses. Viral data were expressed as MPN (infectious viruses, ICC-[RT]-PCR), presence/absence (PCR) or gene copies (qPCR) (Tables 1–4). The most frequently measured protozoan pathogens, *Cryptosporidium* spp. and *Giardia* spp. (oo)cysts, were usually enumerated using immunomagnetic separation, followed by staining, although in some instances, qPCR was also performed (Tables 1–4). *Enterocytozoon bieneusi* was measured using similar detection methods to that of *Cryptosporidium* and *Giardia* (oo)cysts (Table 2), while two pathogenic amoeba species (*Acanthamoeba* spp. and *Naegleria fowleri*) were reported as presence/absence (i.e., PCR) (Table 1). Lastly, *Candida* spp. were enumerated using membrane filtration on selective-differential media and reported as CFU (Table 2). Sections below summarize our results regarding relationships that FIB, alternative indicators and MST markers have with pathogens and waterborne illness occurrence in freshwater, marine/brackish waters and swimming pools.

3. FIB and Pathogens in Freshwater

The relationships between FIB and various pathogens in freshwater, and the individual studies from which they were derived, are summarized in Table 1. Of the 41 studies, approximately one third (*n* = 18) [35–52] did not report any relationship between indicators and pathogens measured.

Of the remaining 23 studies, thirteen reported positive relationship between at least one indicator and one pathogen [53–65], while ten did not find significant relationships [66–75]. Please see Table 1 ("relationship" and "comments" columns) for summary of relationships and other comments regarding studies that found no significant relationship or those that did not report it.

Studies that found significant, positive relationships most commonly reported it for *Cryptosporidium/Giardia* (oo)cysts and pathogenic *E. coli* spp., followed by *Salmonella* spp. and *Campylobacter* spp. (Table 1). Relationships were less frequently noted for *Shigella* spp. and adenoviruses, as well as non-fecal pathogens such as *Legionella* spp. and *Acanthamoeba* spp. (Table 1). *E. coli* was the FIB with the greatest number of significant relationships, followed by enterococci, fecal and total coliforms (Table 1). Significant relationships were reported between *E. coli* and pathogenic *E. coli* spp. ($n = 7$), *Cryptosporidium/Giardia* (oo)cysts ($n = 6$), *Salmonella* spp. ($n = 6$), *Campylobacter* spp. ($n = 4$), and adenoviruses ($n = 2$) (Table 1). Enterococci also had the greatest number of statistically significant relationships with pathogenic *E. coli* spp. ($n = 5$), *Cryptosporidium/Giardia* (oo)cysts ($n = 4$), *Salmonella* spp. ($n = 3$), *Campylobacter* spp. ($n = 2$), and adenoviruses ($n = 1$) (Table 1). Fecal coliforms correlated with pathogenic *E. coli* spp. ($n = 5$), followed by *Salmonella* spp. ($n = 3$), *Cryptosporidium/Giardia* (oo)cysts ($n = 2$), and *Campylobacter* and *Shigella* spp. ($n = 1$ each) (Table 1). Statistically significant relationships between total coliforms and different pathogens (pathogenic *E. coli* spp., *Salmonella* spp., *Campylobacter* spp., *Legionella*, and *Acanthamoeba* spp.) were reported only once for each pathogen (Table 1). The methodology employed did not appear to influence the outcome, as significant relationships were not more likely when both indicator and pathogen were measured by a similar technique (Table 1).

The frequency of significant relationships of FIB with bacterial or protozoan pathogens was similar; however, significant relationships with viral pathogens were less frequent (Fisher's exact test, p: 0.0005–0.0022). While lack of relationship between FIB and pathogenic viruses is not surprising given the enormous differences between the two groups in terms of persistence in the environment and low levels of viral pathogens typically found in ambient waters, correlations between FIB and protozoan pathogens are more difficult to understand. Interestingly, when *Cryptosporidium* and *Giardia* spp. were detected, they were generally present in higher concentrations compared to viral pathogens. Significant relationships were reported more commonly for rivers and streams compared to lakes [58–60,62], but this trend was not statistically significant (Fisher's exact test, two-tailed $p = 0.085$). Correlations appeared to be influenced by weather conditions, as most occurred during wet seasons and/or following rainfall events [53,61,63,67,75]. Not surprisingly, correlations were also more likely following sewage spills and/or wastewater discharges [54,56,57,61] and in waters impacted by agricultural operations [57,61], likely due to elevated FIB concentrations, greater likelihood of pathogen presence and the potential for location to be dominated by single fecal source.

Table 1. Relationships between fecal indicator bacteria and various pathogens in freshwater.

Indicator(s) [1]	Pathogen(s) [1]	Location	Relationship [2]	Comments	Reference
E. coli [a]	V. cholerae [b], Salmonella spp. [b], Shigella spp. [b]	Apies River and tributaries, South Africa	NR	All three pathogens frequently co-detected. Concentrations of E. coli and pathogens higher during wet season.	[35]
E. coli [a]	Cryptosporidium and Giardia (oo)cysts [c]	Sure River and tributaries, Luxembourg	Cryptosporidium and Giardia oo(cysts) correlated with each other and with E. coli.	Cryptosporidium and Giardia oo(cysts) frequently co-detected. Concentrations highest during the wet season.	[53]
E. coli [d]	M. avium [d], P. aeruginosa [d], Salmonella spp. [d]	"Aohai See" Lake, China	No significant correlation.	All three pathogens frequently co-detected. Different seasonal patterns observed for E. coli and all three pathogens.	[66]
E. coli [e]	Campylobacter spp. [a], Giardia and Cryptosporidium (oo)cysts [c]	Avon River, New Zealand	E. coli strongly correlated with the all three pathogens.	All three pathogens frequently detected in samples where E. coli > 550 CFU. Higher concentrations of all pathogens found in samples during a large sewage discharge due to earthquake.	[54]
E. coli [a]	Giardia and Cryptosporidium (oo)cysts [c]	Canals connecting Rapipat and Rangsit canals, Thailand	NR	Highest levels of FIB and pathogens found in the most populated area.	[36]
E. coli [e,d], enterococci [e,d]	Cryptosporidium and Giardia (oo)cysts [c]	Chicago area waterways system, various rivers and lakes, USA states	Stronger correlations between FIB and Giardia spp. than Cryptosporidium spp.	Correlations generally stronger in samples not impacted by the wastewater effluent. Associations between pathogens and enterococci generally stronger than with E. coli	[55]
Fecal coliforms [e], E. coli [e] and enterococci [e]	Pathogenic E. coli [b]	St Joseph River and Galien River watersheds in Michigan and Indiana, USA	No significant correlation.	Two or more virulence genes frequently co-detected. Samples with lower FIB levels, typically had a lower proportion of virulence genes.	[67]
E. coli [e], enterococci [e]	Pathogenic E. coli [b], Cryptosporidium and Giardia (oo)cysts [c]	Various streams in Pennsylvania, USA	FIB correlated with all pathogens.	Samples exceeding recreational water quality guidelines more likely to contain pathogenic E. coli genes but not Cryptosporidium and Giardia (oo)cysts. Affected by non-point source and run-off following snow melt and rain events as well.	[56]
E. coli [d]	S. enterica [d], Aeromonas spp. [d], M. avium [d], P. aeruginosa [d]	Ao, Hong and Tao lakes in Beijing, China	No significant correlation.	E. coli and Aeromonas spp. co-detected in all samples. Higher concentrations of E. coli and pathogens in particle attached fraction of the sample.	[68]
Total coliforms [a], E. coli [a], enterococci [a]	P. aeruginosa [a]	Sauce Grande lagoon, Argentina	NR	Pseudomonas aeruginosa was co-detected with all FIB in all samples. All FIB positively correlated with temperature.	[37]
Total coliforms [a], fecal coliforms [a]	Human enterovinuses [b], adenoviruses [b]	Altamaha River, USA	No significant correlation.	Viruses co-detected in 26% of samples. Presence of viruses directly related to dissolved oxygen and streamflow, but inversely related to temperature, rainfall in the last 30 days.	[69]
Total coliforms [a], fecal coliforms [a], E. coli [a], enterococci [e]	Salmonella spp. [b], S. aureus [b]	Msunduzi River, South Africa	NR	Presence of Salmonella spp., Staphylococcus aureus and enterococci frequently coincided with fecal coliform and E. coli levels above 1000 MPN/100 mL. Salmonella spp. not detected in drier, colder months when fecal coliform and E. coli levels were below 1000 MPN/100 mL.	[38]

Table 1. *Cont.*

Indicator(s) [1]	Pathogen(s) [1]	Location	Relationship [2]	Comments	Reference
Fecal coliforms [e], *E. coli* [e], enterococci [e]	Pathogenic *E. coli* [b]	Various rivers in Georgia, Kansas, Michigan, North Carolina, New Jersey, Ohio, South Dakota, Tennessee, Texas and Virginia, USA	Only eaeA gene positively correlated with FIB.	Multiple pathogenic genes co-detected in samples meeting and exceeding FIB guidelines. Some pathogenic genes also detected in three samples that met FIB guidelines. All sites known to be impacted by human fecal pollution and agricultural operations (upstream).	[57]
Enterococci [e]	*Campylobacter* spp. [d]	Various ponds, rivers and creeks in Florida, USA	No significant correlation.	Enterococci and *Campylobacter* spp. frequently co-detected, but enterococci were also detected in samples negative for *Campylobacter*. Florida DOH guidelines would not indicate *Campylobacter* spp. presence.	[70]
Fecal coliforms [e], enterococci [e]	Infectious enteroviruses [a], total enteroviruses [d], hepatitis A [d], Norwalk I and II [d], astroviruses [d], rotaviruses [d]	Rivers in France	NR	Infectious enteroviruses were not detected in samples with elevated fecal coliforms concentrations. Fecal coliforms, but not enterococci fluctuated seasonally.	[59]
Total coliforms [e]	*Legionella* spp. [d]	Hot spring recreational facilities, Taiwan	NR	Most samples failed to meet Taiwan CDC guidelines of 0 total coliforms per 100 mL. No *Legionella* spp. detected in two samples that met Taiwan CDC coliform guidelines.	[10]
E. coli [a]	Pathogenic *E. coli* [d], *Shigella* spp. [d], *Salmonella* spp. [d], *C. jejuni* [d], *L. pneumophila* [d], *L. monocytogenes* [d], *V. cholerae* [d], and *V. parahaemolyticus* [d]	Various streams around Lake Miyajinnuma, Japan	No significant correlation.	Various pathogen genes frequently co-detected. Temporal variation in pathogen concentration was observed with higher levels detected in colder months and when geese were present (not significant).	[71]
E. coli [d]	Human adenovirus [d], *Giardia* and *Cryptosporidium* (oo)cysts [c]	Rivers in France	NR	Highest concentration of adenovirus found at two urban sites. Generally higher concentration of *Giardia* compared to *Cryptosporidium*.	[11]
Total coliforms [e]	*Acanthamoeba* spp. [b,d], *Naegleria* spp. [b,d], *Legionella* spp. [b,d]	Puzih River and two hot springs recreational facilities, Taiwan	*Acanthamoeba* spp. and *Legionella* spp. significantly associated with total coliforms in hot spring samples but not river. No significant correlation for *Naegleria* spp.	*Legionella* detection was significantly correlated with water temperature and more likely in the presence of *Vermamoeba vermiformis*.	[58]
E. coli [a], enterococci [a]	Human adenoviruses [b,d], noroviruses GII [b], and enteroviruses [b]	Danube, Berettyo, Koros and Tisza Rivers and two rivulets (Koloska and Keki), Hungary	NR	In ~1/3 of samples at least two viral targets were co-detected. ~42%, 12% and 14% of designated recreational waters contained adenoviruses, enteroviruses and noroviruses.	[42]
E. coli [a], enterococci [e]	*Salmonella* spp. [b]	Transitional and inland waters, Portugal	Significant correlation commonly observed in waters classified as "poor" and "sufficient" but also seen in waters classified as "good" or "excellent"	Higher geometric mean of FIB in *Salmonella* spp. positive samples than in *Salmonella* spp. negative samples. Even though significant correlation was reported, *Salmonella* was also detected in water samples with "good" and "excellent" water quality.	[60]

Table 1. *Cont.*

Indicator(s) [1]	Pathogen(s) [1]	Relationship [2]	Location	Comments	Reference
Total coliforms [e], *E. coli* [e]	Pathogenic *E. coli* [b]	NR	Sauce Chico River, El Belisario Stream and San Bernardo Stream, Argentina	Shiga-toxin producing *E. coli* found in samples where *E. coli* counts generally exceeded or were close to the US EPA recommended limits. High *E. coli* counts correlated with rainy season.	[43]
Total coliforms [a], fecal coliforms [e]	Rotavirus [b], human Adenovirus [b], human Astrovirus [b], Norovirus [b]	No significant correlation.	Rivers and streams, Brazil	Rotaviruses detected most frequently, followed by adenoviruses. The majority of samples exceeded recommendations for recreational waters from the standard methods used for the examination of water and wastewater of 5000 and 1000 MPN per 100 mL for total and fecal coliforms.	[73]
E. coli [e], enterococci [e]	*Pseudomonus* spp. [e]	NR	Lake Ma Vallee, Democratic Republic of Congo	Samples met European Directive 2006/7/CE for *E. coli* and enterococci. *Pseudomonus* spp. detected at only one site which coincidentally had the highest *E. coli* and enterococci concentrations.	[44]
E. coli [a]	Pathogenic *E. coli* [d], *C. jejuni* [d], *Shigella* spp. [d], *Salmonella* spp. [d]	Beach seasonal mean *C. jejuni* abundance correlated with beach seasonal *E. coli* concentration and at one beach pathogenic *E. coli* abundance was positively correlated with daily *E. coli* concentrations	Michigan, Superior, Huron and Erie lakes, USA	High degree of beach specific temporal variability in pathogenic gene concentrations.	[60]
Fecal coliforms [a]	Pathogenic *E. coli* [b], *Shigella* spp. [b] and *Salmonella* spp. [b]	The occurrence of pathogenic bacteria associated with fecal coliform densities.	La Paz River basin, Bolivia	Approximately 50% of pathogenic bacteria resistant to at least two antibiotics. Pathogens were frequently detected during rainy season at sites impacted by anthropogenic activities.	[61]
E. coli [a], enterococci [a], fecal coliforms [a]	*Cryptosporidium* spp. [c], *Salmonella* spp. [c], *Campylobacter* spp. [a]	NR	Lake Parramatta, Australia	Only *Salmonella* spp. detected sporadically in waters with relatively low FIB concentrations. FIB concentration higher during wet weather.	[45]
E. coli [e]	*Campylobacter* spp. [d], *Legionella* spp. [d], adenovirus [d], *Cryptosporidium* spp. [d]	NR	River, lake ponds and a wadi in Netherlands	*Campylobacter* spp. detected in all samples, *Cryptosporidium* spp. never detected, other pathogens detected sporadically.	[46]
Fecal coliforms [e], *E. coli* [e], enterococci [e]	*Campylobacter* spp. [b], *Salmonella* spp. [b], *E. coli* O157:H7 [d], *Cryptosporidium* and *Giardia* (oo)cysts [c], astroviruses [b], hepatitis A [b] and E [b] viruses, rotavirus [b], norovirus [b], enterovirus [b]	NR	Canals and lakes, Netherlands	Arboviruses, hepatitis A and E viruses and *E. coli* O157:H7 were not detected in any of the samples. Rotavirus, norovirus, enterovirus *Salmonella* and *Campylobacter* spp. detected sporadically. Infectious enteroviruses found in one sample. Low concentration of *Cryptosporidium* and *Giardia* (oo)cysts detected in samples that complied with the European bathing water legislation.	[47]
Total coliforms [e]	*L. pneumophila* [d]	Total coliforms and *L. pneumophila* significantly correlated.	Puzih River and hot spring recreational areas, Taiwan	*L. pneumophila* detected in > 90% of samples. *L. pneumophila* and total coliforms also correlated with turbidity.	[62]

Table 1. *Cont.*

Indicator(s)[1]	Pathogen(s)[1]	Relationship[2]	Location	Comments	Reference
E. coli[e], enterococci[e]	Shiga toxin genes[d]	No significant correlation.	Lake Erie and tributaries, USA	Abundance and distributions of shiga-toxin genes highly variable. The majority of samples positive for shiga toxin genes were below the advisory threshold levels for *E. coli* and enterococci.	[74]
E. coli[e], enterococci[e], fecal coliforms[e]	Cryptosporidium and Giardia (oo)cysts[c], infectious enteroviruses[a], Salmonella spp[a]	NR	Lake Carroll, Tampa, FL	Higher concentrations of indicators and more frequent pathogen detection following rain events.	[48]
E. coli[e]	Human adenovirus[d], human enterovirus[d], Norovirus GI and GII[d]	No significant correlation.	Delaware Lake, Madison Lake and East Fork Lake, USA	Adenoviruses detected more frequently than enteroviruses, followed by noroviruses. Human adenovirus and enterovirus correlated.	[72]
E. coli[a], total coliforms[a], enterococci[e]	Campylobacter spp.[a], Salmonella spp.[a], P. aeruginosa[a], Cryptosporidium and Giardia (oo)cysts[c], Aeromonas spp.[e]	NR	River Ruhr and barrier lakes, Germany	All sampling sites achieved "sufficient" bathing water quality for enterococci but not *E. coli*. With the exception of *Aeromonas* spp., detection of all other pathogens was sporadic. Precipitation preceding sampling event resulted in elevated concentration of total coliforms, *E. coli*, enterococci, *Aeromonas* spp. and *Cryptosporidium* and *Giardia* (oo)cysts.	[49]
E. coli[e], enterococci[e]	Pseudomonas spp.[e], Norovirus[d]	NR	Geothermal pools, Iceland	High concentrations of *Pseudomonas* spp. detected in samples that also contained high FIB counts. Norovirus was not detected.	[50]
E. coli[d], enterococci[d]	S. aureus[d], Salmonella spp.[d], noroviruses[d]	NR	Prickett Creek, USA	No correlation between *E. coli* and enterococci.	[51]
Total coliforms[e], fecal coliforms[e], E. coli[e], enterococci[e]	L. monocytogenes[b], Salmonella spp.[b], E. coli O157:H7[b], Campylobacter spp.[b], Cryptosporidium and Giardia (oo)cysts[c]	Weak relationships, but mostly positive (except *L. monocytogenes*).	South Nation River basin, Canada	The fraction of samples that contained an indicator when pathogen was detected was highest for the protozoan parasites. Relationships dependent on season and site.	[63]
E. coli[a], enterococci[a]	Human adenoviruses[b]	Concentrations of all indicators correlated with frequency of adenovirus detection.	Various rivers and lakes in France, Germany, Italy, Netherlands, Poland, United Kingdom	> 50% of samples positive for adenovirus. *E. coli* concentrations higher than enterococci.	[64]
E. coli[a], enterococci[a]	Adenoviruses[d], norovirus GI[b] and GII[b]	NR	Various rivers and lakes in France, Germany, Italy, Netherlands, Poland, United Kingdom	Both viruses frequently detected in samples that met "good" water quality guidelines for both *E. coli* and enterococci. Adenoviruses detected more frequently than noroviruses.	[52]
Total coliforms[a], fecal coliforms[a], E. coli[a], enterococci[e]	Salmonella spp.[f], pathogenic E. coli[f], Cryptosporidium and Giardia (oo)cysts[c]	Significant but weak correlations between indicators and *Salmonella* spp. and pathogenic *E. coli*.	Wanzhou watershed, China	*Cryptosporidium* and *Giardia* (oo)cysts detected in samples with low indicator concentrations. Concentrations of indicators influenced by rainfall.	[65]
Total coliforms[a]	Cryptosporidium and Giardia (oo)cysts[c]	No significant correlation	Lake Tianjin, China	Significant correlation between *Cryptosporidium* and *Giardia* (oocysts). *Giardia* detected more frequently.	[75]

[1] Data reporting: most probable number (MPN)[a], Presence/absence[b], total (oo)cysts[c], gene copies[d], colony forming units (CFU)[e], Integrated cell culture (ICC)/MPN PCR[f].
[2] NR (not reported).

141

4. FIB and Pathogens in Marine and Brackish Water

Table 2 lists general FIB and pathogen relationships reported in the datasets analyzed for marine and brackish waters. Of the 29 studies reviewed, almost half ($n = 13$) did not report statistical analysis of the relationships [52,76–87]. Within the remaining studies, ten did not find a relationship [64,70,88–95] while six reported a positive relationship between at least one indicator and one pathogen [59,96–100]. Statistical significance was reported less frequently in marine and brackish waters compared to freshwater (17 vs. 44) and the proportion of statistically significant relationships (compared to non-significant) was considerably higher in freshwater (Fisher's exact test, $p < 0.0001$). Please see Table 2 ("relationship" and "comments" columns) for a summary of relationships and other comments regarding studies that found no significant relationship or those that did not report it.

Significant relationships with FIB were most commonly reported for *Salmonella* spp., followed by adenoviruses, and *Campylobacter* spp., *Vibrio* spp., *S. aureus*, and protozoan pathogens (Table 2). The most significant relationships with pathogens were reported for enterococci ($n = 11$), followed by *E. coli* ($n = 4$), and fecal coliforms ($n = 2$). No statistically significant relationships were reported for total coliforms. Significant relationships were reported between enterococci and adenoviruses ($n = 8$), *Salmonella* spp. ($n = 4$), *Cryptosporidium/Giardia* (oo)cysts ($n = 4$), *Campylobacter* spp. ($n = 3$), and *Candida* spp., *Vibrio* spp., *S. aureus*, noroviruses, and *E. bieneusi* (one observation each) (Table 2). *E. coli* formed significant relationships with *Salmonella* spp. and *Vibrio* spp. ($n = 1$ each) and adenoviruses ($n = 2$). Statistically significant relationships with fecal coliforms were reported only for adenoviruses (28.6%, $n = 7$). The methodology employed did not appear to influence the outcome; significant relationships were not more likely when both indicator and pathogen were measured by a similar technique (Table 2).

As expected, FIB had more significant relationships with bacterial pathogens compared to viral pathogens (Fisher's exact, $p = 0.0069$), but there was no significant difference in other comparisons (i.e., FIB relationships with bacterial compared to protozoan pathogens, or FIB relationships with protozoan compared to viral pathogens). Of note, FIB most likely to correlate with pathogens were enterococci, which supports its recommended use to monitor marine recreational water quality. No clear trend for different marine water types (e.g., brackish waters and coastal beaches) was observed with respect to statistically significant indicator/pathogen relationships [59,96,98–101], suggesting that hydrological factors play less of a role compared to freshwaters. Similar to freshwater, the common trend among the studies reporting significant relationships was that they were conducted in waters impacted by fecal contamination [96,98,99], and when bather numbers were high [97], conditions likely to result in elevated FIB and pathogen levels.

Table 2. Relationships between fecal indicator bacteria and various pathogens in brackish and marine waters.

Indicator(s) [1]	Pathogen(s) [1]	Location	Relationship [2]	Comments	Reference
Fecal coliforms [e], E. coli [e], enterococci [a,d,e]	V. vulnificus [e], S. aureus [e], enterovirus [d], norovirus [d], hepatitis A virus [d], Cryptosporidium and Giardia (oo)cysts [c]	Virginia Key Beach, Florida, USA	NR	When HPyV, V. vulnificus, and Giardia spp. were detected so were all indicators and alternative indicators. When FIB levels exceeded regulatory standards, HPyVs and pathogens also detected.	[77]
Fecal coliforms [e], E. coli [e], enterococci [d,e]	V. vulnificus [e], S. aureus [e], norovirus [d], hepatitis A virus [d], Cryptosporidium and Giardia (oo)cysts [c]	Coastal Beaches, Miami Dade County, Florida, USA	NR	When enterococci levels by qPCR and CS exceeded MDL, Cryptosporidium, Giardia, enteroviruses and V. vulnificus were co-detected.	[76]
Enterococci [e]	Cryptosporidium and Giardia (oo)cysts [c]	Coastal beaches, Venezuela	No significant correlation.	Presence of Cryptosporidium and Giardia were significantly correlated.	[88]
E. coli [e], enterococci [e]	C. albicans [b], Salmonella spp. [b]	Saronicos Gulf, Athens, Greece	Enterococci but not E. coli correlated with Salmonella spp., but not C. albicans.	Pathogens detected in waters of "good" and "excellent" quality.	[16]
Total coliforms [a], fecal coliforms [a]	Salmonella spp. [b]	Canals around Galveston Bay, TX, USA	NR	Salmonella spp. detection occurred (nearly 100%) when FC concentrations >2000/100 mL.	[78]
Enterococci [a]	C. parvum [c], G. lamblia [c], G. duodenalis [c] E. bieneusi [c]	Maryland, US Chesapeake Bay, USA	C. parvum, G. duodenalis and E. bieneusi correlated with enterococci counts.	Correlations observed especially apparent with high bather numbers in water.	[97]
Enterococci [a,d], E. coli [a,d], fecal coliforms [a], total coliforms [a]	L. pneumophila [b], S. aureus [b], MRSA [b], adenovirus [b], enterovirus [d], Hepatitis A [d], Norovirus [d]	Malibu beach, California USA	NR	No indicator used had a significant correlation with GI illness in swimmers or any reference pathogen.	[79]
Enterococci [e]	Campylobacter spp. [d]	Florida, Quietwater Beach, USA	No significant correlation.	Enterococci co-detected with pathogenic Campylobacter spp., but levels of enterococci were not indicative of levels of Campylobacter present.	[70]
E. coli [a], enterococci [a]	Salmonella spp. [b], Campylobacter spp. [a], Cryptosporidium and Giardia (oo)cysts [c], adenoviruses [a] enteroviruses [a]	Estuaries, Melbourne Australia	No significant correlation.	Changes in FIB concentrations associated with changes in temperature, flow, humidity and rainfall.	[89]
Total coliforms [e], fecal coliforms [e], E. coli [e], enterococci [e]	Adenoviruses [a]	Southern California coastal waters, USA	No significant correlation.	5 of 12 sites, FIB exceeded CA recreational water quality limits.	[90]
Total coliforms [e], fecal coliforms [e], enterococci [e]	Adenoviruses [b], enteroviruses [b], hepatitis A [b]	Rivers and creeks in California, USA	No significant correlation.	FIB and viral pathogen detection associated with storm events. Total and fecal coliforms correlated with each other but not enterococci.	[91]
Total coliforms [a], fecal coliforms [a], enterococci [a]	Enterovirus [b], adenoviruses [b]	Newport Bay, California, USA	No significant correlation	FIB concentrations showed strong seasonal pattern, associated with winter storms. Total and fecal coliforms correlated with each other but not enterococci.	[92]

Table 2. *Cont.*

Indicator(s) [1]	Pathogen(s) [1]	Location	Relationship [2]	Comments	Reference
Fecal coliforms [e], E. coli [e], enterococci [e]	Salmonella spp. [b], enteric viruses [b]	Ben T. Davis and Bahia beaches, Florida, USA	NR	Salmonella spp. not detected. Coxsackie B4 detected following major sewage spill FIB correlated with rainfall.	[80]
Fecal coliforms [e], enterococci [e]	Cryptosporidium and Giardia (oo)cysts [c] enteroviruses [a]	Sarasota Bay, Florida, USA	NR	FIB co-detected with all samples positive for enteric pathogens.	[81]
E. coli [e], enterococci [e]	Salmonella spp. [e]	Coastal Waters, Portugal	Levels of FIB correlated with presence of Salmonella spp., especially in waters deemed "poor" or "sufficient" compared to "excellent".	Salmonella spp. also detected in samples classified as "Good" or "Excellent".	[59]
Fecal coliforms [e], E. coli [e], enterococci [e]	Adenovirus [b]	Hillsborough River and St. Johns River, Florida, USA	Presence of adenovirus strongly correlated with concentrations of all three FIB.	Samples collected in waters with known human fecal pollution, all FIB exceeded regulatory standards.	[96]
E. coli [e], fecal coliforms [e], enterococci [e]	Adenovirus [b]	Hillsborough River, FL Tampa Bay Beach, Florida, USA	E. coli, enterococci and fecal coliforms correlated with adenovirus.	All FIB concentrations exceeded regulatory standards in samples.	[99]
Enterococci [e], fecal coliforms [e], total coliforms [e], E. coli [e]	Adenovirus [b]	Avalon and Doheny Beaches, California	No significant correlation.	FIB concentrations frequently exceeded recreational water quality guidelines. Adenoviruses frequently detected at Doheny beach, but not Avalon.	[93]
Total coliforms [e], fecal coliforms [e], enterococci [e], E. coli [e]	Enteroviruses [e]	Coastal beaches, Barcelona, Spain	NR	All samples with elevated FIB levels also had high levels of somatic and F-specific phage present. 55% of samples having infectious virus beach quality was within EU standards for levels of FIB.	[82]
Enterococci [a], fecal coliforms [a], E. coli [a], total coliforms [a]	Enterovirus [a], Cryptosporidium and Giardia (oo)cysts [c]	St. Lucie Estuary, Florida, USA	No significant correlation.	Viruses detected in samples where FIB levels were within regulatory limits.	[94]
Enterococci [a,d]	Adenovirus [b], Norovirus [d], Cryptosporidium and Giardia (oo)cysts [c], C. jejuni, Salmonella spp. [b], S. aureus [b], E. coli O157-H7 [b]	Coastal beaches, Florida, USA	NR	FIB and pathogens co-detected Seawater samples taken near sewage discharges.	[83]
Enterococci [e]	V. vulnificus [e], V. parahaemolyticus [e]	Chesapeake, Bay, MD, USA	NR	Enterococci were co-detected with V. vulnificus and V. parahaemolyticus.	[84]

Table 2. *Cont.*

Indicator(s) [1]	Pathogen(s) [1]	Location	Relationship [2]	Comments	Reference
Enterococci [e]	*V. vulnificus* [e], *V. parahaemolyticus* [e]	Chesapeake, Bay MD, USA	NR	Enterococci were co-detected with *V. vulnificus* and *V. parahaemolyticus*. All *V. vulnificus* isolates susceptible to 14 of 26 antibiotics and *V. parahaemolyticus* to 11 of 26 antibiotics. All samples positive for enterococci and *Vibrio* spp. and within local recreational water quality guidelines.	[85]
Total coliforms [e], fecal coliforms [e], *E. coli* [e], enterococci [e]	Hepatitis A [b], Norovirus GI [b]	Coastal beaches, Lisbon, Portugal	No significant correlation.	All samples considered "good" quality based on local recreational water quality guidelines.	[95]
Enterococci [a,e]	*S. aureus* [e]	Coastal beaches, Miami, Florida, USA	NR	*S. aureus* was found in 37% of total samples, 1.1% positive for MRSA. Enterococci had a positive correlation with reports of skin illness.	[86]
E. coli [e], enterococci [e]	*Salmonella* spp. [a], *Campylobacter* spp. [a], *S. aureus* [e], *V. vulnificus* [e], *V. parahaemolyticus* [e]	Hawaii streams, USA	*Salmonella, Campylobacter* and *C. jejuni* positively associated with enterococci and marginally associated with *S. aureus*. *V. vulnificus* was positively associated with all FIB, *V. parahaemolyticus* with *E. coli*.	Detection of at least one pathogens occurred in 21 of 22 streams tested.	[100]
Fecal coliforms [e], enterococci [e]	Enteroviruses [b]	Florida Keys, Florida, USA	NR	Enterovirus co-detected with fecal coliforms, enterococci. No sites in violation of water quality standards.	[87]
E. coli [a], enterococci [a]	Human Adenovirus [b]	Coastal beaches in Cyprus, Italy, Portugal, Spain and United Kingdom	No significant correlation.	FIB levels significantly lower in seawater than in freshwater samples.	[64]
E. coli [e], enterococci [e]	Human adenovirus [b] norovirus [b] GI and GII	Coastal beaches in Cyprus, Italy, Portugal, Spain and United Kingdom	NR	Beaches considered "clean" based on FIB levels were positive for both adenovirus and noroviruses. Freshwater sites had higher frequency of virus detection than marine sites.	[52]

[1] Data reporting: most probable number (MPN) [a], Presence/absence [b], total (oo)cysts [c], gene copies [d], colony forming units (CFU/PFU) [e], Integrated cell culture (ICC)/MPN PCR [f]. [2] NR (not reported).

5. Alternative Indicators and Pathogens in Marine, Brackish and Freshwater

Ten studies conducted in freshwater and fourteen studies conducted in brackish and marine waters measured at least one alternative indicator and one pathogen. In freshwater, four studies measured *C. perfringens*, five studies measured bacteriophage, and one study measured both (Table 3). In brackish/marine waters, the majority (*n* = 12) of studies measured coliphage (somatic, F-specific), followed by *C. perfringens* (*n* = 7), and phages infecting *Bacteroides thetaiotaomicron* (*n* = 1) (Table 3). Similar to FIB, more statistically significant relationships were reported in freshwater compared to brackish/marine waters (Fisher's exact test, *p* = 0.0057). Please see Table 3 ("relationship" and "comments" columns) for summary of relationships and other comments regarding studies that found no significant relationship or those that did not report it.

In freshwater, half of studies (*n* = 5) did not report statistical analysis [41,45,47,49,102], four reported at least one statistically significant relationship [54,63,64,103], while a single study reported a non-significant relationship [39] (Table 3). Statistically significant relationships were reported more frequently for *C. perfringens*, followed by F-specific and somatic coliphages (Table 3). *C. perfringens* had positive relationships with *Campylobacter* spp. (*n* = 2), and *Listeria* spp., *Salmonella* spp. and pathogenic *E. coli* spp. (one observation each). F-specific coliphage correlated with noroviruses, *Cryptosporidium/Giardia* (oo)cysts, and *Campylobacter* spp. (one observation each) while somatic coliphage correlated only with adenoviruses (*n* = 2). Similar to FIB, the observed correlations occurred in waters affected by sewage discharge [54], following rainfall events [103], and were affected by season and sampling site [63].

In marine and brackish waters, approximately, half of studies (*n* = 6) did not report any statistical analysis [76,77,81,82,87,89], while three reported statistically significant relationships [79,90,100], and five reported non-significant relationships [64,88,91,92,94]. Two studies found significant relationships between F-specific coliphage and pathogens; one reported it with methicillin resistant *S. aureus* (MRSA), and *S. aureus* at a marine beach affected by fecal-impacted freshwater intrusion [79], while a second reported it for adenoviruses in water impacted by urban run-off [90] (Table 3). No studies noted a significant relationship between somatic coliphage and pathogens (Table 3). Only a single study conducted in Hawaii [100], a state that recommends using *C. perfringens* for monitoring ambient waters [104], found a relationship between this indicator, and two pathogens (*Campylobacter* spp., and *V. parahaemolyticus*) (Table 3). The methodology employed did not appear to influence the outcome in marine or freshwaters; significant relationships were not more likely when both indicator and pathogen were measured by a similar technique (Table 3). While there were insufficient data to perform statistical analyses regarding relationship of alternative indicators and different pathogen groups, F-specific coliphage tended to perform better compared to somatic coliphage and *C. perfringens*.

Table 3. Relationship of alternative indicators of fecal pollution and pathogens in freshwater and marine/brackish waters.

Indicator(s) [1]	Pathogen(s) [1]	Location	Relationship [2]	Comments	Reference
			Freshwater		
C. perfringens [e], F-RNA coliphage [e]	Campylobacter spp. [a], Giardia and Cryptosporidium (oo)cysts [c]	Avon River, Christchurch, New Zealand	F-RNA more strongly correlated with all three pathogens than C. perfringens.	F-RNA concentrations typically higher than C. perfringens. Study conducted in river affected by sewage discharge.	[74]
Somatic coliphage [e]	Infectious enteroviruses [a], total enteroviruses [d], hepatitis A [d], Norwalk I and II [d], astroviruses [d], rotaviruses [d]	Rivers in France	No significant correlation.	Enterovirus genomes and somatic coliphage frequently co-detected. Infectious enteroviruses and hepatitis A, Norwalk I and II, astroviruses, rotaviruses detected in only one or two samples.	[39]
C. perfringens [e]	Human adenovirus [d], Giardia and Cryptosporidium (oo)cysts [c]	Rivers in France	NR	Highest concentration of protozoan parasites and C. perfringens found at the site with high proportion of agricultural operations, forests and semi-natural environments.	[41]
Somatic and F+ coliphage [e]	Noroviruses [f], rotaviruses [f], infectious reoviruses and enteroviruses [a]	Maas and Waal Rivers, Netherlands	NR	Both coliphages and all viruses co-detected in all samples. Coliphage concentrations higher than pathogenic virus concentrations.	[102]
Somatic and F+ coliphage [e]	Noroviruses [d], adenoviruses [d], astroviruses [d], rotaviruses [d]	Marine Reservoir and tributaries, Singapore	F+ coliphage positively correlated with norovirus concentrations.	Higher statistical correlation observed between enteric viruses than between enteric viruses and coliphages. Noroviruses most abundant, followed by rotaviruses. Wet weather concentration of coliphage and viruses higher than dry weather concentration, but difference is not statistically significant.	[103]
C. perfringens [e]	Cryptosporidium spp. [c], Salmonella spp. [b], Campylobacter spp. [a]	Lake Parramatta, Australia	NR	No Cryptosporidium detected which coincided with the low C. perfringens concentrations. C. perfringens concentration lower than FIB.	[45]
Somatic and F+ coliphages [e]	Campylobacter spp. [a], Salmonella spp. [b], E. coli O157:H7 [d], Cryptosporidium and Giardia (oo)cysts [c], astroviruses [b], hepatitis A and E viruses [b], rotavirus [b], norovirus [b], enterovirus [a]	Canals and lakes, Netherlands	NR	Somatic coliphage detected more frequently and at higher concentrations compared to F+ coliphage. Highest concentrations of bacteriophages occurred following a heavy rainfall.	[47]
C. perfringens [e]	Campylobacter spp. [a], Salmonella spp. [a], P. aeruginosa [f], Cryptosporidium and Giardia (oo)cysts [c], Aeromonas spp. [e]	River Ruhr and barrier lakes, Germany	NR	Concentrations typically lower and less variable compared to the FIB. No association with precipitation.	[49]

Table 3. *Cont.*

Indicator(s) [1]	Pathogen(s) [1]	Location	Relationship [2]	Comments	Reference
C. perfringens [e]	L. monocytogenes [b], Salmonella spp. [b], E. coli O157:H7 [b], Campylobacter spp. [b], Cryptosporidium and Giardia (oo)cysts [c]	South Nation River basin, Canada	Positive, but weak relationships with pathogens.	Correlations with FIB were also weak but positive.	[63]
Somatic coliphage [e]	Human adenoviruses [b]	Various rivers and lakes in France, Germany, Italy, Netherlands, Poland, United Kingdom	Concentrations of somatic coliphage correlated with frequency of adenovirus detection.	FIB showed better correlation with adenovirus than somatic coliphage. Somatic coliphage concentrations comparable to E. coli concentrations.	[64]
Marine, and brackish waters					
C. perfringens [e]	V. vulnificus [b], S. aureus [e], enterovirus [d], norovirus [d], hepatitis A virus [d], Cryptosporidium and Giardia (oo)cysts [c]	Virginia Key Beach, Florida, USA	NR	Higher concentrations in high tide samples as opposed to low tide. Not correlated with FIB.	[77]
C. perfringens [e], F+ coliphage [e]	V. vulnificus [e], S. aureus [e], enterovirus [d], norovirus [d], hepatitis A virus [d], Cryptosporidium and Giardia (oo)cysts [c]	Coastal Beaches, Miami Dade County, Florida, USA	NR	High levels of C. perfringens also signaled high levels of all FIB.	[76]
C. perfringens [a]	Cryptosporidium and Giardia (oo)cysts [c]	Coastal beaches, Venezuela	No significant correlation.	Detection of C. perfringens coincided with human-associated MST markers.	[88]
F+ coliphage [e]	L. pneumophila [b], S. aureus [b], MRSA [b], adenovirus [b], enterovirus [d], Hepatitis A [d], Norovirus [d]	Malibu beach, California USA	F+ coliphage had strong association with MRSA and S. aureus presence.	F+ coliphage had strong association with GI illness.	[79]
C. perfringens [e] and F+ coliphage [e]	Salmonella spp. [b], Campylobacter spp. [a], Cryptosporidium and Giardia (oo)cysts [c], adenoviruses [a], enteroviruses [a]	Docklands, South Yarra and Abbotsford estuaries, Melbourne Australia	NR	Positive correlation between the presence of C. perfringens and F+ coliphage.	[89]
Somatic [e] and F+ coliphage [e]	Adenoviruses [a]	Southern California coastal waters, USA	Presence of adenovirus was significantly correlated with F-specific coliphage.	No correlation between two coliphage types.	[90]
Somatic [e] and F+ coliphage [e]	Adenoviruses [b], enteroviruses [b], hepatitis A [b]	Rivers and creeks in California, USA	No significant correlation.	Somatic coliphages detected more frequently than F+. Somatic coliphage were not correlated with total coliforms, but F+ coliphage were positively correlated with total/fecal coliforms but not enterococci.	[91]
F+ coliphage [a]	Enterovirus [b], adenoviruses [b]	Newport Bay, California, USA	No significant correlation.	Peak concentrations of FIB and F+ coliphage associated with winter storms.	[92]
C. perfringens [e] and coliphage [e]	Cryptosporidium and Giardia (oo)cysts [c], enteroviruses [a]	Sarasota Bay, Florida, USA	NR	Alternative indicators for co-detected in samples positive for enteric pathogens. Coliphage levels were significantly influenced by salinity and turbidity.	[81]

Table 3. *Cont.*

Indicator(s) [1]	Pathogen(s) [1]	Location	Relationship [2]	Comments	Reference
		Marine, and brackish waters			
Somatic [e] and F+ coliphage [e], phages infecting *Bacteroides thetaiotaomicron* GA17 [e]	Enteroviruses [e]	Coastal Waters, Portugal	NR	Enteroviruses were co-detected with FIB. Genogroup I and II F-specific RNA more common in samples the others. Densities of somatic coliphage were higher than FIB densities and did not correlate with them.	[82]
Somatic [e] and F+ coliphage [e]	Enterovirus [a], *Cryptosporidium* and *Giardia* (oo)cysts [c]	St. Lucie Estuary, Florida, USA	No significant correlation.	Somatic coliphage concentrations higher than F+ coliphage. Somatic coliphage correlated with the total coliform concentrations.	[94]
C. perfringens [e] and F+ coliphage [e]	*Salmonella* spp. [a], *Campylobacter* spp. [a], *S. aureus* [e], *V. vulnificus* [e], *V. parahaemolyticus* [e]	Hawaii streams, USA	*C. perfringens* was marginally associated with *Campylobacter* spp. and *V. parahaemolyticus*.	Concentrations of *C. perfringens* and F+ coliphage comparable.	[100]
C. perfringens [e], F+ coliphage [e]	Enteroviruses [b]	Florida Keys, Florida, USA	NR	Enteroviruses co-detected with *C. perfringens* and coliphage.	[87]
Somatic coliphage [e]	Human Adenovirus [b]	Coastal beaches in Cyprus, Italy, Portugal, Spain and United Kingdom	No significant correlation.	Somatic coliphage concentrations lower than FIB.	[94]

[1] Data reporting: most probable number (MPN) [a], Presence/absence [b], total (oo)cysts [c], gene copies [d], colony forming units or plaque forming units (CFU/PFU) [e], Integrated cell culture (ICC)/MPN (RT)PCR [f]. [2] NR (not reported).

6. MST Markers and Pathogens in Marine, Brackish and Freshwater

The number of studies that measured MST marker(s) along with at least one pathogen is considerably smaller (*n* = 19; eight in freshwater, and 11 in brackish/marine/waters) compared to studies measuring FIB or alternative indicators (Table 4). The majority of MST measurements reported were for human-associated marker(s) (76.1%), followed by general MST markers (7.0%), cattle and dog associated MST markers (5.6%), and seagull and swine-associated MST markers (2.8%) (Table 4). Most frequently measured pathogens were viruses (adenovirus, enterovirus, noroviruses, hepatitis, and infectious enteric viruses) and bacteria (*E. coli*, *Campylobacter* spp., *Salmonella* spp., *V. vulnificus*, *S. aureus*, and *Legionella* spp.) with 22 measurements each, while *Cryptosporidium* and *Giardia* (oo)cysts were reported less frequently (*n* = 6) (Table 4). Irrespective of the water type, nine of these studies did not report statistical analyses for relationships between MST marker(s) and pathogens [51,76,77,79,80,83,86,88,105], and another seven reported non-significant relationship [48,56,57,70,72,98,99]. The remaining two studies reported statistically significant relationship [93,106] (Table 4). Please see Table 4 ("relationship" and "comments" columns) for summary of relationships and other comments regarding studies that found no significant relationship or those that did not report it.

Significant relationships between pathogens and human-associated MST markers were reported for HF183 and adenoviruses, at a marine beach impacted by non-point source(s) [93], and between HF183/HF134 and *Campylobacter* spp. in freshwater affected by livestock operations [106]. In the same freshwater study, cattle-associated MST markers (CF128, CF193) correlated with *E. coli* O157:H7, and *Salmonella* spp., while a general *Bacteroidales* MST marker (Bac32F) correlated with all three pathogens [106]. The methodology employed did not appear to influence the outcome; in other words, significant relationships were not more likely when both indicator and pathogen were measured by a similar technique (Table 4). There were insufficient data regarding relationship of MST markers and different pathogen groups (e.g., bacterial, viral and protozoan) to perform statistical analyses. While it may seem counter-intuitive that MST markers (particularly human-associated subset), were not generally correlated with pathogens, it is important to note that sensitivity and specificity of MST markers varies greatly [14]. Furthermore, many pathogens reported in these studies are zoonotic, making this relationship even more tenuous.

Table 4. Relationships between MST markers and various pathogens in in freshwater and marine/brackish waters.

MST marker [1]	Pathogens [1]	Location	Relationship [2]	Comments	Reference
		Freshwater			
esp [a], LTIIa [a], STII [a]	Pathogenic E. coli spp. [a], Cryptosporidium and Giardia (oo)cysts [b]	Various streams in Pennsylvania, USA	No significant correlation.	All MST markers detected more frequently in samples exceeding recreational water quality guidelines.	[56]
esp [a]	Pathogenic E. coli spp. [a]	Various rivers in Georgia, Kansas, Michigan, North Carolina, New Jersey, Ohio, South Dakota, Tennessee, Texas and Virginia, USA	No significant correlation.	esp was present in nine samples that met exceeding recreational water quality guidelines.	[57]
HPyV [a], nifH [a], HF183 [a]	Campylobacter spp. [c]	Various ponds, rivers and creeks in Florida, USA	No significant correlation.	Campylobacter and MST markers co-detected at only one site. HPyV and nifH were not detected during the study.	[70]
gyrB [c], g-Bfra [c]	Human adenovirus [c], human enterovirus [c], Norovirus GI and GII [c], porcine sapovirus [c]	Delaware Lake, Madison Lake and East Fork Lake, USA	No significant correlation.	g-Bfra detected more frequently and at higher concentrations than gyrB. gyrB and g-Bfra frequently correlated.	[72]
esp [d], HPyV [a], HF183 [a]	Cryptosporidium and Giardia (oo)cysts [b], infectious enteroviruses [d], Salmonella spp. [d]	Lake Carroll, Tampa, FL	No significant correlation.	Higher concentrations of indicators and more frequent pathogen detection following rain events. esp, but not HPyV or HF183 correlated with FIB (E. coli, enterococci, fecal coliforms).	[48]
Bac32F [a], CF128 [a], CF193 [a], HF134 [a], HF183 [a], PF163 [a]	E. coli O157:H7 [a], Salmonella spp. [a], Campylobacter spp. [a]	Little Bow and Oldman Rivers, Canada	Positive relationship between detection of Bac32F and all pathogens. Positive relationship between CF128/193 and E. coli O157:H7 and Salmonella spp. Positive relationship between HF183/134 and Campylobacter spp.	Bac32F detected most frequently, followed by CF128/193, PF163 and HF183/134. Pathogens were detected infrequently with Campylobacter spp. most commonly detected. Water impacted by agricultural operations.	[106]
HPyV [c], HF183 [c], AllBac [c]	S. aureus [c] Salmonella spp. [c], noroviruses [c]	Prickett Creek, USA	NR	Salmonella spp. were most frequently detected pathogen.	[51]
esp [a]	Infectious enteric viruses [a]	Lake Michigan, USA	NR	Precipitation and turbidity positively correlated with viruses.	[105]
		Marine and brackish waters			
HPyV [a], esp [a]	V. vulnificus [c], S. aureus [c], enterovirus [c], norovirus [c], hepatitis A [c] virus, Cryptosporidium and Giardia (oo)cysts [b]	Virginia Key Beach, Florida, USA	NR	HPyV, V. vulnificus, Giardia spp. were co-detected with all FIB and alternative indicators. When FIB levels exceeded regulatory standards, HPyVs and pathogens also detected.	[77]
HPyV [a], esp [a], Bacteroides thetaiotaomicron [a], BacHum-UCD [a] and DogBac [a]	V. vulnificus [c], S. aureus [c], enterovirus [c], norovirus [c], hepatitis A [c] virus, Cryptosporidium and Giardia (oo)cysts [b]	Coastal Beaches, Miami Dade County, Florida, USA	NR	During rain event, DogBac was co-detected with Cryptosporidium, Giardia, enteroviruses and V. vulnificus along with enterococci.	[76]

Table 4. *Cont.*

MST marker [1]	Pathogens [1]	Location	Relationship [2]	Comments	Reference
		Marine and brackish waters			
HF183 [c], *C. coccoides* [c]	*Cryptosporidium* and *Giardia* (oo)cysts [b]	Coastal beaches, Venezuela	NR	The levels of (oo) cysts varied with the extent of sewage pollution and bather density. HF183 and *C. coccoides* correlated with *C. perfringens*.	[88]
GenBac3 [c], HF183 [a,c], BacHum-UCD [c], *B. dorei* [a,c], HumM2 [c], HF134 [a], HumM19 [a], *B. stercoris* [a], *B. uniformis* [c], *nifH* [a,c], *esp* [c], HPyV [a,c], Gull Bacteroides [a], *C. marimammalium* [c], BacCow-UCD [c], BacCan-UCD [c]	*L. pneumophila* [a], *S. aureus* [a], MRSA [a], pathogenic *E. coli* [a], adenovirus [a], enterovirus [c], Hepatitis A [c], Norovirus [a]	Malibu beach, California USA	NR	Human-associated MST markers were only predictive of illness at the site known to be impacted by human sewage from faulty infrastructure.	[79]
HPyV [a], *nifH* [a], HF183 [a]	*Campylobacter* spp. [c]	Quietwater Beach, Florida, USA	No significant correlation.	In some instances, MST markers were co-detected with *Campylobacter* especially following rain events.	[70]
esp [a], HPyV [a]	*Salmonella* spp. [a], enteric viruses [d]	Ben T. Davis and Bahia beaches, Florida, USA	NR	Coxsackie virus B4 and HPyVs were co-detected following a major sewage spill. Fecal coliform concentrations correlated with the *esp* marker HPyV did not correlate with FIB.	[80]
HPyV [c], HF183 [c], *nifH* [a]	Adenovirus [a]	Hillsborough River and St. Johns River, Florida, USA	No significant correlation with HPyV, NR for HF183, *nifH*.	Adenovirus co-detected with HF183 and *nifH*.	[98]
GenBac3 [a], HPyV [c], HF183 [a], *nifH* [a]	Adenovirus [a]	Hillsborough River, St, Johns River, Ben T. Davis beach, Florida, USA	No significant relationship with HPyV, other MST markers NR	All FIB concentrations exceeded regulatory standards HF183 and *nifH* detected in 80% of samples, whereas adenoviruses were detected in 60% of the samples.	[99]
HPyV [c], HF183 [a], *nifH* [a]	Adenovirus [a]	Avalon and Doheny Beaches, California, USA	At Doheny Beach HPyV and HF183 presence correlated with adenovirus.	Adenovirus not detected at Avalon Beach, impacted by non-point source(s).	[93]
PMMoV [c], HF183 [c], BacHum-UCD [c], *esp* [a], *nifH* [c]	Adenovirus [a], Norovirus, *Cryptosporidium* and *Giardia* (oo)cysts [b], *C. jejuni* [a], *Salmonella* spp. [a], *S. aureus* [a], *E. coli* 0157-H7 [a]	Coastal beaches, Florida, USA	NR	PMMoV co-occurred with FIB, other MST markers and pathogens. Seawater samples taken near sewage outfalls.	[53]
BacHum-UCD [c], HF183 [c], DogBac [c], *C. marimammalium* [c]	*S. aureus* [e]	Coastal beaches, Miami, Florida, USA	NR	Co-occurrence with *S. aureus* detection. No correlation found with MST markers and skin illness.	[86]

[1] Data reporting: Presence/absence [a], total (oo)cysts [b], gene copies [c], most probable number (MPN) [d], colony forming units (CFU) [e]; [2] NR (not reported).

7. Various Indicators and Pathogens in Swimming Pools

Our search of literature for paired measurements of indicator(s) and pathogen(s) recorded for swimming pools yielded considerably fewer studies (*n* = 3), compared to ambient waters. None of the studies reported statistical analyses on relationships between indicators and pathogens. Two studies, both conducted in Italy, were performed on pools that were in compliance with microbiological requirements for *E. coli*, enterococci, *P. aeruginosa*, and *S. aureus* [107,108]. However, one study detected infectious *Simkania negevensis*, a bacterium related to *Chlamydia*, in nearly 43% of samples, while the second one measured Papillomaviruses in 64% of samples [108]. Interestingly, HPyVs were co-detected with Papillomaviruses in all the samples [108]. *L. pneumophila* and enteric viruses (adenovirus, norovirus, and enteroviruses) [108] were not detected. Examination of wading pools in Finland during a gastroenteritis outbreak detected Norovirus GII and astrovirus in ~83% and ~33% of samples, respectively [109]. *E. coli* was absent from samples collected ~2 weeks before the outbreak, but high concentrations (370–24,000 CFU/100 mL) were measured in two samples taken during the outbreak [109].

8. Relationship of Indicators with Illness

To identify associations between the presence of general FIB, alternative indicators or MST markers with that of waterborne illness occurrence, various epidemiologic studies were collected from existing literature dating back to the early 1990s. For inclusion, it was required that the study measured at least one FIB, alternative indicator or MST marker (culture or molecular) in combination with an epidemiological survey of resulting illness from the recreational water exposure. In total, 17 studies [76,79,86,110–124] met these criteria and were included in analyses. One study each was conducted in Europe and Africa, and fifteen studies were conducted in the US. Since some of these studies were conducted in more than one water type, this resulted in the inclusion of 20 freshwater sites and 29 brackish/marine sites. Thirteen different microbiological assays were reported including those targeting: enterococci, fecal and total coliforms, *E. coli*, somatic and F+ coliphage, as well as various general and human-associated MST markers (Figure 2). In addition to gastrointestinal illnesses characterized by symptoms of diarrhea, vomiting, and stomach cramps, other waterborne illnesses included skin, ear and sinus infection [76,79,86,110–113,115–122,124]. For epidemiological studies, assays targeting enterococci were the most commonly recorded, with 25 instances of measurements of either culture based or molecular enterococci targets, followed by human-associated MST markers, F+ coliphage, fecal coliforms, general MST markers, total coliforms, culturable *E. coli*, somatic coliphage and finally *E. coli* qPCR signal (Figure 2).

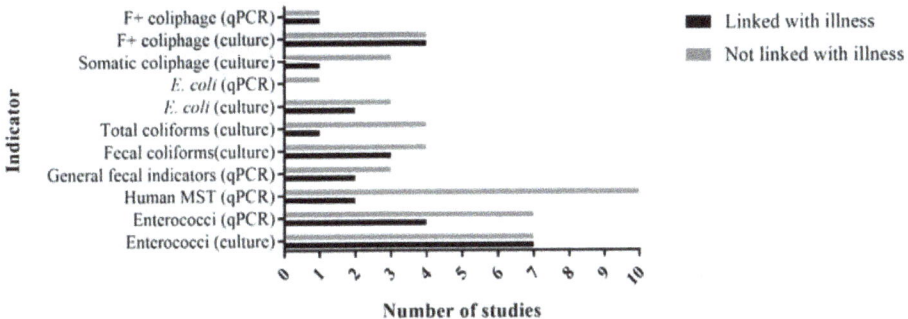

Figure 2. Summary of epidemiological studies reporting on linkage between illness and various indicator types.

Correlations between observed illness in these studies were most common with enterococci (10 studies out of 17) [79,86,110,111,113,114,116,117,120,121], followed by F+ coliphage (5 studies) [79,113,118,119,123] (Figure 2), suggesting that these two indicators may be better predictors of waterborne illness occurrence. Fecal coliforms, human-associated MST markers (Bsteri, BuniF2, and HF134), general MST marker (GenBac3), culturable *E. coli*, total coliforms, and somatic coliphage were correlated with illness less frequently (Figure 2). Twenty-seven indicator measurements across all studies were correlated with human illness, and 93% of these studies were conducted in waters with known point or non-point source contamination, contaminated surface/ground water flow or following wet weather events. Only six studies [79,86,117–119,124], all of which found relationship between indicator and illness, measured pathogens, in addition to recording illness information, and indicator organism concentrations. Only one of the six studies found a relationship between pathogens and illness or indicator concentrations. This is not surprising since, in these studies, pathogens were detected infrequently and at low concentrations. This illustrates the potential challenges of detecting relationships between indicators and pathogens in the field even when health relationships were observed with fecal indictors.

9. Factors that Influence Indicator and Pathogen Relationships

Most recreational waters at any given time are impacted by many different sources of fecal contamination (e.g., treated and untreated wastewater, agricultural operations, stormwater, and domestic and wildlife animals) and these influences can change depending on many different factors including precipitation, tidal flow and wind direction. In addition, each fecal source has its own set of indicators and the potential for different types of pathogens. Therefore, the more fecal sources a recreational water is impacted by, the more challenging it will be to show correlations between indicators and pathogens. Preceding sections described our findings regarding relationships between indicators and pathogens in recreational waters, as well as relationships between indicators and illness. Overall, FIB were better predictors of bacterial and protozoan pathogen presence (compared to viral), relationships were more probable under scenarios where both indicator and pathogen were likely to be present at higher concentrations, and enterococci and F-specific coliphage tended to be better predictors of waterborne illness occurrence compared to other indicators. The following sections examine various factors that are likely to influence the observed trends.

10. Detection Frequency and Concentrations of Indicators and Pathogens in Marine, Brackish and Freshwaters

The observed relationships between indicators and pathogens can be influenced by logistical factors that may confound determination of actual relationships, including study design and methodological limitations. Study design determines the frequency at which a target (FIB, alternative indicator, MST marker or pathogen) was measured (per study or cumulative multiple studies), while methodology employed influences likelihood of detection. We compiled studies that reported frequency of detection (or data that allowed calculation of frequency detection such as total number of samples and samples positive) for at least one FIB/alternative indicator/MST marker and at least one pathogen per sample(s), resulting in inclusion of 49 studies (Table 5). Microbial data collected were first grouped according to indicator (FIB, alternative or MST) or pathogen type (bacterial, viral or protozoan), and further organized according to the detection format employed (different types of culture-based or molecular). Table 5 describes the detection frequency (per study and per total cumulative samples) for microorganism targets (FIB, alternative indicators, MST, and pathogens) for both freshwater and brackish/marine waters.

Table 5. Frequency (%) of detection of microorganisms over all eligible studies (those that included data on individual observations). Detection frequency is expressed per study and for cumulative samples across all studies. Studies with least one sample positive for the organism were scored positive in the "per study" column.

Organism	Detection Frequency per Study (%) and n [2]	Detection Frequency per Sample [2]	Detection Frequency per Study (%) and n [2]	Detection Frequency per Sample [2]
	Freshwater		Brackish/Marine	
	FIB			
Total coliforms (MPN)	100% (4)	100% (275)	N/A	N/A
Total coliforms (CFU)	100% (3)	97.2% (1988)	100% (5)	99.7% (317)
Fecal coliforms (MPN)	100% (4)	100% (147)	N/A	N/A
Fecal coliforms (CFU)	100% (6)	96.7% (1726)	100% (11)	98.3% (524)
E. coli (MPN)	100% (8)	97.7% (1846)	100% (5)	100% (55)
E. coli (CFU)	100% (10)	90% (2530)	100% (8)	94.1% (406)
E. coli (Q)	100% (5)	89.6% (221)	N/A	N/A
Enterococci (MPN)	100% (2)	81.7% (301)	100% (5)	61.7% (162)
Enterococci (CFU)	100% (13)	96.6% (2584)	100% (13)	97.6% (705)
Enterococci (Q)	100% (2)	100% (302)	100% (3)	100% (34)
	Alternative indicators			
C. perfringens (CFU)	100% (4)	83.2% (1843)	100% (5)	61.6% (73)
C. perfringens (Q)	100% (2)	73.2% (56)	N/A	N/A
Somatic coliphage (PFU)	100% (4)	85.5% (394)	100% (1)	100% (20)
F+ coliphage (PFU)	100% (2)	93.2% (73)	100% (7)	34.4% (90)
F- coliphage (PFU)	N/A	N/A	100% (3)	28% (25)
B. fragilis phage (PFU)	N/A	N/A	100% (1)	16.7% (12)
B. thetaiotaomicron phage (PFU)	N/A	N/A	100% (1)	30% (20)
	MST markers			
GenBac3 (Q)	100% (1)	75% (8)	N/A	N/A
HF183 (E)	N/A	N/A	100% (3)	31.8% (255)
HF183 (Q)	N/A	N/A	100% (4)	25.5% (105)
BacHum-UCD (Q)	N/A	N/A	100% (1)	95.45% (22)
HPyV (E)	100% (1)	0% (18)	100% (4)	51.08% (204)
HPyV (Q)	100% (1)	100% 98)	100% (2)	12.2% (255)
C. coccoides Human (Q)	N/A	N/A	100% (1)	69.2% (13)
B. thetaiotamicron (E)	N/A	N/A	100% (1)	26.7% (15)
nifH (E)	100% (1)	0% (18)	100% (2)	2.8% (255)
nifH (Q)	N/A	N/A	100% (1)	100% (7)
gyrB (Q)	100% (1)	50.8% (65)	N/A	N/A
g-Bfra	100% (1)	92.3% (65)	N/A	N/A
esp (E)	100% (3)	6.2% (649)	80% (5)	19.12% (204)
LTII (E)	100% (1)	7.4% (217)	N/A	N/A
STII (E)	100% (1)	4.6% (217)	N/A	N/A
DogBac (Q)	N/A	N/A	100% (1)	86.7% (15)
	Bacterial pathogens			
E. coli O157:H7 (MPN)	100% (1)	0.6% (823)	N/A	N/A
E. coli O157:H7 (E)	100% (1)	13.4% (67)	0% (1)	0% (7)
Pathogenic *E. coli* (*eae*) (E)	100% (4)	53.7% (350)	N/A	N/A
Pathogenic *E. coli* (*eae*) (Q)	100% (1)	31.3% (32)	N/A	N/A
Pathogenic *E. coli* (*stx1*) (E)	100% (4)	7.9% (302)	N/A	N/A
Pathogenic *E. coli* (*stx2*) (E)	100% (3)	29.7% (350)	N/A	N/A
Salmonella spp. (MPN)	100% (6)	14% (1076)	33% (3)	8.7% (196)
Salmonella spp. (E)	N/A	N/A	100% (1)	28.6% (7)
Salmonella spp. (Q)	100% (4)	27.3% (1188)	N/A	N/A
S. aureus (MPN)	100% (1)	44.6% (112)	100% (2)	70.4% (27)
S. aureus (E)	N/A	N/A	100% (1)	57.1% (7)
S. aureus (Q)	100% (1)	37.5% (8)	N/A	N/A
Campylobacter spp. (MPN)	100% (3)	24.7% (1009)	100% (1)	30.9% (55)
Campylobacter spp. (E)	N/A	N/A	100% (1)	14.3% (7)
Campylobacter spp. (Q)	100% (3)	81.3% (80)	100% (1)	18.2% (11)
Pseudomonas spp. (MPN)	100% (2)	80.6% (191)	N/A	N/A
P. aeruginosa (Q)	100% (2)	39.6% (53)	N/A	N/A
Shigella spp. (E)	100% (1)	6.3% (48)	N/A	N/A
Shigella spp. (Q)	100% (2)	14.5% (1148)	N/A	N/A
Legionella spp. (E)	100% (2)	41.9% (217)	N/A	N/A
Legionella spp. (Q)	100% (1)	20% (30)	N/A	N/A
Listeria spp. (MPN)	100% (1)	18.7% (395)	N/A	N/A
V. cholerae (Q)	100% (2)	52.5% (1148)	N/A	N/A
V. vulnificus (Q)	N/A	N/A	100% (2)	44.4% (27)
Aeromonas spp. (Q)	100% (3)	100% (248)	N/A	N/A
M. avium (Q)	100% (2)	34.4% (64)	N/A	N/A

Table 5. *Cont.*

Organism	Detection Frequency per Study (%) and n [2]	Detection Frequency per Sample [2]	Detection Frequency per Study (%) and n [2]	Detection Frequency per Sample [2]
	Freshwater		Brackish/Marine	
	Viral pathogens			
Infectious enterovirus (MPN)	100% (3)	18.4% (158)	100% (3)	0% (27)
Enterovirus (E)	100% (3)	14.4% (222)	100% (3)	37.8% (45)
Enterovirus (Q)	100% (4)	29.1% (103)	33% (3)	14.8% (27)
Infectious reovirus (MPN)	100% (1)	21.9% (32)	N/A	N/A
Reovirus (Q)	100% (1)	100% (8)	N/A	N/A
Human adenovirus (MPN)	N/A	N/A	100% (1)	0% (27)
Human adenovirus (E)	100% (4)	42.2% (1118)	100% (6)	16.5% (309)
Human adenovirus (Q)	100% (5)	40.7% (214)	100% (1)	33.3% (12)
Astrovirus (E)	100% (1)	15.4% (52)	N/A	N/A
Astrovirus (Q)	100% (2)	17.3% (133)	N/A	N/A
Norovirus (E)	100% (3)	29.5% (112)	100% (1)	27.3% (22)
Norovirus (Q)	100% (1)	100% (8)	50% (2)	26.3% (19)
Norovirus GI (Q)	50% (4)	7.5% (213)	N/A	N/A
Norovirus GII (Q)	66.7% (3)	16.2% (198)	N/A	N/A
Rotavirus (E)	100% (3)	18.4% (141)	N/A	N/A
Rotavirus (Q)	66.7% (3)	33.8% (142)	N/A	N/A
Hepatitis A (E)	N/A	N/A	100% (1)	80% (10)
Hepatitis A (Q)	100% (1)	1.5% (68)	0% (1)	0% (12)
Bovine adenovirus (Q)	100% (1)	56.7% (30)	N/A	N/A
	Protozoan pathogens			
Acanthamoeba spp. (E)	100% (1)	24.6% (126)	N/A	N/A
Naegleria spp. (E)	100% (1)	13.5% (126)	N/A	N/A
Cryptosporidium spp. (M)	88.9% (9)	36.5% (1456)	60% (5)	23.2% (112)
Cryptosporidium spp. (E)	N/A	N/A	0% (1)	0% (12)
Cryptosporidium spp. (Q)	N/A	N/A	100% (1)	26.7% (15)
Giardia spp. (M)	100% (8)	63.7% (1426)	80% (5)	22.3% (112)
Giardia spp. (E)	N/A	N/A	100% (2)	16.7% (12)
Giardia spp. (Q)	N/A	N/A	100% (1)	33.3% (15)
	Fungal pathogens			
C. albicans (MPN)	N/A	N/A	100% (1)	45.4% (152)

[1] MPN, most probable number; CFU, colony forming units; PFU, plaque forming units; E, end-point PCR; Q, qPCR; M, microscopy; [2] N/A, not available.

Each FIB was detected at least once in 100% of studies, which was true for most of the microbial targets. General FIB were also the most frequently detected on a per sample basis, as they were found in 94.2% of samples across 13,823 measurements in marine and freshwaters (Table 5). In freshwater, detection frequency of FIB per sample was 95% across 11,920 measurements and it was somewhat lower in brackish/marine waters (93% across 2203 measurements) (Table 5). Detection frequency of alternative indicators per sample, irrespective of the water type, was considerably less than FIB, averaging 60.6% (across 2606 measurements); the difference between water types was also more pronounced than for FIB (freshwater detection frequency 83.7%/2366 measurements vs. marine 45.1%/240 samples) (Table 5). While the 2705 samples analyzed for MST markers in marine and freshwaters were similar to alternative indicators, the overall detection frequency average (42.9%) was considerably lower (Table 5). The frequency of detection and total number of samples collected in each water type (37.4%/1355 in freshwater vs. 47.3%/1350 in marine water) was similar (Table 5).

Irrespective of the water type, bacterial pathogens were measured more often (9280 total samples), compared to viral (3462) and protozoan (3400) pathogens, although the frequency of detection across different pathogen groups was similar (33.8%, bacterial; 29.6%, viral; and 28.9%, protozoan (Table 5)). There also appeared to be no appreciable difference in detection frequency between the water types for any of the pathogen groups, although considerably more samples were collected in freshwater (Table 5). For bacterial pathogens, frequency of detection across 8936 total samples collected in freshwater was 35.2%, compared to 30.3% in 344 marine/brackish water samples (Table 5). Similarly, viral pathogens were detected in 33.1% freshwater samples (out of 2952) and 23.6% of 510 marine water samples (Table 5). Lastly, protozoan pathogens were detected in 34.6% of 3,134 freshwater samples and 24.4% of 266 marine water samples (Table 5).

A subset of studies examined ($n = 33$) reported concentration data in the body of the manuscript, tables or supplemental materials, allowing graphs to be created displaying average densities per organism and water type (Figures 3 and 4). Concentrations of indicators were on average 1–3 $\log_{10}$ higher than pathogen concentrations for both water types. Both indicators and pathogens in marine waters were found at slightly lower levels (0.5–1 $\log_{10}$) than those observed in freshwater (Figures 3 and 4 and Table 6). Within an indicator group, concentrations of FIB ranged from not detected (ND (observed only for enterococci)) to 5.39 $\log_{10}$ per 100 mL (Table 6), and total coliform levels were the highest, followed by fecal coliforms, *E. coli*, and enterococci (Figures 3 and 4). Alternative indicator concentrations were lower than FIB (ranging from ND–3.29 $\log_{10}$ per 100 mL (Table 6)), and *C. perfringens* levels were higher than somatic and F-specific coliphage (Figures 3 and 4). MST marker concentrations were reported less frequently and were more variable, ranging from ND–2.50 $\log_{10}$ copies per 100 mL (Table 6 and Figures 3 and 4). Bacterial pathogen concentrations (range: ND–5.09 $\log_{10}$ per 100 mL) were higher than viral (range: ND–1.58 $\log_{10}$ per 100 mL) and protozoan pathogens (range: ND–1.93 $\log_{10}$ per 100 mL), in both marine and freshwater (Table 6, Figures 3 and 4).

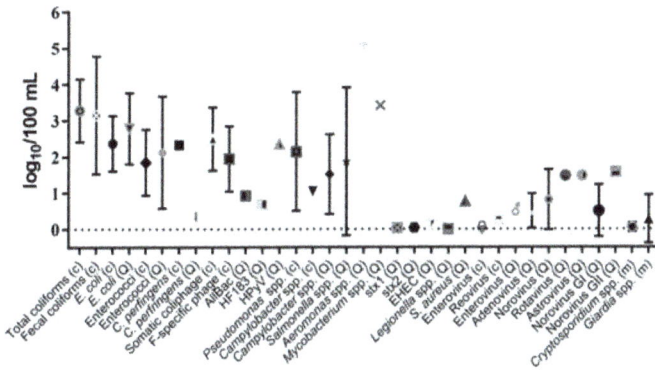

Figure 3. Mean concentration of FIB, alternative indicators, MST markers, bacterial, viral and protozoan pathogens in freshwater. Error bars represent standard deviation (c, culture-based; Q, qPCR; m, microscopy).

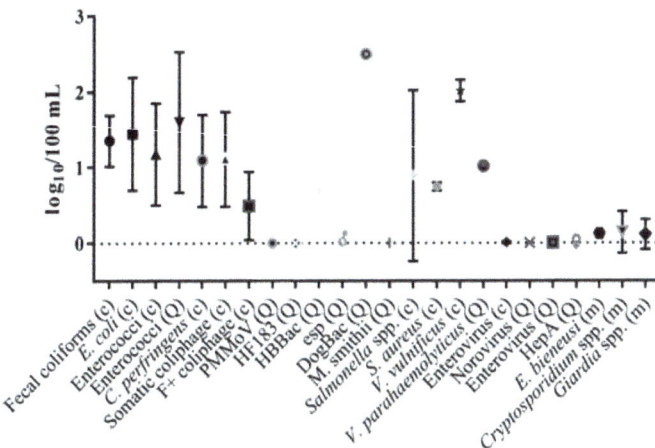

Figure 4. Mean concentration of FIB, alternative indicators, MST markers, bacterial, viral and protozoan pathogens in marine and brackish waters. Error bars represent standard deviation (c, culture-based; Q, qPCR; m, microscopy).

Table 6. Concentrations of various indicators and pathogens from select studies in marine/brackish and freshwaters.

Organism [1]	Range or Average per Study (log$_{10}$ per 100 mL) [2,3]	Marine References [4]	Freshwater References [4]
FIB			
Total coliforms (c)	2.67–3.89	N/A	[37,75]
Fecal coliforms (c)	0.93–5.39	[76,77,80,87,94]	[39,57,65,125]
E. coli (c)	0.59–3.51	[76,77,80,82,89,94,96,100]	[36,37,44,46,50,51,54–57,65,75,125]
E. coli (q)	1.75–3.97	N/A	[41,51,55,68]
Enterococci (c)	ND–3.62	[70,76,77,80,82–85,87–89,94,96,100,101]	[37,39,44,47,50,51,55–57,65,70]
Enterococci (q)	0.63–3.21	[76,77,83]	[51,55]
Alternative indicators			
C. perfringens (c)	0.20–2.33	[76,77,87–89,100]	[54]
C. perfringens (q)	0.35	N/A	[41]
Somatic coliphage (c)	0.61–3.29	[82,90,94]	[39,102,103,126]
F-specific coliphage (c)	ND–2.76	[76,82,89,90,94,100]	[47,54,102,103]
MST markers			
AllBac(q)	0.93	[83]	[51]
PMMoV (q)	ND	[83]	N/A
HF183 (q)	ND–0.69	N/A	[51]
HBBac (q)	0.72	[83]	N/A
HPyV (q)	2.36	N/A	[51]
esp (q)	0.06	[76]	N/A
nifH (q)	ND	[83]	N/A
DogBac (q)	2.50	[76]	N/A
Bacterial pathogens			
Campylobacter spp. (c)	1.05	N/A	[54]
Campylobacter spp. (q)	0.74–2.29	N/A	[46,70]
EHEC (q)	0.13	N/A	[65]
Salmonella spp. (c)	ND–2.36	[80,84,89,100]	N/A
Salmonella spp. (q)	0.06–4.08	N/A	[51,65,68]
S. aureus (c)	0.70–0.77	[76,77]	N/A
S. aureus (q)	0.78	N/A	[51]
Aeromonas spp. (q)	5.09	N/A	[68]
Stx1 (q)	0.03	N/A	[57]
Stx2 (q)	0.03	N/A	[57]
Mycobacterium spp. (q)	3.41	N/A	[68]
Pseudomonas spp. (c)	0.37–3.72	N/A	N/A
Legionella spp (q)	ND	N/A	[46]
V. vulnificus (c)	1.91–2.11	[84,100]	N/A
V. parahaemolyticus (q)	1.01	[85]	N/A
Viral pathogens			
Enterovirus (c)	ND–0.04	[80,82,87,89,94]	[39,47,102]
Enterovirus (q)	ND–0.56	[76,77]	[39]
Adenovirus (q)	0.08–1.02	N/A	[41,46,103]
Astrovirus (q)	1.48	N/A	[103]
Norovirus (q)	ND–1.40	[77,94]	[51,102]
Norovirus GI (q)	ND–1.02	N/A	[50,103]
Norovirus GII (q)	1.58	N/A	[103]
Rotavirus (q)	1.41–1.53	N/A	[102,103]
Reovirus (c)	0.18–0.31	N/A	[47,102]
Hepatitis A (q)	ND	[77]	N/A
Protozoan pathogens			
E. bieneusi (m)	0.12	[101]	N/A
Giardia spp.(m)	ND–1.93	[76,83,88,89,94,96,127]	[36,41,47,54–56,65,75]
Cryptosporidium spp. (m)	ND–0.73	[76,77,83,88,89,94,96,127]	[36,41,47,54–56,65,75]

[1] c, culture; q, qPCR; m, microscopy. [2] Range is provided when more than one study measured a given parameter, while average per study is provided when a single study measured a given parameter. Units include: CFU, MPN, PFU, gene copies or total (oo)cysts. [3] ND, not detected; [4] N/A, not available.

As evidenced by the examples above, readily detected microorganisms are more likely to be measured and frequency of detection of a given microorganism is influenced by the concentration and distribution of the target in the sample types tested, as well as the limit of detection of the method used. Culture methods such as membrane filtration can have a low limit of detection, e.g., 1 CFU/100 mL, and can reliably detect FIB in water samples with minimal contamination. Conversely, pathogens are generally present sporadically and in lower levels than fecal indicators. These types of targets require high-throughput filtration methods that can achieve large concentration factors, with the tradeoff that limits of detection are generally quite high. In addition, the volumes sampled, and the concentration strategy used can vary between studies and can affect the sensitivity of a given method. These logistical factors frequently result in unbalanced comparisons in which the indicator organism is frequently detected, but the pathogen is not. Therefore, the disconnect between indicators and pathogens may not be due to a true lack of relationship in many cases, but to methodology that is much more suited to detecting indicators than pathogens.

11. Microbial Levels in Fecal Material

The observed relationships between indicators and pathogens can also be affected by factors intrinsic to the organisms themselves, including levels in various hosts, as well as shedding frequencies and duration. FIB are commensal inhabitants of the GI tract of humans and other animals and as such are shed continually in feces. Levels of fecal coliforms, *E. coli*, and enterococci typically found in human feces range 10^5–10^9 CFU per gram [13], while levels detected in untreated wastewater are somewhat lower (10^5–10^8 CFU per 100 mL) [13,128]. The concentration of FIB in animal excreta is lower still, ranging from 10^4 to 10^7 CFU per gram, depending on the animal host [13]. Alternative indicators are also commensal organisms of the GI tract but are typically found in lower concentrations and are more influenced by diets and physiologies of the host [13,14,128]. For example, *C. perfringens* levels in animal and human feces range from undetectable to 10^8 CFU per gram [13], while coliphages were absent from some animal feces and primary wastewater effluents [128,129] and typically did not exceed ~10^3 PFU/mL of untreated wastewater [128]. MST markers target different fecal microorganisms that are strongly associated with particular hosts [14] and the human-associated subset is reported to range from 10^3 to 10^{10} gene copies per gram of feces or 100 mL of untreated wastewater, while animal-associated MST markers range from 10^4–10^9 gene copies per gram of feces depending on the sensitivity of individual markers and geographic region [13].

Pathogens may cause symptomatic or asymptomatic infection of their human and animal hosts. Shedding rates can vary widely, although levels found in the wastewater are typically several orders of magnitude lower than any indicator species [128,130–133] likely due to the sporadic nature of pathogen occurrence and detection compared to indicators. Additionally, only a small part of the population is infected with pathogens at any given time, resulting in considerable variation in the levels of pathogens, particularly when originating from relatively small populations. Differential shedding of pathogens from infected hosts is also contributing to the occurrence of pathogens in recreational waters. For example, shedding rates for human viral pathogens can be as high as 10^{11} viral particles per gram of feces in the case of adenoviruses [134], while shedding rates of bacterial pathogens are typically lower [133], as cattle excreting >10^4 CFU per gram of feces *E. coli* O157:H7 are considered to be "super-shedders" [135]. *Cryptosporidium* and *Giardia* (oo)cyst shedding rates by the infected individuals can range from 10^6 to 10^{11} per gram of feces [132] and are typically higher in animal hosts compared to human [131,136], although not all (oo)cysts excreted by animals are zoonotic [131,137].

Shedding duration of viruses can vary from weeks to months [133], and some viruses display distinct seasonal trends (e.g., infectious enteroviruses are more prevalent in wastewater in summer and early fall) [134]. Similar to pathogenic viruses, excretion of (oo)cysts is typically long term [132]. Shedding duration of bacterial pathogens is shorter with median values typically reported to be ~2 weeks, although in some instances it can last considerably longer [138,139]. Similar to viral and protozoan pathogens, shedding is affected by many different factors including diet and age of the host [140,141], temperature [140], as well as composition of gut microbiome [142]. Infectious dose of different pathogens is also variable and typically the lowest for viruses [134,143], medium range for protozoan pathogens and generally highest for bacterial pathogens [143], although *E. coli* O157:H7, with a low infectious dose, is an exception [144]. The infectious dose of viral, bacterial and protozoan pathogens is dependent on many factors, including individual strains and health status of the host [134,143].

12. Susceptibility to Environmental Stressors

While wastewater treatment processes generally result in some removal of indicators and pathogens [128,145], sanitary sewer and combined sewer overflows, along with other infrastructure failures can result in release of indicators and pathogens into ambient waters. In addition, different indicator and pathogen groups exhibit variable susceptibilities to disinfection strategies. Bacteria are generally susceptible to chlorination and UV treatment [146]. Protozoa and viruses are typically most susceptible to UV treatment [146,147], with the notable exception of adenoviruses [148]. Once indicators and pathogens are released into ambient waters, a new panoply of biotic and abiotic environmental factors affects fate and transport characteristics, including ambient sunlight, indigenous microbiota (i.e., predation and competition interactions), temperature, salinity, nutrient levels, location (water column vs. sediment), source of fecal pollution and resilience of individual organisms.

Ambient sunlight and associated UV radiation typically act to increase the decay rates, although the magnitude of this effect is influenced by the environmental conditions [149] and measurement strategies [150,151]. For example, viable cells and culturable/infectious organisms typically display the effects of UV damage more readily than their corresponding nucleic acids. Interactions with indigenous microbiota also increase decay rates, although this was predominantly shown for FIB, MST markers and some bacterial pathogens, (e.g., [152–155]) with inconclusive data for other organisms (e.g., various bacteriophages and *C. parvum* [156,157]). Influx of nutrients (in the form of organic carbon, nitrogen and phosphorus) can result in extended persistence [158–160], and potentially mitigate the effects of biotic interactions [161] but this assertion was not tested in detail for organisms other than culturable FIB. Temperature and location affect decay rates of most organisms tested (e.g., FIB, bacteriophage, viral pathogens, MST markers) almost unilaterally with greater persistence at lower temperatures [150,162–166] and in the sediments and sands compared to the water column (recently reviewed in [167]).

Similar to the effect of ambient sunlight, salinity (and the associated ionic content of brackish and marine waters) affected the decay rates of culturable/infectious FIB, alternative indicators, MST markers and pathogens more so than their corresponding nucleic acids [168–174]. The effect of source of fecal pollution has been studied on FIB and MST markers, and indicators originating from ruminants are more persistent compared to those from other fecal sources (e.g., dog, seagull, and human) [169,175–179], although different human sources (e.g., feces, septage, and sewage) elicit different decay rates [152]; analogous information for alternative indicators and pathogens is still missing. Finally, studies that compared decay of various indicators to pathogens directly under the same experimental conditions are rare and report conflicting results. For instance, in one study, *E. coli* O157:H7 persisted longer than FIB (e.g., *E. coli* and enterococci) in freshwater [180], but another group reported similar trend in the freshwater sediments but not the water column [181]. Another group reported no difference in decay between FIB, various MST markers and *C. jejuni, S. enterica* and adenovirus in freshwater [151]. Others reported considerably faster decay of *C. jejuni* (but not *C. coli* or *Salmonella* spp.) than FIB and MST markers, irrespective of the water type [171]. As exemplified above, variable responses of different indicator and pathogen groups to these stressors and the resulting differential decay rates further confound the indicator paradigm.

13. Conclusions

FIB and alternative indicator organisms (*C. perfringens* and coliphages) have been used for over a century, and continue to be used today as indicators of general fecal pollution in many applications, including the assessment of sanitary quality of recreational waters [8]. MST markers are used to identify source(s) of fecal pollution and are a more recent addition to the monitoring toolbox available to water quality managers and other practitioners in the field [14]. The goal of this review is to two-fold. Our primary objective was to examine reported relationships between various indicators and pathogens in recreational waters to determine the value of different indicators as surrogates for pathogen presence. Secondly, we aimed to more closely inspect different factors that may have an impact on this relationship.

The majority of the studies either did not report a relationship, or they reported a statistically non-significant relationship. Among the studies that observed statistically significant relationships, it was considerably more common in freshwater compared to marine waters. General FIB tended to form statistically significant relationships more commonly with bacterial and protozoan pathogens, (compared to viral pathogens) and this difference was statistically significant. Alternative indicators and MST markers correlated with pathogens less frequently, although it occurred more in freshwater than marine/brackish waters. Overall, statistically significant relationships were detected more frequently in waters known to be impacted by fecal pollution and following wet weather events, both scenarios under which indicators and pathogens are more likely to be co-detected.

Among factors influencing these relationships frequency of detection and variable concentrations of indicators and pathogens were identified as major contributing factor. Not surprisingly, general FIB were measured and detected more frequently than any other indicator or pathogen (generally in >90% of samples) and were also reported at higher concentrations, irrespective of the water type. Alternative indicators were also frequently detected in samples (>70%), while MST markers were measured and detected less frequently, and in lower concentrations than FIB or alternative markers (frequently in <10% of samples). Pathogen detection frequencies were similarly low. Low frequency of detection affects the ability to establish relationships between the frequently-detected and infrequently-detected analytes, as the dataset becomes left-censored (biased toward non-detects values). What looks like "absence" is frequently an artifact of comparing an analyte with high density (e.g., FIB) with one of low density (e.g., pathogen). Better concentration and recovery methods for the infrequently-detected analytes may provide a more realistic picture of the relationships among these various microorganisms in environmental waters. Finally, concentrations in feces and wastewater, shedding rates and patterns of various indicator and pathogen groups differ, as do their fate and transport characteristics in secondary habitats. Indicators are typically present in higher concentrations than any of the pathogen groups, and are also shed constantly, or more frequently, compared to pathogens. Upon entry into the secondary habitats, a host of biotic and abiotic factors differentially affects persistence of indicators and pathogens, further confounding the indicator–pathogen paradigm. Lastly, another important factor impacting the ability to establish relationships between indicators and pathogens is the realization that most locations are impacted by multiple sources of fecal contamination. Although it is difficult to measure the impact of multiple fecal inputs, tools such as sanitary surveys and GIS mapping have the ability to indicate potential point and non-point sources of fecal pollution and future MST studies should improve our understanding of the impacts of multiple fecal sources.

To further our understanding of indicator and pathogen relationships, future studies measuring these microorganisms in recreational waters should evaluate and report the existence (or lack thereof) of such relationships. Other considerations include careful selection of targeted pathogens and methodology used to quantify them. Furthermore, providing the data on a per sample basis (rather than descriptive statistics of a dataset) in at least supplementary materials, will enable metanalyses, which may yield a more robust estimate of a true state of indicator/pathogen paradigm. Lastly, while standardized and sensitive methods exist for FIB detection and enumeration in recreational waters, analogous procedures for alternative indicators, MST markers and pathogens are still missing. Standardization of detection and quantification methods suitable for each indicator/pathogen group can enable more accurate evaluation of any statistically significant relationships between these two groups.

Author Contributions: Conceptualization, A.K., B.R.M. and V.J.H.; Investigation, A.K. and B.R.M.; Data Curation, A.K. and B.R.M.; Writing-Original Draft Preparation, A.K. and B.R.M.; Writing-Reviewing & Editing, A.K. and V.J.H.; Visualization, A.K.

Funding: This research received no external funding.

Conflicts of Interest: The authors declare no conflict of interest.

References

1. Kummu, M.; de Moel, H.; Ward, P.J.; Varis, O. How close do we live to water? A global analysis of population distance to freshwater bodies. *PLoS ONE* **2011**, *6*, e20578. [CrossRef] [PubMed]
2. National Oceanic and Atmospheric Administration. *State of the Coast: National Coastal Population Report. Population Trends from 1970 to 2020*; National Oceanic and Atmospheric Administration: Silver Springs, MD, USA, 2013.
3. Dorfman, M.H.; Stoner, N.; Rosselot, K.S. *Testing the Waters: A Guide to Water Quality at Vacation Beaches*; Natural Resources Defense Council: New York, NY, USA, 2014.
4. Rabinovici, S.J.; Bernknopf, R.L.; Wein, A.M.; Coursey, D.L.; Whitman, R.L. Economic and health risk trade-offs of swim closures at a lake Michigan beach. *Environ. Sci. Technol.* **2004**, *38*, 2737–2745. [CrossRef] [PubMed]
5. Devine, J. *The Impacts of Beach Pollution*; Natural Resources Defense Council: New York, NY, USA, 2014.
6. Penn, J.; Hu, W.; Cox, L.; Kozloff, L. Values for recreational beach quality in Oahu, Hawaii. *Mar. Resour. Econ.* **2016**, *31*, 47–62. [CrossRef]
7. European Environment Agency. *European Bathing Water Quality in 2017*; European Environment Agency: Luxembourg, Luxembourg, 2018.
8. American Water Works Association. *Water Quality and Treatment: A Handbook of Community Water Supplies*, 4th ed.; McGraw-Hill: New York, NY, USA, 1990.
9. World Health Organization. *Guidelines for Safe Recreational Water Environments—Volume 2 Swimming Pools and Similar Environments*; World Health Organization: Geneva, Switzerland, 2006.
10. World Health Organization. *Gudelines for Safe Recreational Water Environments, Volume 1: Coastal and Fresh Waters*; World Health Organization: Geneva, Switzerland, 2003.
11. Environmental Protection Department. *Water Quality Criteria/Standards Adopted in the Asia Pacific Region*; Asia Pacific Economic Cooperation Secretariat: Singapore, 2003.
12. European Environment Agency. *Directive 2006/7/EC of the European Parliament and of the Council of February 2006 Concerning the Management of Bathing Water Quality and Repealing Directive 76/160/EEC*; European Environment Agency: Geneva, Switzerland, 2006.
13. Harwood, V.; Shanks, O.; Korajkic, A.; Verbyla, M.; Ahmed, W.; Iriate, M. *General and Host-Associated Bacterial Indicators of Faecal Pollution*; Global Water Pathogen Project; Michigan State University: E. Lansing, MI, USA, 2017.
14. Harwood, V.J.; Staley, C.; Badgley, B.D.; Borges, K.; Korajkic, A. Microbial source tracking markers for detection of fecal contamination in environmental waters: Relationships between pathogens and human health outcomes. *FEMS Microbiol. Rev.* **2014**, *38*, 1–40. [CrossRef] [PubMed]
15. Department of Environment and Conservation. *Western Australian Guidelines for Biosolids Management*; European Environment Agency: Geneva, Switzerland; Perth, Australia, 2012.
16. North Carolina Environmental Quality. *North Carolina Adm. Code 15A NCAC 2U Reclaimed Water*; North Carolina Department of Environment and Natural Resources: Raleigh, NC, USA, 2011.
17. Queensland Government Environmental Protection Agency. *Queensland Water Recycling Guidelines*; Queensland Government Environmental Protection Agency: Brisbane, Australia, 2005.
18. United States Environmental Protection Agency. *Review of Coliphages as Possible Indicators of Fecal Contamination for Ambient Water Quality*; United States Environmental Protection Agency: Washington, DC, USA, 2015.
19. United States Environmental Protection Agency. *2016 Coliphage Experts Workshop: Discussion Topics and Findings*; United States Environmental Protection Agency: Washington, DC, USA, 2016.
20. Nguyen, K.H.; Senay, C.; Young, S.; Nayak, B.; Lobos, A.; Conrad, J.; Harwood, V.J. Determination of wild animal sources of fecal indicator bacteria by microbial source tracking (MST) influences regulatory decisions. *Water Res.* **2018**, *144*, 424–434. [CrossRef] [PubMed]

21. Soller, J.A.; Schoen, M.E.; Varghese, A.; Ichida, A.M.; Boehm, A.B.; Eftim, S.; Ashbolt, N.J.; Ravenscroft, J.E. Human health risk implications of multiple sources of faecal indicator bacteria in a recreational waterbody. *Water Res.* **2014**, *66*, 254–264. [CrossRef] [PubMed]

22. Forni, D.; Cagliani, R.; Clerici, M.; Sironi, M. Origin and dispersal of hepatitis E virus. *Emerg. Microbes Infect.* **2018**, *7*, 11. [CrossRef] [PubMed]

23. Salines, M.; Andraud, M.; Rose, N. Combining network analysis with epidemiological data to inform risk-based surveillance: Application to hepatitis E virus (HEV) in pigs. *Prev. Vet. Med.* **2018**, *149*, 125–131. [CrossRef] [PubMed]

24. Lama, J.K.; Bachoon, D.S. Detection of *Brucella suis*, *Campylobacter jejuni*, and *Escherichia coli* strains in feral pig (*Sus scrofa*) communities of Georgia. *Vector-Borne Zoonot. Dis.* **2018**, *18*, 350–355. [CrossRef]

25. Migura-Garcia, L.; Ramos, R.; Cerda-Cuellar, M. Antimicrobial resistance of *salmonella* serovars and *campylobacter* spp. Isolated from an opportunistic gull species, yellow-legged gull (*Larus michahellis*). *J. Wildl. Dis.* **2017**, *53*, 148–152. [CrossRef] [PubMed]

26. Valeriani, F.; Giampaoli, S.; Romano Spica, V. The molecular enrichment approach for the identification of microbiological indicators in recreational waters. *Microchem. J.* **2014**, *112*, 70–74. [CrossRef]

27. Graciaa, D.S.; Cope, J.R.; Roberts, V.A.; Cikesh, B.L.; Kahler, A.M.; Vigar, M.; Hilborn, E.D.; Wade, T.J.; Backer, L.C.; Montgomery, S.P.; et al. Outbreaks associated with untreated recreational water—United States, 2000–2014. *Am. J. Transplant.* **2018**, *18*, 2083–2087. [CrossRef] [PubMed]

28. Hlavsa, M.C.; Roberts, V.A.; Anderson, A.R.; Hill, V.R.; Kahler, A.M.; Orr, M.; Garrison, L.E.; Hicks, L.A.; Newton, A.; Hilborn, E.D.; et al. Surveillance for waterborne disease outbreaks and other health events associated with recreational water—United States, 2007–2008. *MMWR Surveill. Summ.* **2011**, *60*, 1–32. [PubMed]

29. Hlavsa, M.C.; Roberts, V.A.; Kahler, A.M.; Hilborn, E.D.; Wade, T.J.; Backer, L.C.; Yoder, J.S. Recreational water-associated disease outbreaks—United States, 2009–2010. *MMWR Morb. Mortal. Wkly. Rep.* **2014**, *63*, 6–10. [PubMed]

30. Hlavsa, M.C.; Roberts, V.A.; Kahler, A.M.; Hilborn, E.D.; Mecher, T.R.; Beach, M.J.; Wade, T.J.; Yoder, J.S. Outbreaks of illness associated with recreational water—United States, 2011–2012. *MMWR Morb. Mortal. Wkly. Rep.* **2015**, *64*, 668–672. [PubMed]

31. Dale, K.; Kirk, M.; Sinclair, M.; Hall, R.; Leder, K. Reported waterborne outbreaks of gastrointestinal disease in Australia are predominantly associated with recreational exposure. *Aust. N. Z. J. Public Health* **2010**, *34*, 527–530. [CrossRef]

32. Guzman-Herrador, B.; Carlander, A.; Ethelberg, S.; Freiesleben de Blasio, B.; Kuusi, M.; Lund, V.; Lofdahl, M.; MacDonald, E.; Nichols, G.; Schonning, C.; et al. Waterborne outbreaks in the Nordic countries, 1998 to 2012. *Eurosurveillance* **2015**, *20*, 21160. [CrossRef]

33. Sinclair, R.G.; Jones, E.L.; Gerba, C.P. Viruses in recreational water-borne disease outbreaks: A review. *J. Appl. Microbiol.* **2009**, *107*, 1769–1780. [CrossRef]

34. Ahmed, W.; Goonetilleke, A.; Gardner, T. Alternative indicators for detection and quantification of faecal pollution. *Water* **2008**, *39*, 46–49.

35. Abia, A.L.K.; Ubomba-Jaswa, E.; Genthe, B.; Momba, M.N.B. Quantitative microbial risk assessment (QMRA) shows increased public health risk associated with exposure to river water under conditions of riverbed sediment resuspension. *Sci. Total Environ.* **2016**, *566–567*, 1143–1151. [CrossRef]

36. Diallo, M.B.; Anceno, A.J.; Tawatsupa, B.; Houpt, E.R.; Wangsuphachart, V.; Shipin, O.V. Infection risk assessment of diarrhea-related pathogens in a tropical canal network. *Sci. Total Environ.* **2008**, *407*, 223–232. [CrossRef] [PubMed]

37. Fernandez, C.; Salerno, C.M.; Paoloni, J.D.; Laurent, G.C. Water quality in a lagoon in the southeast pampa region of Argentina. *Rev. Argent. Microbiol.* **2007**, *39*, 51–56. [PubMed]

38. Gemmell, M.E.; Schmidt, S. Is the microbiological quality of the Msunduzi River (KwaZulu-Natal, South Africa) suitable for domestic, recreational, and agricultural purposes? *Environ. Sci. Pollut. Res. Int.* **2013**, *20*, 6551–6562. [CrossRef] [PubMed]

39. Hot, D.; Legeay, O.; Jacques, J.; Gantzer, C.; Caudrelier, Y.; Guyard, K.; Lange, M.; Andreoletti, L. Detection of somatic phages, infectious enteroviruses and enterovirus genomes as indicators of human enteric viral pollution in surface water. *Water Res.* **2003**, *37*, 4703–4710. [CrossRef]

40. Hsu, B.M.; Chen, C.H.; Wan, M.T.; Cheng, H.W. *Legionella* prevalence in hot spring recreation areas of Taiwan. *Water Res.* **2006**, *40*, 3267–3273. [CrossRef] [PubMed]

41. Jacob, P.; Henry, A.; Meheut, G.; Charni-Ben-Tabassi, N.; Ingrand, V.; Helmi, K. Health risk assessment related to waterborne pathogens from the river to the tap. *Int. J. Environ. Res. Public Health* **2015**, *12*, 2967–2983. [CrossRef] [PubMed]

42. Kern, A.; Kadar, M.; Szomor, K.; Berencsi, G.; Kapusinszky, B.; Vargha, M. Detection of enteric viruses in hungarian surface waters: First steps towards environmental surveillance. *J. Water Health* **2013**, *11*, 772–782. [CrossRef]

43. Marucci, P.L.; Olivera, N.L.; Brugnoni, L.I.; Sica, M.G.; Cubitto, M.A. The occurrence of Shiga toxin-producing *Escherichia coli* in bathing water of the Sierra de la Ventana region, Buenos Aires Province, Argentina. *Environ. Monit. Assess.* **2011**, *175*, 1–8. [CrossRef]

44. Mwanamoki, P.M.; Devarajan, N.; Thevenon, F.; Atibu, E.K.; Tshibanda, J.B.; Ngelinkoto, P.; Mpiana, P.T.; Prabakar, K.; Mubedi, J.I.; Kabele, C.G.; et al. Assessment of pathogenic bacteria in water and sediment from a water reservoir under tropical conditions (Lake Ma Vallee), Kinshasa Democratic Republic of Congo. *Environ. Monit. Assess.* **2014**, *186*, 6821–6830. [CrossRef]

45. Roser, D.J.; Davies, C.M.; Ashbolt, N.J.; Morison, P. Microbial exposure assessment of an urban recreational lake: A case study of the application of new risk-based guidelines. *Water Sci. Technol.* **2006**, *54*, 245–252. [CrossRef]

46. Sales-Ortells, H.; Agostini, G.; Medema, G. Quantification of waterborne pathogens and associated health risks in urban water. *Environ. Sci. Technol.* **2015**, *49*, 6943–6952. [CrossRef] [PubMed]

47. Schets, F.M.; van Wijnen, J.H.; Schijven, J.F.; Schoon, H.; de Roda Husman, A.M. Monitoring of waterborne pathogens in surface waters in Amsterdam, the Netherlands, and the potential health risk associated with exposure to *Cryptosporidium* and *Giardia* in these waters. *Appl. Environ. Microbiol.* **2008**, *74*, 2069–2078. [CrossRef] [PubMed]

48. Staley, C.; Reckhow, K.H.; Lukasik, J.; Harwood, V.J. Assessment of sources of human pathogens and fecal contamination in a florida freshwater lake. *Water Res.* **2012**, *46*, 5799–5812. [CrossRef] [PubMed]

49. Strathmann, M.; Horstkott, M.; Koch, C.; Gayer, U.; Wingender, J. The River Ruhr—An urban river under particular interest for recreational use and as a raw water source for drinking water: The collaborative research project "Safe Ruhr"—Microbiological aspects. *Int. J. Hyg. Environ. Health* **2016**, *219*, 643–661. [CrossRef] [PubMed]

50. Thorolfsdottir, B.O.; Marteinsson, V.T. Microbiological analysis in three diverse natural geothermal bathing pools in iceland. *Int. J. Environ. Res. Public Health* **2013**, *10*, 1085–1099. [CrossRef]

51. Weidhaas, J.; Anderson, A.; Jamal, R. Elucidating waterborne pathogen presence and aiding source apportionment in an impaired stream. *Appl. Environ. Microbiol.* **2018**, *84*, AEM-02510. [CrossRef]

52. Wyn-Jones, A.P.; Carducci, A.; Cook, N.; D'Agostino, M.; Divizia, M.; Fleischer, J.; Gantzer, C.; Gawler, A.; Girones, R.; Holler, C.; et al. Surveillance of adenoviruses and noroviruses in European recreational waters. *Water Res.* **2011**, *45*, 1025–1038. [CrossRef]

53. Burnet, J.B.; Penny, C.; Ogorzaly, L.; Cauchie, H.M. Spatial and temporal distribution of *Cryptosporidium* and *Giardia* in a drinking water resource: Implications for monitoring and risk assessment. *Sci. Total Environ.* **2014**, *472*, 1023–1035. [CrossRef]

54. Devane, M.L.; Moriarty, E.M.; Wood, D.; Webster-Brown, J.; Gilpin, B.J. The impact of major earthquakes and subsequent sewage discharges on the microbial quality of water and sediments in an urban river. *Sci. Total Environ.* **2014**, *485–486*, 666–680. [CrossRef]

55. Dorevitch, S.; Doi, M.; Hsu, F.C.; Lin, K.T.; Roberts, J.D.; Liu, L.C.; Gladding, R.; Vannoy, E.; Li, H.; Javor, M.; et al. A comparison of rapid and conventional measures of indicator bacteria as predictors of waterborne protozoan pathogen presence and density. *J. Environ. Monit.* **2011**, *13*, 2427–2435. [CrossRef]

56. Duris, J.W.; Reif, A.G.; Krouse, D.A.; Isaacs, N.M. Factors related to occurrence and distribution of selected bacterial and protozoan pathogens in pennsylvania streams. *Water Res.* **2013**, *47*, 300–314. [CrossRef] [PubMed]

57. Haack, S.K.; Duris, J.W.; Fogarty, L.R.; Kolpin, D.W.; Focazio, M.J.; Furlong, E.T.; Meyer, M.T. Comparing wastewater chemicals, indicator bacteria concentrations, and bacterial pathogen genes as fecal pollution indicators. *J. Environ. Qual.* **2009**, *38*, 248–258. [CrossRef]

58. Ji, W.T.; Hsu, B.M.; Chang, T.Y.; Hsu, T.K.; Kao, P.M.; Huang, K.H.; Tsai, S.F.; Huang, Y.L.; Fan, C.W. Surveillance and evaluation of the infection risk of free-living amoebae and *Legionella* in different aquatic environments. *Sci. Total Environ.* **2014**, *499*, 212–219. [CrossRef] [PubMed]

59. Mansilha, C.R.; Coelho, C.A.; Reinas, A.; Moutinho, A.; Ferreira, S.; Pizarro, C.; Tavares, A. *Salmonella*: The forgotten pathogen: Health hazards of compliance with European bathing water legislation. *Mar. Pollut. Bull.* **2010**, *60*, 819–826. [CrossRef] [PubMed]

60. Oster, R.J.; Wijesinghe, R.U.; Haack, S.K.; Fogarty, L.R.; Tucker, T.R.; Riley, S.C. Bacterial pathogen gene abundance and relation to recreational water quality at seven Great Lakes beaches. *Environ. Sci. Technol.* **2014**, *48*, 14148–14157. [CrossRef] [PubMed]

61. Poma, V.; Mamani, N.; Iniguez, V. Impact of urban contamination of the La Paz River basin on thermotolerant coliform density and occurrence of multiple antibiotic resistant enteric pathogens in river water, irrigated soil and fresh vegetables. *Springerplus* **2016**, *5*, 499. [CrossRef] [PubMed]

62. Shen, S.M.; Chou, M.Y.; Hsu, B.M.; Ji, W.T.; Hsu, T.K.; Tsai, H.F.; Huang, Y.L.; Chiu, Y.C.; Kao, E.S.; Kao, P.M.; et al. Assessment of *Legionella pneumophila* in recreational spring water with quantitative PCR (Taqman) assay. *Pathog. Glob. Health* **2015**, *109*, 236–241. [CrossRef] [PubMed]

63. Wilkes, G.; Edge, T.; Gannon, V.; Jokinen, C.; Lyautey, E.; Medeiros, D.; Neumann, N.; Ruecker, N.; Topp, E.; Lapen, D.R. Seasonal relationships among indicator bacteria, pathogenic bacteria, *Cryptosporidium* oocysts, *Giardia* cysts, and hydrological indices for surface waters within an agricultural landscape. *Water Res.* **2009**, *43*, 2209–2223. [CrossRef] [PubMed]

64. Wyer, M.D.; Wyn-Jones, A.P.; Kay, D.; Au-Yeung, H.K.; Girones, R.; Lopez-Pila, J.; de Roda Husman, A.M.; Rutjes, S.; Schneider, O. Relationships between human adenoviruses and faecal indicator organisms in European recreational waters. *Water Res.* **2012**, *46*, 4130–4141. [CrossRef] [PubMed]

65. Xiao, G.; Wang, Z.; Chen, J.; Qiu, Z.; Li, Y.; Qi, J.; Liu, W.; Shu, W. Occurrence and infection risk of waterborne pathogens in Wanzhou watershed of the Three Gorges Reservoir, China. *J. Environ. Sci.* **2013**, *25*, 1913–1924. [CrossRef]

66. Cui, Q.; Fang, T.; Huang, Y.; Dong, P.; Wang, H. Evaluation of bacterial pathogen diversity, abundance and health risks in urban recreational water by amplicon next-generation sequencing and quantitative PCR. *J. Environ. Sci.* **2017**, *57*, 137–149. [CrossRef] [PubMed]

67. Duris, J.W.; Haack, S.K.; Fogarty, L.R. Gene and antigen markers of Shiga-toxin producing *E. coli* from Michigan and Indiana river water: Occurrence and relation to recreational water quality criteria. *J. Environ. Qual.* **2009**, *38*, 1878–1886. [CrossRef] [PubMed]

68. Fang, T.; Cui, Q.; Huang, Y.; Dong, P.; Wang, H.; Liu, W.T.; Ye, Q. Distribution comparison and risk assessment of free-floating and particle-attached bacterial pathogens in urban recreational water: Implications for water quality management. *Sci. Total Environ.* **2018**, *613–614*, 428–438. [CrossRef] [PubMed]

69. Fong, T.T.; Griffin, D.W.; Lipp, E.K. Molecular assays for targeting human and bovine enteric viruses in coastal waters and their application for library-independent source tracking. *Appl. Environ. Microbiol.* **2005**, *71*, 2070–2078. [CrossRef] [PubMed]

70. Hellein, K.N.; Battie, C.; Tauchman, E.; Lund, D.; Oyarzabal, O.A.; Lepo, J.E. Culture-based indicators of fecal contamination and molecular microbial indicators rarely correlate with *Campylobacter* spp. in recreational waters. *J. Water Health* **2011**, *9*, 695–707. [CrossRef] [PubMed]

71. Ishii, S.; Nakamura, T.; Ozawa, S.; Kobayashi, A.; Sano, D.; Okabe, S. Water quality monitoring and risk assessment by simultaneous multipathogen quantification. *Environ. Sci. Technol.* **2014**, *48*, 4744–4749. [CrossRef] [PubMed]

72. Lee, C.S.; Lee, C.; Marion, J.; Wang, Q.H.; Saif, L.; Lee, J. Occurrence of human enteric viruses at freshwater beaches during swimming season and its link to water inflow. *Sci. Total Environ.* **2014**, *472*, 757–766. [CrossRef]

73. Miagostovich, M.P.; Ferreira, F.F.; Guimaraes, F.R.; Fumian, T.M.; Diniz-Mendes, L.; Luz, S.L.; Silva, L.A.; Leite, J.P. Molecular detection and characterization of gastroenteritis viruses occurring naturally in the stream waters of manaus, central Amazonia, Brazil. *Appl. Environ. Microbiol.* **2008**, *74*, 375–382. [CrossRef] [PubMed]

74. Smith, C.J.; Olszewski, A.M.; Mauro, S.A. Correlation of shiga toxin gene frequency with commonly used microbial indicators of recreational water quality. *Appl. Environ. Microbiol.* **2009**, *75*, 316–321. [CrossRef]

75. Xiao, S.; Zhang, Y.; Zhao, X.; Sun, L.; Hu, S. Presence and molecular characterization of *Cryptosporidium* and *Giardia* in recreational lake water in Tianjin, China: A preliminary study. *Sci. Rep.* **2018**, *8*, 2353. [CrossRef]

76. Abdelzaher, A.M.; Wright, M.E.; Ortega, C.; Hasan, A.R.; Shibata, T.; Solo-Gabriele, H.M.; Kish, J.; Withum, K.; He, G.; Elmir, S.M.; et al. Daily measures of microbes and human health at a non-point source marine beach. *J. Water Health* **2011**, *9*, 443–457. [CrossRef] [PubMed]

77. Abdelzaher, A.M.; Wright, M.E.; Ortega, C.; Solo-Gabriele, H.M.; Miller, G.; Elmir, S.; Newman, X.; Shih, P.; Bonilla, J.A.; Bonilla, T.D.; et al. Presence of pathogens and indicator microbes at a non-point source subtropical recreational marine beach. *Appl. Environ. Microbiol.* **2010**, *76*, 724–732. [CrossRef] [PubMed]

78. Goyal, S.M.; Gerba, C.P.; Melnick, J.L. Occurrence and distribution of bacterial indicators and pathogens in canal communities along the Texas coast. *Appl. Environ. Microbiol.* **1977**, *34*, 139–149. [PubMed]

79. Griffith, J.F.; Weisberg, S.B.; Arnold, B.F.; Cao, Y.; Schiff, K.C.; Colford, J.M., Jr. Epidemiologic evaluation of multiple alternate microbial water quality monitoring indicators at three California beaches. *Water Res.* **2016**, *94*, 371–381. [CrossRef] [PubMed]

80. Korajkic, A.; Brownell, M.J.; Harwood, V.J. Investigation of human sewage pollution and pathogen analysis at Florida Gulf coast beaches. *J. Appl. Microbiol.* **2011**, *110*, 174–183. [CrossRef] [PubMed]

81. Lipp, E.K.; Farrah, S.A.; Rose, J.B. Assessment and impact of microbial fecal pollution and human enteric pathogens in a coastal community. *Mar. Pollut. Bull.* **2001**, *42*, 286–293. [CrossRef]

82. Moce-Llivina, L.; Lucena, F.; Jofre, J. Enteroviruses and bacteriophages in bathing waters. *Appl. Environ. Microbiol.* **2005**, *71*, 6838–6844. [CrossRef] [PubMed]

83. Rosario, K.; Symonds, E.M.; Sinigalliano, C.; Stewart, J.; Breitbart, M. Pepper mild mottle virus as an indicator of fecal pollution. *Appl. Environ. Microbiol.* **2009**, *75*, 7261–7267. [CrossRef] [PubMed]

84. Shaw, K.S.; Rosenberg Goldstein, R.E.; He, X.; Jacobs, J.M.; Crump, B.C.; Sapkota, A.R. Antimicrobial susceptibility of *Vibrio vulnificus* and *Vibrio parahaemolyticus* recovered from recreational and commercial areas of Chesapeake Bay and Maryland Coastal Bays. *PLoS ONE* **2014**, *9*, e89616. [CrossRef]

85. Shaw, K.S.; Sapkota, A.R.; Jacobs, J.M.; He, X.; Crump, B.C. Recreational swimmers' exposure to *Vibrio vulnificus* and *Vibrio parahaemolyticus* in the Chesapeake Bay, Maryland, USA. *Environ. Int.* **2015**, *74*, 99–105. [CrossRef]

86. Sinigalliano, C.D.; Fleisher, J.M.; Gidley, M.L.; Solo-Gabriele, H.M.; Shibata, T.; Plano, L.R.; Elmir, S.M.; Wanless, D.; Bartkowiak, J.; Boiteau, R.; et al. Traditional and molecular analyses for fecal indicator bacteria in non-point source subtropical recreational marine waters. *Water Res.* **2010**, *44*, 3763–3772. [CrossRef] [PubMed]

87. Wetz, J.J.; Lipp, E.K.; Griffin, D.W.; Lukasik, J.; Wait, D.; Sobsey, M.D.; Scott, T.M.; Rose, J.B. Presence, infectivity, and stability of enteric viruses in seawater: Relationship to marine water quality in the Florida keys. *Mar. Pollut. Bull.* **2004**, *48*, 698–704. [CrossRef] [PubMed]

88. Betancourt, W.Q.; Duarte, D.C.; Vasquez, R.C.; Gurian, P.L. *Cryptosporidium* and *Giardia* in tropical recreational marine waters contaminated with domestic sewage: Estimation of bathing-associated disease risks. *Mar. Pollut. Bull.* **2014**, *85*, 268–273. [CrossRef] [PubMed]

89. Henry, R.; Schang, C.; Kolotelo, P.; Coleman, R.; Rooney, G.; Schmidt, J.; Deletic, A.; McCarthy, D.T. Effect of environmental parameters on pathogen and faecal indicator organism concentrations within an urban estuary. *Estuar. Coast. Shelf Sci.* **2016**, *174*, 18–26. [CrossRef]

90. Jiang, S.; Noble, R.; Chu, W. Human adenoviruses and coliphages in urban runoff-impacted coastal waters of southern California. *Appl. Environ. Microbiol.* **2001**, *67*, 179–184. [CrossRef] [PubMed]

91. Jiang, S.C.; Chu, W. Pcr detection of pathogenic viruses in southern California urban rivers. *J. Appl. Microbiol.* **2004**, *97*, 17–28. [CrossRef]

92. Jiang, S.C.; Chu, W.; He, J.W. Seasonal detection of human viruses and coliphage in Newport Bay, California. *Appl. Environ. Microbiol.* **2007**, *73*, 6468–6474. [CrossRef]

93. McQuaig, S.; Griffith, J.; Harwood, V.J. Association of fecal indicator bacteria with human viruses and microbial source tracking markers at coastal beaches impacted by nonpoint source pollution. *Appl. Environ. Microbiol.* **2012**, *78*, 6423–6432. [CrossRef]

94. Ortega, C.; Solo-Gabriele, H.M.; Abdelzaher, A.; Wright, M.; Deng, Y.; Stark, L.M. Correlations between microbial indicators, pathogens, and environmental factors in a subtropical estuary. *Mar. Pollut. Bull.* **2009**, *58*, 1374–1381. [CrossRef]

95. Silva, A.M.; Vieira, H.; Martins, N.; Granja, A.T.; Vale, M.J.; Vale, F.F. Viral and bacterial contamination in recreational waters: A case study in the Lisbon bay area. *J. Appl. Microbiol.* **2010**, *108*, 1023–1031. [CrossRef]

96. Efstratiou, M.A.; Tsirtsis, G. Do 2006/7/EC European Union Bathing Water Standards exclude the risk of contact with *Salmonella* or *Candida albicans*? *Mar. Pollut. Bull.* **2009**, *58*, 1039–1044. [CrossRef] [PubMed]

97. Graczyk, T.K.; Sunderland, D.; Awantang, G.N.; Mashinski, Y.; Lucy, F.E.; Graczyk, Z.; Chomicz, L.; Breysse, P.N. Relationships among bather density, levels of human waterborne pathogens, and fecal coliform counts in marine recreational beach water. *Parasitol. Res.* **2010**, *106*, 1103–1108. [CrossRef] [PubMed]

98. McQuaig, S.M.; Scott, T.M.; Harwood, V.J.; Farrah, S.R.; Lukasik, J.O. Detection of human-derived fecal pollution in environmental waters by use of a PCR-based human polyomavirus assay. *Appl. Environ. Microbiol.* **2006**, *72*, 7567–7574. [CrossRef] [PubMed]

99. McQuaig, S.M.; Scott, T.M.; Lukasik, J.O.; Paul, J.H.; Harwood, V.J. Quantification of human polyomaviruses JC virus and BK virus by taqman quantitative pcr and comparison to other water quality indicators in water and fecal samples. *Appl. Environ. Microbiol.* **2009**, *75*, 3379–3388. [CrossRef] [PubMed]

100. Viau, E.J.; Goodwin, K.D.; Yamahara, K.M.; Layton, B.A.; Sassoubre, L.M.; Burns, S.L.; Tong, H.I.; Wong, S.H.; Lu, Y.; Boehm, A.B. Bacterial pathogens in Hawaiian coastal streams—Associations with fecal indicators, land cover, and water quality. *Water Res.* **2011**, *45*, 3279–3290. [CrossRef] [PubMed]

101. Graczyk, T.K.; Sunderland, D.; Tamang, L.; Shields, T.M.; Lucy, F.E.; Breysse, P.N. Quantitative evaluation of the impact of bather density on levels of human-virulent microsporidian spores in recreational water. *Appl. Environ. Microbiol.* **2007**, *73*, 4095–4099. [CrossRef] [PubMed]

102. Lodder, W.J.; de Roda Husman, A.M. Presence of noroviruses and other enteric viruses in sewage and surface waters in the Netherlands. *Appl. Environ. Microbiol.* **2005**, *71*, 1453–1461. [CrossRef] [PubMed]

103. Rezaeinejad, S.; Vergara, G.G.; Woo, C.H.; Lim, T.T.; Sobsey, M.D.; Gin, K.Y. Surveillance of enteric viruses and coliphages in a tropical urban catchment. *Water Res.* **2014**, *58*, 122–131. [CrossRef]

104. Fung, D.Y.C.; Fujioka, R.; Vijayavel, K.; Sato, D.; Bishop, D. Evaluation of fung double tube test for *Clostridium perfringens* and Easyphage test for F-specific RNA coliphages as rapid screening tests for fecal contamination in recreational waters of Hawaii (vol 15, pg 217, 2007). *J. Rapid Methods Autom. Microbiol.* **2007**, *15*, 411. [CrossRef]

105. Wong, M.; Kumar, L.; Jenkins, T.M.; Xagoraraki, I.; Phanikumar, M.S.; Rose, J.B. Evaluation of public health risks at recreational beaches in Lake Michigan via detection of enteric viruses and a human-specific bacteriological marker. *Water Res.* **2009**, *43*, 1137–1149. [CrossRef]

106. Walters, S.P.; Gannon, V.P.; Field, K.G. Detection of *Bacteroidales* fecal indicators and the zoonotic pathogens *E. coli* 0157:H7, *Salmonella*, and *Campylobacter* in river water. *Environ. Sci. Technol.* **2007**, *41*, 1856–1862. [CrossRef] [PubMed]

107. Donati, M.; Cremonini, E.; Di Francesco, A.; Dallolio, L.; Biondi, R.; Muthusamy, R.; Leoni, E. Prevalence of *Simkania negevensis* in chlorinated water from spa swimming pools and domestic supplies. *J. Appl. Microbiol.* **2015**, *118*, 1076–1082. [CrossRef] [PubMed]

108. La Rosa, G.; Della Libera, S.; Petricca, S.; Iaconelli, M.; Briancesco, R.; Paradiso, R.; Semproni, M.; Di Bonito, P.; Bonadonna, L. First detection of papillomaviruses and polyomaviruses in swimming pool waters: Unrecognized recreational water-related pathogens? *J. Appl. Microbiol.* **2015**, *119*, 1683–1691. [CrossRef] [PubMed]

109. Maunula, L.; Kalso, S.; Von Bonsdorff, C.H.; Ponka, A. Wading pool water contaminated with both noroviruses and astroviruses as the source of a gastroenteritis outbreak. *Epidemiol. Infect.* **2004**, *132*, 737–743. [CrossRef] [PubMed]

110. Wade, T.J.; Calderon, R.L.; Brenner, K.P.; Sams, E.; Beach, M.; Haugland, R.; Wymer, L.; Dufour, A.P. High sensitivity of children to swimming-associated gastrointestinal illness: Results using a rapid assay of recreational water quality. *Epidemiology* **2008**, *19*, 375–383. [CrossRef]

111. Yau, V.M.; Schiff, K.C.; Arnold, B.F.; Griffith, J.F.; Gruber, J.S.; Wright, C.C.; Wade, T.J.; Burns, S.; Hayes, J.M.; McGee, C.; et al. Effect of submarine groundwater discharge on bacterial indicators and swimmer health at Avalon Beach, CA, USA. *Water Res.* **2014**, *59*, 23–36. [CrossRef]

112. Napier, M.D.; Haugland, R.; Poole, C.; Dufour, A.P.; Stewart, J.R.; Weber, D.J.; Varma, M.; Lavender, J.S.; Wade, T.J. Exposure to human-associated fecal indicators and self-reported illness among swimmers at recreational beaches: A cohort study. *Environ. Health* **2017**, *16*, 103. [CrossRef]

113. Benjamin-Chung, J.; Arnold, B.F.; Wade, T.J.; Schiff, K.; Griffith, J.F.; Dufour, A.P.; Weisberg, S.B.; Colford, J.M., Jr. Coliphages and gastrointestinal illness in recreational waters: Pooled analysis of six coastal beach cohorts. *Epidemiology* **2017**, *28*, 644–652. [CrossRef]

114. Arnold, B.F.; Wade, T.J.; Benjamin-Chung, J.; Schiff, K.C.; Griffith, J.F.; Dufour, A.P.; Weisberg, S.B.; Colford, J.M., Jr. Acute gastroenteritis and recreational water: Highest burden among young US children. *Am. J. Public Health* **2016**, *106*, 1690–1697. [CrossRef]

115. Wade, T.J.; Sams, E.A.; Beach, M.J.; Collier, S.A.; Dufour, A.P. The incidence and health burden of earaches attributable to recreational swimming in natural waters: A prospective cohort study. *Environ. Health* **2013**, *12*, 67. [CrossRef]

116. Colford, J.M., Jr.; Schiff, K.C.; Griffith, J.F.; Yau, V.; Arnold, B.F.; Wright, C.C.; Gruber, J.S.; Wade, T.J.; Burns, S.; Hayes, J.; et al. Using rapid indicators for enterococcus to assess the risk of illness after exposure to urban runoff contaminated marine water. *Water Res.* **2012**, *46*, 2176–2186. [CrossRef] [PubMed]

117. Wade, T.J.; Sams, E.; Brenner, K.P.; Haugland, R.; Chern, E.; Beach, M.; Wymer, L.; Rankin, C.C.; Love, D.; Li, Q.; et al. Rapidly measured indicators of recreational water quality and swimming-associated illness at marine beaches: A prospective cohort study. *Environ. Health* **2010**, *9*, 66. [CrossRef] [PubMed]

118. Colford, J.M., Jr.; Wade, T.J.; Schift, K.C.; Wright, C.; Griffith, J.F.; Sandhu, S.K.; Weisberg, S.B. *Recreational Water Contact and Illness in Mission Bay, California*; Southern California Coastal Water Research Project: Costa Mesa, CA, USA, 2005.

119. Colford, J.M., Jr.; Wade, T.J.; Schiff, K.C.; Wright, C.C.; Griffith, J.F.; Sandhu, S.K.; Burns, S.; Sobsey, M.; Lovelace, G.; Weisberg, S.B. Water quality indicators and the risk of illness at beaches with nonpoint sources of fecal contamination. *Epidemiology* **2007**, *18*, 27–35. [CrossRef] [PubMed]

120. Wade, T.J.; Calderon, R.L.; Sams, E.; Beach, M.; Brenner, K.P.; Williams, A.H.; Dufour, A.P. Rapidly measured indicators of recreational water quality are predictive of swimming-associated gastrointestinal illness. *Environ. Health Perspect.* **2006**, *114*, 24–28. [CrossRef]

121. Arnold, B.F.; Schiff, K.C.; Ercumen, A.; Benjamin-Chung, J.; Steele, J.A.; Griffith, J.F.; Steinberg, S.J.; Smith, P.; McGee, C.D.; Wilson, R.; et al. Acute illness among surfers after exposure to seawater in dry- and wet-weather conditions. *Am. J. Epidemiol.* **2017**, *186*, 866–875. [CrossRef] [PubMed]

122. Vonschirnding, Y.E.R.; Kfir, R.; Cabelli, V.; Franklin, L.; Joubert, G. Morbidity among bathers exposed to polluted seawater—A prospective epidemiologic-study. *S. Afr. Med. J.* **1992**, *81*, 543–546.

123. Lee, J.V.; Dawson, S.R.; Ward, S.; Surman, S.B.; Neal, K.R. Bacteriophages are a better indicator of illness rates than bacteria amongst users of a white water course fed by a lowland river. *Water Sci. Technol.* **1997**, *35*, 165–170. [CrossRef]

124. Van Asperen, I.A.; Medema, G.; Borgdorff, M.W.; Sprenger, M.J.W.; Havelaar, A.H. Risk of gastroenteritis among triathletes in relation to faecal pollution of fresh waters. *Int. J. Epidemiol.* **1998**, *27*, 309–315. [CrossRef]

125. Schets, F.M.; Schijven, J.F.; de Roda Husman, A.M. Exposure assessment for swimmers in bathing waters and swimming pools. *Water Res.* **2011**, *45*, 2392–2400. [CrossRef]

126. Schets, F.M.; De Roda Husman, A.M.; Havelaar, A.H. Disease outbreaks associated with untreated recreational water use. *Epidemiol. Infect.* **2011**, *139*, 1114–1125. [CrossRef]

127. Grenier, J.L.; Davis, J.A. Water quality in south San Francisco Bay, California: Current condition and potential issues for the South Bay Salt Pond Restoration Project. *Rev. Environ. Contam. Toxicol.* **2010**, *206*, 115–147. [PubMed]

128. McMinn, B.R.; Ashbolt, N.J.; Korajkic, A. Bacteriophages as indicators of faecal pollution and enteric virus removal. *Lett. Appl. Microbiol.* **2017**, *65*, 11–26. [CrossRef] [PubMed]

129. McMinn, B.R.; Korajkic, A.; Ashbolt, N.J. Evaluation of *Bacteroides fragilis* GB-124 bacteriophages as novel human-associated faecal indicators in the United States. *Lett. Appl. Microbiol.* **2014**, *59*, 115–121. [CrossRef] [PubMed]

130. Eftim, S.E.; Hong, T.; Soller, J.; Boehm, A.; Warren, I.; Ichida, A.; Nappier, S.P. Occurrence of norovirus in raw sewage—A systematic literature review and meta-analysis. *Water Res.* **2017**, *111*, 366–374. [CrossRef]

131. Li, J.; Wang, H.; Wang, R.; Zhang, L. *Giardia duodenalis* infections in humans and other animals in China. *Front. Microbiol.* **2017**, *8*, 2004. [CrossRef]

132. Rose, J.B.; Huffman, D.E.; Gennaccaro, A. Risk and control of waterborne cryptosporidiosis. *FEMS Microbiol. Rev.* **2002**, *26*, 113–123. [CrossRef]

133. Sinclair, R.G.; Choi, C.Y.; Riley, M.R.; Gerba, C.P. Pathogen surveillance through monitoring of sewer systems. *Adv. Appl. Microbiol.* **2008**, *65*, 249–269.

134. Ganesh, A.; Lin, J. Waterborne human pathogenic viruses of public health concern. *Int. J. Environ. Health Res.* **2013**, *23*, 544–564. [CrossRef]

135. Matthews, L.; Low, J.C.; Gally, D.L.; Pearce, M.C.; Mellor, D.J.; Heesterbeek, J.A.; Chase-Topping, M.; Naylor, S.W.; Shaw, D.J.; Reid, S.W.; et al. Heterogeneous shedding of *Escherichia coli* O157 in cattle and its implications for control. *Proc. Natl. Acad. Sci. USA* **2006**, *103*, 547–552. [CrossRef]

136. Daniels, M.E.; Shrivastava, A.; Smith, W.A.; Sahu, P.; Odagiri, M.; Misra, P.R.; Panigrahi, P.; Suar, M.; Clasen, T.; Jenkins, M.W. *Cryptosporidium* and *Giardia* in humans, domestic animals, and village water sources in rural india. *Am. J. Trop. Med. Hyg.* **2015**, *93*, 596–600. [CrossRef]

137. Oates, S.C.; Miller, M.A.; Hardin, D.; Conrad, P.A.; Melli, A.; Jessup, D.A.; Dominik, C.; Roug, A.; Tinker, M.T.; Miller, W.A. Prevalence, environmental loading, and molecular characterization of *Cryptosporidium* and *Giardia* isolates from domestic and wild animals along the central California Coast. *Appl. Environ. Microbiol.* **2012**, *78*, 8762–8772. [CrossRef] [PubMed]

138. Vonberg, R.P.; Hohle, M.; Aepfelbacher, M.; Bange, F.C.; Campos, C.B.; Claussen, K.; Christner, M.; Cramer, J.P.; Haller, H.; Hornef, M.; et al. Duration of fecal shedding of shiga toxin-producing *Escherichia coli* O104:H4 in patients infected during the 2011 outbreak in Germany: A multicenter study. *Clin. Infect. Dis.* **2013**, *56*, 1132–1140. [CrossRef] [PubMed]

139. Lanzas, C.; Warnick, L.D.; James, K.L.; Wright, E.M.; Wiedmann, M.; Grohn, Y.T. Transmission dynamics of a multidrug-resistant *Salmonella typhimurium* outbreak in a dairy farm. *Foodborne Pathog. Dis.* **2010**, *7*, 467–474. [CrossRef]

140. Venegas-Vargas, C.; Henderson, S.; Khare, A.; Mosci, R.E.; Lehnert, J.D.; Singh, P.; Ouellette, L.M.; Norby, B.; Funk, J.A.; Rust, S.; et al. Factors associated with Shiga toxin-producing *Escherichia coli* shedding by dairy and beef cattle. *Appl. Environ. Microb.* **2016**, *82*, 5049–5056. [CrossRef]

141. Procter, T.D.; Pearl, D.L.; Finley, R.L.; Leonard, E.K.; Janecko, N.; Reid-Smith, R.J.; Weese, J.S.; Peregrine, A.S.; Sargeant, J.M. A cross-sectional study examining *Campylobacter* and other zoonotic enteric pathogens in dogs that frequent dog parks in three cities in south-western ontario and risk factors for shedding of *Campylobacter* spp. *Zoonoses Public Health* **2014**, *61*, 208–218. [CrossRef] [PubMed]

142. Xu, Y.; Dugat-Bony, E.; Zaheer, R.; Selinger, L.; Barbieri, R.; Munns, K.; McAllister, T.A.; Selinger, L.B. *Escherichia coli* O157:H7 super-shedder and non-shedder feedlot steers harbour distinct fecal bacterial communities. *PLoS ONE* **2014**, *9*, e98115. [CrossRef]

143. Leclerc, H.; Schwartzbrod, L.; Dei-Cas, E. Microbial agents associated with waterborne diseases. *Crit. Rev. Microbiol.* **2002**, *28*, 371–409. [CrossRef] [PubMed]

144. Hara-Kudo, Y.; Takatori, K. Contamination level and ingestion dose of foodborne pathogens associated with infections. *Epidemiol. Infect.* **2011**, *139*, 1505–1510. [CrossRef] [PubMed]

145. Harwood, V.J.; Levine, A.D.; Scott, T.M.; Chivukula, V.; Lukasik, J.; Farrah, S.R.; Rose, J.B. Validity of the indicator organism paradigm for pathogen reduction in reclaimed water and public health protection. *Appl. Environ. Microbiol.* **2005**, *71*, 3163–3170. [CrossRef]

146. Hijnen, W.A.; Beerendonk, E.F.; Medema, G.J. Inactivation credit of uv radiation for viruses, bacteria and protozoan (oo)cysts in water: A review. *Water Res.* **2006**, *40*, 3–22. [CrossRef]

147. Nasser, A.M. Removal of *Cryptosporidium* by wastewater treatment processes: A review. *J. Water Health* **2016**, *14*, 1–13. [CrossRef] [PubMed]

148. Eischeid, A.C.; Meyer, J.N.; Linden, K.G. Uv disinfection of adenoviruses: Molecular indications of DNA damage efficiency. *Appl. Environ. Microbiol.* **2009**, *75*, 23–28. [CrossRef] [PubMed]

149. Nelson, K.L.; Boehm, A.B.; Davies-Colley, R.J.; Dodd, M.C.; Kohn, T.; Linden, K.G.; Liu, Y.; Maraccini, P.A.; McNeill, K.; Mitch, W.A.; et al. Sunlight-mediated inactivation of health-relevant microorganisms in water: A review of mechanisms and modeling approaches. *Environ. Sci. Process. Impacts* **2018**, *20*, 1089–1122. [CrossRef] [PubMed]

150. Bae, S.; Wuertz, S. Decay of host-associated bacteroidales cells and DNA in continuous-flow freshwater and seawater microcosms of identical experimental design and temperature as measured by PMA-qPCR and qPCR. *Water Res.* **2015**, *70*, 205–213. [CrossRef] [PubMed]

151. Bae, S.; Wuertz, S. Survival of host-associated bacteroidales cells and their relationship with *Enterococcus* spp., *Campylobacter jejuni*, *Salmonella enterica* serovar typhimurium, and adenovirus in freshwater microcosms as measured by propidium monoazide-quantitative pcr. *Appl. Environ. Microbiol.* **2012**, *78*, 922–932. [CrossRef] [PubMed]

152. Wanjugi, P.; Sivaganesan, M.; Korajkic, A.; Kelty, C.A.; McMinn, B.; Ulrich, R.; Harwood, V.J.; Shanks, O.C. Differential decomposition of bacterial and viral fecal indicators in common human pollution types. *Water Res.* **2016**, *105*, 591–601. [CrossRef]

153. Korajkic, A.; McMinn, B.R.; Shanks, O.C.; Sivaganesan, M.; Fout, G.S.; Ashbolt, N.J. Biotic interactions and sunlight affect persistence of fecal indicator bacteria and microbial source tracking genetic markers in the upper Mississippi River. *Appl. Environ. Microbiol.* **2014**, *80*, 3952–3961. [CrossRef]

154. Kreader, C.A. Persistence of pcr-detectable bacteroides distasonis from human feces in river water. *Appl. Environ. Microbiol.* **1998**, *64*, 4103–4105.

155. Dick, L.K.; Stelzer, E.A.; Bertke, E.E.; Fong, D.L.; Stoeckel, D.M. Relative decay of bacteroidales microbial source tracking markers and cultivated *Escherichia coli* in freshwater microcosms. *Appl. Environ. Microbiol.* **2010**, *76*, 3255–3262. [CrossRef]

156. Booncharoen, N.; Mongkolsuk, S.; Sirikanchana, K. Comparative persistence of human sewage-specific enterococcal bacteriophages in freshwater and seawater. *Appl. Microbiol. Biotechnol.* **2018**, *102*, 6235–6246. [CrossRef]

157. Chauret, C.; Nolan, K.; Chen, P.; Springthorpe, S.; Sattar, S. Aging of *Cryptosporidium parvum* oocysts in river water and their susceptibility to disinfection by chlorine and monochloramine. *Can. J. Microbiol.* **1998**, *44*, 1154–1160. [CrossRef] [PubMed]

158. McCrary, K.J.; Case, C.L.H.; Gentry, T.J.; Aitkenhead-Peterson, J.A. *Escherichia coli* regrowth in disinfected sewage effluent: Effect of doc and nutrients on regrowth in laboratory incubations and urban streams. *Water Air Soil Pollut.* **2013**, *224*, 1412. [CrossRef]

159. Shelton, D.R.; Pachepsky, Y.A.; Kiefer, L.A.; Blaustein, R.A.; McCarty, G.W.; Dao, T.H. Response of coliform populations in streambed sediment and water column to changes in nutrient concentrations in water. *Water Res.* **2014**, *59*, 316–324. [CrossRef] [PubMed]

160. Gregory, L.F.; Karthikeyan, R.; Aitkenhead-Peterson, J.A.; Gentry, T.J.; Wagner, K.L.; Harmel, R.D. Nutrient loading impacts on culturable *E. coli* and other heterotrophic bacteria fate in simulated stream mesocosms. *Water Res.* **2017**, *126*, 442–449. [CrossRef] [PubMed]

161. Wanjugi, P.; Fox, G.A.; Harwood, V.J. The interplay between predation, competition, and nutrient levels influences the survival of *Escherichia coli* in aquatic environments. *Microb. Ecol.* **2016**, *72*, 526–537. [CrossRef] [PubMed]

162. Sinton, L.W.; Davies-Colley, R.J.; Bell, R.G. Inactivation of enterococci and fecal coliforms from sewage and meatworks effluents in seawater chambers. *Appl. Environ. Microbiol.* **1994**, *60*, 2040–2048. [PubMed]

163. Sinton, L.W.; Finlay, R.K.; Lynch, P.A. Sunlight inactivation of fecal bacteriophages and bacteria in sewage-polluted seawater. *Appl. Environ. Microbiol.* **1999**, *65*, 3605–3613.

164. Sokolova, E.; Astrom, J.; Pettersson, T.J.; Bergstedt, O.; Hermansson, M. Decay of bacteroidales genetic markers in relation to traditional fecal indicators for water quality modeling of drinking water sources. *Environ. Sci. Technol.* **2012**, *46*, 892–900. [CrossRef]

165. Ngazoa, E.S.; Fliss, I.; Jean, J. Quantitative study of persistence of human norovirus genome in water using TaqMan real-time RT-PCR. *J. Appl. Microbiol.* **2008**, *104*, 707–715. [CrossRef]

166. Wait, D.A.; Sobsey, M.D. Comparative survival of enteric viruses and bacteria in Atlantic ocean seawater. *Water Sci. Technol.* **2001**, *43*, 139–142. [CrossRef]

167. Whitman, R.; Harwood, V.J.; Edge, T.A.; Nevers, M.; Byappanahalli, M.; Vijayavel, K.; Brandao, J.; Sadowsky, M.J.; Alm, E.W.; Crowe, A.; et al. Microbes in beach sands: Integrating environment, ecology and public health. *Rev. Environ. Sci. Biotechnol.* **2014**, *13*, 329–368. [CrossRef] [PubMed]

168. Green, H.C.; Shanks, O.C.; Sivaganesan, M.; Haugland, R.A.; Field, K.G. Differential decay of human faecal bacteroides in marine and freshwater. *Environ. Microbiol.* **2011**, *13*, 3235–3249. [CrossRef] [PubMed]

169. Korajkic, A.; McMinn, B.R.; Harwood, V.J.; Shanks, O.C.; Fout, G.S.; Ashbolt, N.J. Differential decay of enterococci and *Escherichia coli* originating from two fecal pollution sources. *Appl. Environ. Microbiol.* **2013**, *79*, 2488–2492. [CrossRef] [PubMed]

170. Jeanneau, L.; Solecki, O.; Wery, N.; Jarde, E.; Gourmelon, M.; Communal, P.Y.; Jadas-Hecart, A.; Caprais, M.P.; Gruau, G.; Pourcher, A.M. Relative decay of fecal indicator bacteria and human-associated markers: A microcosm study simulating wastewater input into seawater and freshwater. *Environ. Sci. Technol.* **2012**, *46*, 2375–2382. [CrossRef] [PubMed]

171. Nayak, B.; Weidhaas, J.; Harwood, V.J. LA35 poultry fecal marker persistence is correlated with that of indicators and pathogens in environmental waters. *Appl. Environ. Microbiol.* **2015**, *81*, 4616–4625. [CrossRef]

172. Hurst, C.J.; Gerba, C.P. Stability of simian rotavirus in fresh and estuarine water. *Appl. Environ. Microbiol.* **1980**, *39*, 1–5.

173. Lo, S.; Gilbert, J.; Hetrick, F. Stability of human enteroviruses in estuarine and marine waters. *Appl. Environ. Microbiol.* **1976**, *32*, 245–249.

174. Fayer, R.; Graczyk, T.K.; Lewis, E.J.; Trout, J.M.; Farley, C.A. Survival of infectious *cryptosporidium parvum* oocysts in seawater and eastern oysters (*Crassostrea virginica*) in the chesapeake bay. *Appl. Environ. Microbiol.* **1998**, *64*, 1070–1074.

175. Korajkic, A.; McMinn, B.R.; Ashbolt, N.J.; Sivaganesan, M.; Harwood, V.J.; Shanks, O.C. Extended persistence of general and cattle-associated fecal indicators in marine and freshwater environment. *Sci. Total Environ.* **2019**, *65*, 1292–1302. [CrossRef]

176. Perkins, T.L.; Perrow, K.; Rajko-Nenow, P.; Jago, C.F.; Jones, D.L.; Malham, S.K.; McDonald, J.E. Decay rates of faecal indicator bacteria from sewage and ovine faeces in brackish and freshwater microcosms with contrasting suspended particulate matter concentrations. *Sci. Total Environ.* **2016**, *572*, 1645–1652. [CrossRef]

177. Curtis, K.; Michael Trapp, J. Examining the colonization and survival of *E. coli* from varying host sources in drainage basin sediments and stormwater. *Arch. Environ. Contam. Toxicol.* **2016**, *71*, 183–197. [CrossRef] [PubMed]

178. Cloutier, D.D.; McLellan, S.L. Distribution and differential survival of traditional and alternative indicators of fecal pollution at freshwater beaches. *Appl. Environ. Microbiol.* **2017**, *83*, e02881-16. [CrossRef] [PubMed]

179. Anderson, K.L.; Whitlock, J.E.; Harwood, V.J. Persistence and differential survival of fecal indicator bacteria in subtropical waters and sediments. *Appl. Environ. Microbiol.* **2005**, *71*, 3041–3048. [CrossRef] [PubMed]

180. Jenkins, M.B.; Fisher, D.S.; Endale, D.M.; Adams, P. Comparative die-off of *Escherichia coli* O157:H7 and fecal indicator bacteria in pond water. *Environ. Sci. Technol.* **2011**, *45*, 1853–1858. [CrossRef] [PubMed]

181. Wanjugi, P.; Harwood, V.J. The influence of predation and competition on the survival of commensal and pathogenic fecal bacteria in aquatic habitats. *Environ. Microbiol.* **2013**, *15*, 517–526. [CrossRef] [PubMed]

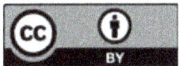

International Journal of
Environmental Research and Public Health

MDPI

Article

Validation of Questionnaire Methods to Quantify Recreational Water Ingestion

Laura M. Suppes [1,*] [iD], **Kacey C. Ernst** [2], **Leif Abrell** [3] [iD] and **Kelly A. Reynolds** [2] [iD]

1   Environmental Public Health Program, The University of Wisconsin-Eau Claire, 105 Garfield Avenue,
     Eau Claire, WI 54702, USA
2   Mel and Enid Zuckerman College of Public Health, The University of Arizona, P.O. Box 245163,
     Tucson, AZ 85724, USA; Kernst@email.arizona.edu (K.C.E.); Reynolds@email.arizona.edu (K.A.R.)
3   Department of Soil, Water & Environmental Science, The University of Arizona, Gould-Simpson Building
     Room 611, 1040 East 4th Street, Tucson, AZ 85721, USA; Abrell@email.arizona.edu
*   Correspondence: suppeslm@uwec.edu; Tel.: +1-715-836-5977

Received: 8 September 2018; Accepted: 19 October 2018; Published: 1 November 2018

Abstract: Swimming pool water ingestion volumes are necessary for assessing infection risk from swimming. Pool water ingestion volumes can be estimated by questionnaire or measuring a chemical tracer in swimmer urine. Questionnaires are often preferred to the chemical tracer method because surveys are less time consuming, but no research exists validating questionnaires accurately quantify pool water ingestion volumes. The objective of this study was to explore if questionnaires are a reliable tool for collecting pool water ingestion volumes. A questionnaire was issued at four pool sites in Tucson, Arizona to 46 swimmers who also submitted a urine sample for analyzing cyanuric acid, a chemical tracer. Perceived ingestion volumes reported on the questionnaire were compared with pool water ingestion volumes, quantified by analyzing cyanuric acid in swimmer urine. Swimmers were asked if they swallowed (1) no water or only a few drops, (2) one to two mouthfuls, (3) three to five mouthfuls, or (4) six to eight mouthfuls. One mouthful is the equivalent of 27 mL of water. The majority (81%) of swimmers ingested <27 mL of pool water but reported ingesting >27 mL ("one mouthful") on the questionnaire. More than half (52%) of swimmers overestimated their ingestion volume. These findings suggest swimmers are over-estimating pool water ingestion because they perceive one mouthful is <27 mL. The questionnaire did not reliably collect pool water ingestion volumes and should be improved for future exposure assessment studies. Images of the ingestion volume categories should be included on the questionnaire to help swimmers visualize the response options.

Keywords: pool water ingestion; recreational water; swimming pool; risk assessment

1. Introduction

The annual number of Recreational Water Illness (RWI) outbreaks associated with treated recreational water venues ("pools") in the U.S. has increased since 1978 when reporting was initiated (pools are defined as swimming pools, spas, interactive fountains, wading pools and dive pools) [1–3]. RWIs range from acute gastrointestinal illness (AGI), skin infection or rash to acute respiratory illness (ARI). The majority of outbreaks are associated with AGI, which accounted for 81% of outbreaks during summer months in 2011–2012 [4]. Most AGI outbreaks in treated recreational water are associated with ingesting *Cryptosporidium*. *Cryptosporidium* has been detected in treated recreational water and associated with outbreaks internationally [5–8]. From 2000–2014, *Cryptosporidium* caused 58% of treated recreational water outbreaks in the U.S. [9]. The volume of pool water ingested by swimmers is necessary to quantify infection risk from enteric pathogens like *Cryptosporidium* [10]. Risk assessment can help identify unsafe swimming behaviors, at-risk populations, and priority hazards to direct the development of pool safety guidelines. Recognizing the need for accurate data collection tools for swimming pool risk assessment, this study compared perceived ingestion volumes reported on a questionnaire to pool water ingestion volumes quantified by analyzing cyanuric acid in swimmer urine. The questionnaire merged information and survey questions collected and developed by the Centers for Disease Control and Prevention (CDC), the U.S. Environmental Protection Agency (USEPA), and academic researchers to assess a variety of swimmer exposures. The objective was to determine if questionnaires are a reliable tool for collecting pool water ingestion volumes.

One primary exposure related to risk of RWI is ingestion of water. Previously, the World Health Organization (WHO) used questionnaires to estimate swimming ingestion rates and found swimmers reported swallowing 20–50 mL/h [11]. These self-reported values, however, are underestimated when compared to ingestion ranges found in other studies applying quantitative measurement techniques. Thus, the WHO questionnaire may not accurately capture pool water ingestion magnitudes among swimmers.

Ingestion can be quantified using methods that compare cyanuric acid in urine and pool water. Cyanuric acid is added as a chlorine stabilizer to outdoor pool water, and when ingested, passes through the human body unmetabolized [12]. Controlled studies show 98% of cyanuric acid ingested is excreted in a 24 h period [12]. Using this technique, researchers Dufour et al. and Suppes et al. showed swimmers ingested between 0–154 mL/h and 0–105.5 mL/h, respectively [13,14]. Information on perceived ingestion by study participants was not collected in the Dufour study, but was collected by Suppes et al. using the questionnaire discussed in this article (see Supplementary Materials). The questionnaire asked swimmers how much pool water was ingested during a timed swim. The current article is one part of the Suppes et al. study and describes how accurately swimmers perceive pool water ingestion by comparing reported to measured volumes. Our findings demonstrate swimmers perceive higher ingestion exposures than in reality, which explains why self-reported ingestion estimates are different than measured estimates.

2. Materials and Methods

2.1. Questionnaire Development

The CDC and USEPA websites and peer-reviewed literature were searched for pool outbreak survey tools, tools developed in response to outbreaks, and tools designed to capture swimmer exposures [15,16]. The CDC National Outbreak Reporting System (NORS) is available for reporting nationwide waterborne disease outbreaks and includes exposure questions related to recreational water. In-depth survey tools are also available through the CDC that collect data on swimmer activity, gastrointestinal symptoms, confounding exposures, pool operations and maintenance, and are designed to be administered by outbreak investigators [15]. Surveys intended to collect additional exposure information, such as potential disinfection by-product exposures, were reviewed from the USEPA assessment tool SWIMODEL among others [15].

Exposure risk factors relative to swimmer behavior and pool maintenance from the CDC surveys, SWIMODEL, and peer-reviewed literature were compiled and organized into a draft questionnaire. Three panels were assembled to review the draft for comprehensiveness and to recommend formatting and included (1) six experts from the swimming pool industry; (2) an international group of nine microbiologists, exposure scientists, and epidemiologists; and (3) an internal University of Arizona panel of six respiratory health, epidemiology, exposure science, and public health specialists. Meetings with each panel were held once and lasted 1–2 h following advance reviews of the questionnaire. Individual communication with panel members by email or phone occurred throughout the questionnaire development process. Questions from the draft were entered into DatStat Illume Survey Developer Gateway Version 5.1.1.17347 (Seattle, WA, USA). The questionnaire was further evaluated by the external review panel for errors and comprehensiveness prior to use. A modified version of the questionnaire can be viewed in Table S1 of the Supplementary Materials.

The question used in this study to estimate pool water ingestion by "mouthfuls/swim" was developed by Schets et al. and was selected over other surveys based on recommendations from the expert questionnaire review committees [17]. Other surveys used specific volume classifications, like "teaspoon", that may have been difficult for younger participants in this study to interpret. The Schets study quantified the average volume in one mouthful (27 mL), which allowed measured volumes in the present study to be categorized into "mouthfuls/swim". Swimmers were asked on our questionnaire if they swallowed (1) no water or only a few drops, (2) one to two mouthfuls, (3) three to five mouthfuls, or (4) six to eight mouthfuls. Using data from the Schets study indicating an average mouthful is 27 mL, qualitative variables from our questionnaire were converted to quantitative volumes. Despite the Schets study defining "no water to a few drops" as 0–5 mL, swimmers with measured ingestion between 0–26 mL were categorized as: "1: no water or only a few drops". There was no qualitative ingestion category in the Schets study representing 6–26 mL. The other categories were: 27–54 mL (one to two mouthfuls), 55–135 mL (three to five mouthfuls), and 136–216 mL (six to eight mouthfuls).

2.2. Data Collection

This research was approved by the University of Arizona Human Subjects Research and Institutional Review Board (project number: 12-0272-12). The questionnaire was issued to 46 swimmers June–September 2013 in Tucson, Arizona, recruited at two outdoor public pools and two outdoor private pools. Swimmers arriving at the pools on data collection days were approached by a member of the research team, given details of the study's objectives, and asked if they would participate by completing a questionnaire after swimming and submitting a 24 h urine sample to quantify pool water ingestion. Urine samples were preserved then cleaned by solid phase extraction and analyzed using ultra-high-pressure liquid chromatography tandem mass spectrometry (UHPLC-MS/MS) for cyanuric acid. Pool water samples were collected at each pool site on the day swimmers were recruited, transferred on ice, and preserved along with urine samples. Cyanuric acid was quantified in pool water using UHPLC-MS/MS. Pool water ingestion volumes were calculated using cyanuric acid concentrations in urine and pool water [13] (Equation (1)). Detailed results from the 24 h urine sample portion of this study are published elsewhere [14].

$$\text{water ingestion (L)} = ([\text{cyanuric acid}]_{\text{urine}}(\tfrac{\mu g}{L}) \div [\text{cyanuric acid}]_{\text{pool water}}(\tfrac{\mu g}{L})) \times \text{urine volume (L)} \qquad (1)$$

All swimmers, regardless of age, gender, or other factors, were approached and asked to participate. Swim duration for all participants was recorded on the questionnaire. Participants accessed the questionnaire either on-site using tablets, electronic or smart phones, or on a personal computer through email. Questionnaires were completed within six hours of swimming.

3. Results

Thirty-eight of 46 participants had usable water ingestion values for analysis. Four did not submit a questionnaire, one submitted a urine sample less than the accepted volume threshold, and three urine samples had signal-to-noise ratios <3, which indicates a measurement below the analytical equipment limit of detection (UHPLC-MS/MS). The percent recoveries of cyanuric acid from urine and pool water were 6% and 112%, respectively. Table 1 summarizes the study population.

Table 2 illustrates the number of swimmers who correctly and incorrectly reported the volume range of pool water ingested during swimming. Sixteen of 38 swimmers (42%) correctly reported their ingestion volume, 20/38 (52%) overestimated the amount of pool water ingested and 2/38 (5%) underestimated their ingestion volume. Thirty-one of 38 swimmers (81%) actually ingested 0–26 mL of water, but only 11/38 swimmers (29%) correctly reported ingesting 0–26 mL. All swimmers (11/11) who reported ingesting "no water to a few drops" did ingest water within the volume range categorized as "no water to a few drops" (0–26 mL). Four of 20 swimmers who reported ingesting "one to two mouthfuls" actually ingested pool water within the volume range "one to two mouthfuls" (27–54 mL). Only one swimmer reported ingesting "three to five mouthfuls", but six actually did ingest pool water within this volume range (55–135 mL). No swimmers ingested or reported ingesting 136–216 mL.

Table 1. Age and gender distributions of study participants.

	Participant Demographics n = 38 (%)
Age	
≤18 years	17 (44.7)
>18 years	21 (55.2)
Gender	
Male	25 (65.7)
Female	13 (34.2)

Table 2. Number of swimmers reporting and actually ingesting pool water amounts within each volume range listed on the questionnaire (n = 38).

		No Water–Few Drops (0–26 mL)	One to Two Mouthfuls (27–54 mL)	Three to Five Mouthfuls (55–135 mL)	Six to Eight Mouthfuls (136–216 mL)
Measured Ingestion *	No water–few drops	11 †	14	6	0
	One to two mouthfuls	0	4 †	0	0
	Three to five mouthfuls	0	2	1 †	0
	Six to eight mouthfuls	0	0	0	0

* Measured ingestion values have been categorized using mouthful volumes characterized by Schets et al. [17].
† Study participants correctly reporting ingestion volume.

4. Discussion

Developers of the question used on our survey found the average volume of one mouthful to be 27 mL, which was used in this study to categorize measured ingestion volumes to mouthfuls. The majority (81%) of swimmers actually ingested <27 mL of pool water but reported ingesting >27 mL (one mouthful) on the questionnaire. More than half (52%) of swimmers overestimated their ingestion volume across all volume categories. These findings suggest swimmers are overestimating pool water ingestion because they perceive one mouthful to be <27 mL. The lack of accurate reporting of ingestion volumes using a question recommended by experts suggests a need for improving questionnaire techniques to assess recreational water ingestion. Since there is uncertainty about the volume of water in one mouthful, the questionnaire can be improved by including images of a one-cup/250 mL measuring glass with one to eight mouthfuls of liquid (Figure 1). Eight was the maximum number of mouthfuls on the questionnaire. The questionnaire can also be improved by changing the "no water to a few drops" category to "less than one mouthful" for consistency in questionnaire response options. Including Figure 1 would help swimmers visualize the ingestion volume categories to reduce inaccurate reporting.

Inconsistencies in method performance between this study and similar studies [13,18] and low recoveries of cyanuric acid in urine indicate a need for improving techniques to quantify pool water ingestion. Using comparable methods, Dorevitch et al. recovered 32.7% of cyanuric acid from swimmer urine and 96.5–99% of cyanuric acid from pool water [18]. Dufour et al. did not report recovery efficiencies for cyanuric acid in urine or pool water using a similar method [13]. Recovery of cyanuric acid in urine and pool water was 6% and 112%, respectively, in the current study. Like this study, Dorevitch et al. calculated pool water ingestion using Equation (1) and did not adjust cyanuric acid in pool water to account for the lower recovery in urine. Self-reported pool water ingestion quantities from a questionnaire by Dorevitch et al. were also compared to measured pool water ingestion quantities. To be consistent with Dorevitch and Dufour, no percent recovery adjustments were made to cyanuric acid in urine or pool water before analyzing measured and self-reported pool water ingestion in this study. Measured ingestion estimates could be higher than reported in all three studies, but exact pool water ingestion quantities cannot be estimated without a method that consistently recovers 100% of cyanuric acid in urine. Cyanuric acid extraction efficiencies are dependent on the solid phase extraction technique and analytical instrument. A more detailed comparison and discussion of method performance and limitations between this study and others is published elsewhere [14].

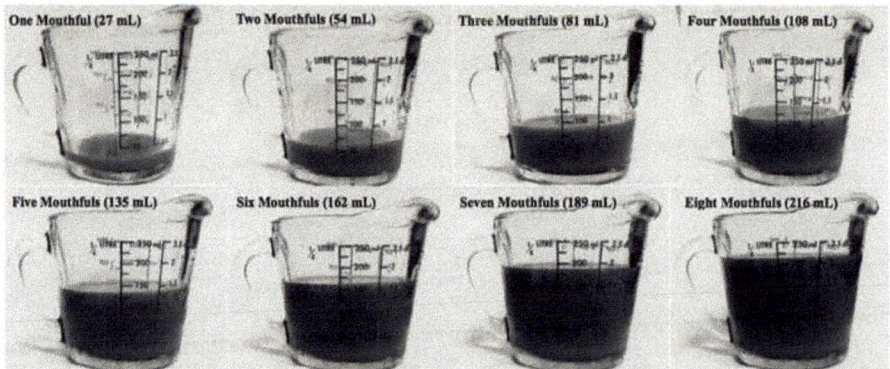

Figure 1. The figure illustrates one to eight mouthfuls of liquid in a one-cup/250 mL measuring glass, assuming one mouthful is equal to 27 mL of liquid [17].

5. Conclusions

This study highlights the need for improved questionnaire techniques to assess recreational water ingestion. Our findings demonstrate swimmers perceive higher ingestion exposures than in reality, which explains why self-reported ingestion estimates are different than measured estimates from previous studies. Since there is uncertainty about the volume of water in one mouthful, researchers who use this question technique in the future should include images of a one-cup/250 mL measuring glass with one to eight mouthfuls of liquid to help swimmers visualize the ingestion volume categories. The questionnaire category "no water to a few drops" should be changed to "less than one mouthful" to be consistent with other response options on the questionnaire. The altered questionnaire should be validated to ensure ingestion volumes are accurately reported.

Supplementary Materials: The following are available online at http://www.mdpi.com/1660-4601/15/11/2435/s1.

Author Contributions: Conceptualization, K.A.R.; methodology, K.A.R.; software, K.C.E. and L.A.; validation, L.M.S., K.C.E., L.A., and K.A.R.; formal analysis, L.M.S.; investigation, K.A.R. and L.M.S.; resources, L.M.S., K.C.E., L.A., and K.A.R.; data curation, L.M.S.; writing—original draft preparation, L.M.S.; writing—review and editing, L.M.S. and K.A.R.; visualization, K.A.R.; supervision, K.A.R.; project administration, K.A.R.; funding acquisition, K.A.R.

Funding: Funding for this research was provided by the National Swimming Pool Foundation and Research Foundation for Health and Environmental Effects.

Acknowledgments: Questionnaire development was made possible with assistance from Kristen Pogreba-Brown from the University of Arizona's Foodborne Illness Outbreak Investigation Team. Training in video surveillance methods was provided by Paloma Beamer at the University of Arizona's College of Public Health. Meredith Lisse and Leena Patel in the Mel and Enid Zuckerman College of Public Health assisted with water sample collection and analysis, site and participant recruitment, and urine processing. Analyses in the Arizona Laboratory for Emerging Contaminants were supported by NSF CBET 0722579. The researchers would also like to thank all those who assisted in the questionnaire review and all volunteers who donated their time to participate in this study.

Conflicts of Interest: The authors declare no conflicts of interest.

References

1. Craun, G.F.; Calderon, R.L.; Craun, M.F. Outbreaks associated with recreational water in the United States. *Int. J. Environ. Health Res.* **2005**, *15*, 243–262. [CrossRef] [PubMed]
2. Hlavsa, M.C.; Roberts, V.A.; Hill, V.R.; Kahler, A.M.; Hilborn, E.D.; Wade, T.J.; Backer, L.C.; Yoder, J.S. Recreational water-associated disease outbreaks—United States, 2009–2010. *Morb. Mortal. Wkly. Rep.* **2014**, *63*, 6–10.
3. Yoder, J.S.; Hlavsa, M.C.; Craun, G.F.; Hill, V.; Roberts, V.; Yu, P.A.; Hicks, L.A.; Alexander, N.T.; Calderon, P.L.; Roy, S.L.; et al. Surveillance for waterborne disease and outbreaks associated with recreational water use and other aquatic facility-associated health events—United States, 2005–2006. *Morb. Mortal. Wkly. Rep.* **2008**, *57*, 1–29.
4. Hlavsa, M.C.; Roberts, V.A.; Kahler, A.M.; Hilborn, E.D.; Mecher, T.R.; Beach, M.J.; Wade, T.J.; Yoder, J.S. Outbreaks of illness associated with recreational water—United States, 2011–2012. *Morb. Mortal. Wkly. Rep.* **2015**, *64*, 668–672.
5. Abd El-Salam, M.M. Assessment of water quality of some swimming pools: A case study in Alexandria, Egypt. *Environ. Monit. Assess.* **2012**, *12*, 7395–7406. [CrossRef] [PubMed]
6. Ehsan, M.A.; Casaert, S.; Levecke, B.; Van Rooy, L.; Pelicaen, J.; Smis, A.; Claerebout, E. *Cryptosporidium* and *Giardia* in recreational water in Belgium. *J. Water Health* **2015**, *13*, 870–878. [CrossRef] [PubMed]
7. Lemmon, J.M.; McAnulty, J.M.; Bawden-Smith, J. Outbreak of cryptosporidiosis linked to an indoor swimming pool. *Med. J. Aust.* **1996**, *165*, 613–616. [PubMed]
8. Polus, M. The occurrence of parasitic intestinal protozoa in swimming pools and other water recreation facilities in Cracow. *Przem. Chem.* **2006**, *95*, 107–109.
9. Hlavsa, M.C.; Cikesh, B.L.; Roberts, V.A.; Kahler, A.M.; Vigar, M.; Hilborn, E.D.; Wade, T.J.; Roellig, D.M.; Murphy, J.L.; Xiao, L.; et al. Outbreaks of illness associated with treated recreational water—United States, 2000–2014. *Morb. Mortal. Wkly. Rep.* **2018**, *67*, 547–551. [CrossRef] [PubMed]
10. Suppes, L.M.; Canales, R.A.; Gerba, C.P.; Reynolds, K.A. Cryptosporidium risk from swimming pool exposures. *Int. J. Hyg. Environ. Health* **2016**, *219*, 915–919. [CrossRef] [PubMed]
11. World Health Organization Guidelines for Safe Recreational Water Environments, Volume 2: Swimming Pool and Similar Environments. Available online: www.who.int/water_sanitation_health/bathing/srwe2full.pdf (accessed on 29 November 2016).
12. Allen, L.M.; Briggle, T.V.; Pfaffenberger, C.D. Absorption and excretion of cyanuric acid in long distance swimmers. *Drug Metab. Rev.* **1982**, *13*, 499–516. [CrossRef] [PubMed]
13. Dufour, A.P.; Evans, O.; Behymer, T.D.; Cantu, R. Water ingestion during swimming activities in a pool: A pilot study. *J. Water Health* **2006**, *4*, 425–430. [CrossRef] [PubMed]
14. Suppes, L.M.; Abrell, L.; Dufour, A.P.; Reynolds, K.A. Assessment of swimmer behaviors on pool water ingestion. *J. Water Health* **2014**, *112*, 150–152. [CrossRef] [PubMed]
15. Centers for Disease Control and Prevention Recreational Water Illness Response Toolkit. Available online: http://www.cdc.gov/healthywater/emergency/toolkit/rwi-outbreak-toolkit.html (accessed on 29 November 2016).
16. United States Environmental Protection Agency Swimmer Exposure Assessment Model. Available online: https://www.epa.gov/pesticide-science-and-assessing-pesticide-risks/swimmer-exposure-assessment-model-swimodel (accessed on 29 November 2016).
17. Schets, F.M.; Schijven, J.F.; Husman, A.M.D. Exposure assessment for swimmers in bathing waters and swimming pools. *Water Res.* **2011**, *45*, 2392–2400. [CrossRef] [PubMed]
18. Dorevitch, S.; Panthi, S.; Huang, Y.; Li, H.; Michalek, A.M.; Pratap, P.; Wroblewski, M.; Liu, L.; Scheff, P.A.; Li, A. Water ingestion during water recreation. *Water Res.* **2011**, *45*, 2020–2028. [CrossRef] [PubMed]

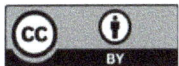

International Journal of
Environmental Research and Public Health

MDPI

Review

Recreational Use of Spa Thermal Waters: Criticisms and Perspectives for Innovative Treatments

Federica Valeriani, Lory Marika Margarucci and Vincenzo Romano Spica *

Public Health Unit, University of Rome "Foro Italico", Rome 00135, Italy; federica.valeriani@uniroma4.it (F.V.);
lory.margarucci@tiscali.it (L.M.M.)
* Correspondence: vincenzo.romanospica@uniroma4.it

Received: 26 October 2018; Accepted: 23 November 2018; Published: 27 November 2018

Abstract: Natural spa springs are diffused all over the world and their use in pools is known since ancient times. This review underlines the cultural and social spa context focusing on hygiene issues, public health guidelines and emerging concerns regarding water management in wellness or recreational settings. The question of the "untouchability" of therapeutic natural waters and their incompatibility with traditional disinfection processes is addressed considering the demand for effective treatments that would respect the natural properties. Available strategies and innovative treatments are reviewed, highlighting potentials and limits for a sustainable management. Alternative approaches comprise nanotechnologies, photocatalysis systems, advanced filtration. State of the art and promising perspectives are reported considering the chemical-physical component and the biological natural complexity of the spa water microbiota.

Keywords: recreational water; spa; thermal water; innovative treatment

---

1. Introduction

Natural spa springs are used for recreational purposes or wellness applications and are available globally [1–3]. Especially in the Mediterranean basin, these waters have been exploited and valorized for health and recreational purposes since ancient times [4–7]. After inheriting the approach to health and well-being from the Greek culture, the Romans magnified this opportunity of personal and social care through the realization of the monumental *thermae publicae*, with major spa buildings that included areas for baths, gardens, stadiums, gyms, restrooms and spaces for massages or health-related activities [7]. Over the centuries and different cultures, spas have maintained a significant role for promoting health in the community. Nowadays, the increase in wellness awareness and fitness expectations has led to the exploitation of thermal waters and extended spa businesses, based on the notion of a joint interaction between natural resources and manmade enterprises [8]. Collectively, the spa economy is estimated at $94 billion, with a consistent growth perspective in the coming decades [9]. Indeed, the global wellness economy had amplified the demand and the offer of products or services based on mineral waters, sea and hot spring resources [8,9]. Specifically, the spa and recreational thermal water tourism mainly flows towards Europe, mostly in German-speaking and Mediterranean countries, but also in North America and Southeast Asia [8–11]. The application of thermal waters in swimming pools, spa and wellness centers represents a renewed and promising tool for prevention, rehabilitation, and health promotion, providing possible physical, mental or social benefits to patients and several groups of people [1,12]. The general context of spa environments can support a holistic approach to health promotion, also through the exposure to natural open-spaces, the presence of water itself, the access to physical activities, physiotherapies, and health education opportunities. Even if additional evidence-based data are needed, several studies have shown the therapeutic role of mineral elements and other chemical compounds present in thermal waters [13]. The treatments with mineral thermal water or mud proved effective in pain relief and function restoration, impacting also on quality of life: several parameters of clinical interest, and other key issues were reported to play a role in several rheumatologic diseases e.g., knee and hand osteoarthritis, chronic low back pain, rheumatoid arthritis, and osteoporosis) compared to baseline and non-mineral similar treatments [14–16]. The thermal waters and spas have ancient roots in history and still today represent a promising opportunity for physical and social well-being but require surveillance to assure appropriate hygiene standards to the final aim of reducing hazards and maximizing benefits.

The water of natural spas should be of satisfactory microbiological quality and must be adequately managed to control the exposure of bathers and personnel to infectious agents. Indeed, the literature describes individual cases or outbreaks associated with the use of swimming/spa pools or similar environments, such as hot springs, hot tubs, whirlpools, natural spas, for recreational, wellness or therapeutic purposes [17–21]. Knowledge on pool uses and on composition of the water that supplies the spa is needed for an effective and appropriate management. Indeed, the peculiar and typical composition of each thermal water represents an interesting richness and a potentially beneficial property for health, but it also implies additional difficulties in defying the correct management, treatment and monitoring of that specific water in a defined application, such as aerosol, beverages lavender or in pool [22,23]. Based on their geological composition, natural waters may be enriched with several salts and ions, such as sulfur, halogens from group 17 of the periodic table, e.g., chlorine (Cl), bromine (Br), iodine (I), or alkaline earth metals comprising group 2 of the periodic table, e.g., magnesium (Mg) or calcium (Ca) [23,24]. Therefore, in natural spa pools, the water should be left untreated for assuring the specific composition, maintaining the original properties and the potential health benefits [10,11,24–27]. However, it is well known that pools and spas can present a considerable source of infection and other threats to human health [22,28,29]. In particular, several bacteria such as *Legionella, Pseudomonas, Mycobacteria*, as well as protozoa such as amoebae, algae and other microorganisms can naturally proliferate in the conditions characteristic of thermal waters and, if not managed properly, can become a hazard for users [17–21]. This problem represents a dilemma between treating or not treating natural spa waters and induces several pool managers to add disinfectants into the natural solutions highly rich in salts, resigning the original water properties in favor of safety, even if there is a lack of knowledge on the chemical risks related to the use of disinfectants in these waters. Several alternative strategies have been proposed and the recent progress in nanotechnologies is contributing to the field, leading to the introduction of innovative water treatment strategies for thermal waters and spa contexts [30]. The objective of this review is to consider issues related to thermal spa waters within the field of the recreational uses in pools, showing homologies and differences from a public health point of view and perspectives for innovative treatments.

2. Spa Trends in the World

The last century saw massive changes and new trends in international health-tourism, where, alongside the traditional health services, thermal-tourism and wellness-fitness became increasingly popular [31,32]. The spa industry has grown by 7.7% annually, from $60 billion in 2007 to $94 billion in 2013, representing the fastest growing subsector in health tourism and leisure sector [33,34]. Several countries reported an increase in spa economy; the spa services in Europe are mostly related to health and healing while spa tourism in the US is more oriented towards the affirmation of a healthy lifestyle [8,31,34]. In this area, Europe maintains a clear leadership; however, the Asia-Pacific region, particularly Thailand, China and Australia, have great potentials and resources for the growth of the wellness spa tourism market, especially due to the price reasonableness of the exclusive services [34–36]. Exposure to spa waters and related environments is involving a growing number of people all over the world, posing new question related to safety and public health issues.

The increasing interest in thermal waters and spa resources is also reflected in the scientific literature. Indeed, research related to "thermal waters" or "medicinal waters" or "spa salus per aquam" has increased over the last 50 years (Figure 1). The first publication dated 1853 and it already underlined how thermal water properties cannot be not altered in any way by treatments [37]. Later, several authors have investigated the application of thermal water medicine and the nature of spa waters [38,39]. The use of thermal waters for therapeutic purposes has always aroused a continuous interest and debate all over the world, being dependent on the detailed physicochemical pattern of the water joined with the specific indication for a treatment in a defined pathological condition [40,41]. Following the number of publications from different regions, it can be noticed how the interest in this topic is mainly concentrated in Europe (42.3%), Asia (26.3) and Africa (21.7%). Regardless the complex and heterogeneous debate on evidence-based therapeutic applications, spa waters represent a current major approach to wellness worldwide. Their frequent use in pools often is a challenge for public health authorities, both at cultural and technological level.

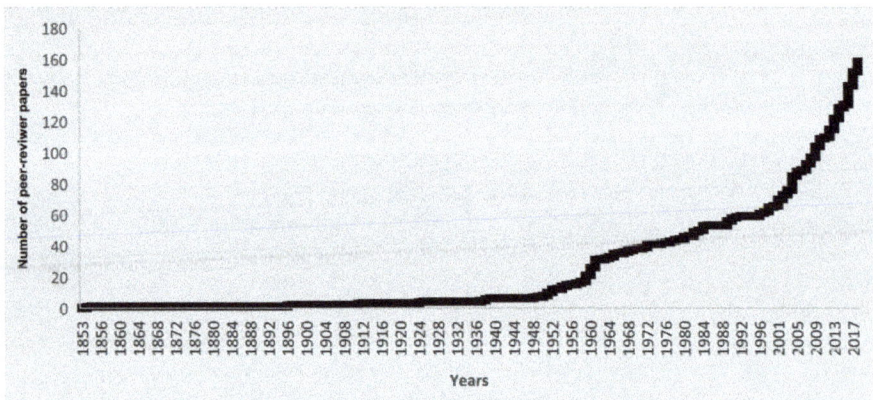

Figure 1. Number of publication entries in Medline (PubMed trend from 1853 to 2018, last access 10/2018). Publication entries were searched with the query: "thermal waters" OR "medicinal waters" OR "spa salus per aquam".

3. The Question about "Identity" and "Untouchability" of Spa and Medicinal Natural Waters

The growing popularity of swimming and other water activities for sports, fitness, therapy, wellness or relaxation and amusement has increased the diffusion of swimming pools as well as specific-use pools, such as spa pools, hot tubs, whirlpool bath, and natural spa pools [22,25,42]. The term "spa" is an acronym for *salus per aquam*, meaning health through water [5]. The common terms associated with spa pools include hot tubs, whirlpool bath, and natural spa pools; all these types of pools imply different water management and are designed for different wellness, therapeutic or recreational purposes. Most spa pools (>98%) resigned their natural properties, being disinfected by the addition of traditional chemicals with high oxidation potential, such as chlorine [25]. The treatment choice as well as the risk assessment process must consider the nature of the water that supplies the pool plant [25]. In natural spa pools, indeed, the water should remain untreated because the claimed beneficial effects are supposed to derive from their unique chemical-physical properties (Table 1) [22,25,43].

Moreover, in order to characterize these spring waters, also the biological component plays a role. Spa waters, indeed, contain a metabolically versatile microflora that is characterized by specialized bacteria belonging to that ecological niche, within a defined range of chemical and physical parameters [43,44]. The biotic and abiotic components of these ecological niches have been deeply studied, representing a mine for the identification of unknown and/or extremophile species within the complex microbial community [44–47]. Today, it is possible to characterize this microbial community by a massive-sequencing approach, describing a spa water microbiota and defining a "microbial signature" that can be sampled and typed from the original spring source up to the pool facility and final user's applications [48–50]. This approach was already applied in different spa pools and can provide further perspectives for the characterization of spa waters in recreational or wellness uses, adding a candidate new biological parameter to the traditional chemical-physical ones: the microbiota as a novel marker for public health [49–52]. Interestingly, it is now possible to associate water properties to its microflora component, e.g., presence of H_2S and communities of sulphate reducing bacteria, temperature and thermophiles, iron (Fe) and iron (III)-reducing bacteria, unravelling biochemical pathways and considering water as an active biological fluid [24,53,54]. The microbiota itself and the analysis of microflora biodiversity by Next Generation Sequencing (NGS), can support the proposal of a modern classification of waters and their properties, opening up new perspectives for the development of appropriate strategies for managing hygiene by respecting chemical, physical and also microbiological natural components [10,50,53–56]. This approach is very promising but still limited not just by the need of wet-laboratory equipment, protocols or qualified personnel because several external services are available and more and more affordable. Most of all the bottleneck is determined by the requirement of dedicated bioinformatic tools, such as database driven software to analyze the data obtained from massive sequencing and transfer information in an appropriate form to address public health questions. In order to collect and map information from different springs, a dedicated database for spa microbiota was developed and made accessible online to the collaborative research network at www.mfATLAS.it [50]. This tool was designed within a project focused on studying the biological component in spa water springs and pools (Figure 2). It is open to collaborations to analyze and host data from additional sampling points all over the world and the relative metadata, further expanding the atlas-map and database. The availability of this massive sequencing approach and bioinformatic support can improve knowledge on the natural microflora inhabiting thermal spring waters, their geographical distribution, providing also information for the identification of new species and their potential role in the field of wellness, therapeutics in that spa facility, or for other biotechnology applications [11–15,55]. Based on the available version of the mfAtlas database and in according with the observations from other studies and the Earth Microbiome Project, the percentage of unknown species in is still high, covering about 10–70% of the spa water microbiota component [50,56]. Previously, the access to unravelling these complex environmental communities was strongly restricted by the available culture-based methods or classical sequencing of libraries after cloning steps, rather than the massive sequencing approach that today is rapidly and successfully diffusing in different fields [56–60]. NGS revealed as a promising strategy not only in characterizing the natural microflora of spa waters, but also the presence of microbiological markers, pathogens or the effectiveness of disinfection and other water treatments [56–59]. This novel approach to solve hygiene questions is based on the genetic analysis of water biodiversity, starting from the DNA of its microflora (mfDNA) [52]. It is opening promising perspectives for understanding the beneficial potentials of spa waters, their fingerprint and their "untouchability" based on the respect of chemical, physical, and also biological components.

Table 1. Classification of natural mineral waters based on fixed residue at 180 °C and chemical composition, according the 2009/54/EC Directive [43].

Classification of Mineral Waters	
Classification according to fixed residue at 180°	Classification according to chemical composition
Very low mineral content waters (Fixed residue <50 mg/L)	Bicarbonate waters (>600 mg/L)
Low mineral content waters (Fixed residue 50–500 mg/L)	Calcic waters (>150 mg/L)
Medium mineral content waters (Fixed residue 500–1500 mg/L)	Chloride waters (>200 mg/L)
Rich mineral content water (Fixed residue <1500 mg/L)	Ferrous waters (>1 mg/L)
	Fluorurate waters (>1 mg/L)
	Magnesiac waters (>50 mg/L)
	Sulphated waters (>200 mg/L)
	Sodium-Rich waters (>200 mg/L)

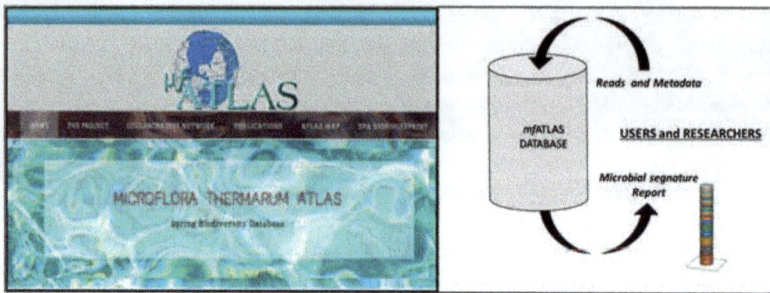

Figure 2. The mfAtlas database: presently, the database is accessible to the research network at www.mfATLAS.it. The database is designed to be further extended to harbour information such as water management, environmental and epidemiological data, international legislations.

Treatments for Spa and Medicinal Natural Waters: Limits and Perspectives

Several alternative water treatments were considered to assure the original properties and composition of the water, reducing the adverse effects on bathers and environments, to the final aim of offering sustainable solutions for spa waters in pools [61–63]. This challenging objective shares principles and problems also with the management of other kinds of waters, so that a success in this field can impact in other areas of water hygiene and conversely.

Otherwise, traditional disinfection approaches, e.g., chlorine, not only affect the harmful microorganisms present in the pool but also destroy the beneficial chemical-physical composition and the natural microflora, adulterating the therapeutic proprieties of these waters. The organic and inorganic compounds present in these waters can react with chemical substances used for disinfection, such as chloride/bromide-based chemicals, generating potentially toxic secondary products [24,63–66]. Nonetheless, the equilibrium between maintaining the natural proprieties of the thermal waters in pools and minimizing the microbial risk for people is not easy and can be achieved by considering several candidate approaches [22,54,66]. Firstly, a possible solution can be based on a personalization of the hygiene approach. The waters for natural spas, indeed, should be carefully tested for satisfactory microbiological quality before designing and constructing the water-plant, adopting a kind of individualized strategy based on the specific composition and destination use of that water in that plant, following a dedicated water safety plan [10,22,25,66–69]. In vitro models and protocols can prove useful in comparing materials or treatment methods [70]. The main task of water management is to achieve a satisfactory control on exposure of the bathers to infectious agents or other health risks, realizing an effective prevention of disease and accidents [22]. The high salinity or high temperature of spa waters represents an additional challenge for the pipeline plant and its maintenance, e.g., due to corrosion and concretion. Managing natural spa pools should follow the guidelines for traditional pools, but additional concerns have to be highlighted, so that alternative strategies may also be considered if proven to be effective and acceptable [25,47,68–70].

Even if spa waters should not be treated in order to try to maintain their original properties, however, sometimes they are used as a common source of water for just filling a pool for recreational purposes. Regarding the use of traditional pool disinfection of spa waters e.g., by chlorination, several inconveniences can occur in addition to the generation of known but also of unexpected Disinfection by-products (DBP) [65,66,69]. DBP are derived after the interaction with organic materials following an already well-known process, but the scenario is complicated by the presence of other chemicals naturally presents in the spa water or introduced by the bathers [22,65,71]. Oxidation in presence of an already high salinity can favor precipitates and concretions or induce unexpected toxic DBP with undesired -and often unpredictable-effects on bathers [71]. Moreover, the high temperature and the intense aeration due to frequent bubbling in this kind of pools, considerably can increase the evaporation of the active chemicals. Therefore, the disinfectant active doses are often poorly quantified, and "classic" chemicals generally may show a very irregular efficiency in spa pools. The type, form and use of each disinfectant need to be chosen with respect to the specific requirements of the pool [68,71–74]. Pool size itself may represent a critical parameter [22,25]. The choice of the disinfection strategy must be made after consideration of the efficacy of the specific product under the specific circumstances of use and the feasibility of a monitoring of the disinfectant levels in that pool [22,25,75–77]. Table 2 lists the several types of disinfecting agents and their advantages and limits of use in swimming pools as well as their applications in spa pools. Chlorine is inexpensive and relatively convenient to produce, store, transport, and apply. It provides rapid and long-lasting bactericidal effects but is limited mainly because of the formation of potentially toxic DBPs, such as trihalomethanes, halomethanes (THMs), haloacetic acids, halonitromethanes, haloacetonitriles, chloramines, and chlorophenols [22,25,65,72–80]. For example, the levels of potentially toxic DBPs tend to be higher in hot tubs, due to recirculation and smaller volumes but also because acceptable thresholds tend to be more elevated than in swimming pools [73–75]. However, when treating natural spring waters with chemical disinfection, whatever the final use, their natural characteristics are modified [22,25]. In order to avoid adulteration of the natural properties of spa pools, a commonly adopted alternative is based on dilution of pollutants by the frequent replacement of pool water. This may be feasible for small pools and when a large reservoir is available, but it can become unsustainable on the long term, due to the risk of depleting the aquifer.

Ozonation or ultraviolet (UV) irradiation represent additional solutions that are known and already well engineered and tested. Even if effective they can be demanding to maintain during time and both methods have no residual disinfection activity in the pool water [80–89]. Recently, advanced oxidation processes (AOPs) have shown a demonstrated efficacy in the treatment of organic pollutants in aquatic environments, but AOP technologies involve the generation of nonspecific hydroxyl radicals and the production of activated compounds involved in THM formation in the post-chlorination step, thus increasing the potential for DBPs formation [61,76,77,81]. UV irradiation is effective for controlling resistant microorganisms, such as *Cryptosporidium parvum* and *Giardia lamblia* [83–85]. This physical treatment seems cost-competitive in terms of improving the quality of swimming pool water; however, it has several limitations, including the life spam of the lamp and the potential formation of nitrogenous-based DBPs [61,82–91]. Bromine-based disinfectants may provide rapid and long-lasting disinfection effects, but they are more difficult to manage [61,92]. Several studies raised the problem of DBPs and reported eye or skin irritation due to bromine-based disinfectants [92]. The use of bromine-based disinfectants is generally not very feasible for outdoor pools and spas also because the bromine residue can get rapidly depleted in sunlight [25,92]. Copper/silver ionization was also proposed based on experimental observations on the effectiveness of silver nanoparticles (NPs) on harmful microorganisms, but several limits were reported including toxicity [61,92]. Hydrogen peroxide is a broad-spectrum disinfectant usually supplied as a solution to be dosed or added to spa pools; it is generally prepared by stabilizing ion-based chemistry [93]. The limitation in using hydrogen peroxide is the requirement of high concentrations depending on the condition of the facility; therefore, hydrogen peroxide disinfection was suggested only for small pools [25].

The World Water Development Report 2018 has outlined innovative natural treatments [94]. In this document nature-based solutions (NBS) are defined as a potential contribution to solving or overcoming the major water management problems or technical challenges [22,25,95–98]. A revolution in water treatment technologies is occurring and novel treatments based on physical methods are now considered and studied [96,97]. Membrane filtration has largely replaced granular filtration, and UV irradiation is enabling reduction in the use of or even elimination of classic disinfection chemicals, such as chlorine and its derivatives [97,99,100]. Ultrafiltration membranes are widely used in water treatment because of their favourable characteristics, such as easy modularization and improvement in water quality. A main limitation is membrane fouling that induces a reduction of membrane flux, an increase in energy consumption and in the consequent costs for water treatment [98].

Table 2. Several types of antimicrobial agents and their candidate applications in SPA pools: main advantages and limits for swimming pool uses.

Disinfection Solution	Advantages	Limits	SPA Pool Applications	References
Chlorine-based disinfectant	Inexpensive and relatively convenient to produce, store, transport and use. Provides rapid and long-lasting disinfection effects. Residual disinfectant activity in pool.	The formation of potentially toxic DBPs, such as THMs, HAAs, HANs, THAs and CAMs. Presence of chlorine-resistant microorganisms such as *Cryptosporidium parvum* and *Giardia lamblia*.	In hot tubs, acceptable free chlorine levels tend to be higher than in swimming pools. Moreover, due to the chemical characteristics of thermal water, the reaction between chemical compound and disinfection agents can lead the increase the potentially toxic DBPs.	[22,25,65,72–80]
Ozone	Highly effective, no smell. Can reduced the formation of potentially toxic disinfection by-products (DBPs).	Toxic and explosive; heavier than air. Risks and adverse health effects for the operator. Lack of residual disinfection proprieties; (usually joined with chlorine). Production of activated compounds suitable for THMs formation in the post-chlorination step.	AOPs have recently shown successes in the treatment of organic pollutants in aquatic environments, involving the generation of non-specific OH radicals. A de-ozonization step is needed.	[61,81]
Ultraviolet (UV) irradiation	Physical treatment without adding chemicals to the water. Effective for the control of resistant microorganisms including protozoa such as *Cryptosporidium parvum* and *Giardia lamblia*.	The formation of nitrogenous-based DBPs (HANs) Lack of residual disinfection proprieties.	UV radiation can be proposed to reduce the risk of infection by dermatophytes eventually present in swimming pools that use thermal water. Cost-competitive with chlorine to improve the quality of swimming pool water.	[61,81–90]
Bromine-based disinfectant	Inexpensive and relatively convenient to apply. Provides rapid and long-lasting disinfection effects.	It is difficult to dissolve and must be inserted into the pool through an automatic feeder. DBP There are reports that is associated with eye and skin irritation.	The use of bromine-based disinfectants is generally not practical for outdoor pools and spas because the bromine residual is depleted rapidly in sunlight.	[25,61,92]
Stabilised silver/copper	Copper/silver ionization was proposed for treatment of swimming pool water: protocols and devices are available. No pH adjustment is required.	Low effectiveness. Limited information on toxicity of ion forms and interaction with other chemicals.	Silver is a broad-spectrum disinfectant usually supplied as a solution to be dosed or added to the spa-pool system. Higher concentrations may be required depending on the condition of the facility.	[25,61,92]
Hydrogen peroxide	Effective. Low pollution on water.	With hydrogen peroxide the by-products are not problematic but it can generate toxic radical compounds.	Hydrogen peroxide can be used with silver and copper ions (low levels of the silver and copper); proper consideration to replacement of water for preventing excessive build-up of the ions.	[25,93]

Note: Disinfection byproducts (DBPs); Hypochlorous acid (HOCl); Trihalomethanes (THMs); Haloacetonitriles (HANs); Hydroxyl radical (OH); Advanced oxidation processes (AOPs).

Rapid advances in nanotechnologies have encouraged the development of industrial applications of manufactured nanoparticles (NPs) in a wide range of commercial products, such as drugs, paints, electronics, foods, or cosmetics [101]. However, laws or guidelines regarding the applications of NPs still are lacking and additional research on safety performance standards is required [101,102]. Table 3 summarizes the main innovative strategies and the possible applications of NPs in spa pools. For example, nanoscale chitosan and its derivatives were proposed also in water treatment, because of their antimicrobial effects on bacteria, viruses, fungi, and bacteriophages, through damaging cell membrane or chelating trace metals [101–106]. Chitosan is currently used in personal care products and biomedical products, as microbicide in agriculture and food wraps, and as a flocculant in water and wastewater treatments [102–106]. It is a promising compound for low-cost and low-tech disinfection applications and it was suggested for applications in developing countries, but it has several limitations including its deterioration under different conditions [107]. A promising scenario is coming from the use of light of different wavelength through photocatalysis processes [108]. In principle, this approach can allow water treatment just by light and air, through the production of free radicals. Metal oxide semiconductor NPs with a wide band gap are the basic materials used in heterogeneous photocatalysis method. They can accelerate the degradation of pollutants under solar illumination [108]. Titanium dioxide (TiO_2) and zinc oxide (ZnO) NPs are among the most extensively used metal NPs [107,108]. TiO_2 is already present in different products including foods additives and cosmetics, paints and also coating for pools [70,109]. Silver and copper metals have been also considered for their antibacterial properties within nanotechnological applications. Other kind of nanoparticles, Silver NPs (AgNPs), have been developed since late 1800s and have been registered with the Environmental Protection Agency for use as swimming pool algaecides since 1954 and as drinking water filters since 1970s [108–111].

AgNPs exhibit a strong and broad-spectrum antimicrobial activity and showed no harmful effects on humans [112]. They are currently being used in the development of point-of-use water disinfection systems and antibiofouling surfaces [113]. An innovative scenario is offered by the availability of Carbon nanotubes (CNTs), that have been reported to induce DNA damages and cytotoxic effects in prokaryotic cells, consequently disrupting the microbial diversity and community structure [114]. Several possible toxicological mechanisms of CNTs on microorganisms have been proposed, among which the disruption of the cell membrane integrity, that is considered a key mechanism in this antimicrobial process [114–116]. In the 21st century, advances made in the synthesis of carbon-based nanomaterials have resulted in the development of graphene–carbon nanotubes [117]. Notably, the three-dimensional graphene and graphene oxide-based nanostructures exhibit a large surface area and sorption sites that provide a high adsorption capacity to efficiently extract pollutants and inactivate viruses or bacteria in water [118,119].

In conclusion, advancements in the field are in continuous progress and several alternatives have been proposed for water treatments, opening promising perspectives also for thermal spa pools. Due to the heterogeneity of thermal spa waters and their peculiar requirements for the therapeutic use in spa facilities, presently it seems still difficult to find a single strategy for all different situations. Therefore, more than a unique ideal solution, the optimal strategy should be searched in the combination of different methods, following an individualized approach based on water properties, plant characteristics, destination use of the spa pool.

Table 3. Current and potential applications of antimicrobial nanomaterials.

Nanomaterials	CAS NUMBER	Nature of Disinfection Type		Antimicrobial Mechanism	Current Applications	Potential Future Applications in SPA Pools	References
		Physical	Chemical				
Silver nanoparticles (AgNPs)	7440-22-4		☑	AgNPs can disrupt the outer membrane of target cells.	Portable water filters, clothing, medical devices, coatings for washing machines, refrigerators, and food containers	An alternative to traditional chemical disinfectants that are prone to generate harmful disinfection by-products	[101,108–111]
Chitosan	9012-76-4		☑	Membrane damage, chelation of trace metals. Nano-scale chitosan and derivatives exhibit antimicrobial effects towards bacteria, viruses, fungi.	Personal care products, microbicide in agriculture and biomedical products, food wraps, biomedical, flocculants in water and wastewater treatment	They are promising for low-cost and low-tech disinfection applications. In water filtration, chitosan combined with sand filtration removes up to 99% of turbidity.	[101–106]
Graphene oxide	1034343-98-0	☑	☑	DNA damages and cytotoxic effects towards prokaryotic cells and detrimentally change the microbial diversity and community structures	Graphene oxide (GO) and silver-graphene oxide (Ag-GO) are used in various fields, such as biotechnology and environmental engineering, due to their unique material properties, including hydrophilicity, high surface area, mechanical strength, and antibacterial activity	In aquatic ecosystems, the stability of nanomaterials is affected by the water chemistry parameters of the receiving aquatic environments such as ionic strength, natural organic matters and pH	[114–119]
H$_2$S	7783-06-4		☑	H$_2$S killed microorganisms through inducing oxidative stress by inhibiting antioxidant enzymes	None	Restore the normal bacteriostatic nature of the thermal water	[24]
Nano TiO$_2$	13463-67-7		☑	Production of Reactive Oxygen Species (ROS), cell membrane and cell wall damage	Air purifiers, water treatment systems for organic contaminant degradation.	The applicability is in evaluation. The presence of some inorganic ions can be problem, because reduce the performance of TiO$_2$ in water treatment.	[108,109]
Ultrafiltration	-	☑		Ultrafiltration allowed the removal of suspended matter, as well as a part of the organic matter	Water treatment, swimming pool	Ultrafiltration can be selected as an alternative treatment process because of its ability to remove bacteria and viruses.	[97–100]
ZnO	1314-13-2	☑	☑	Intracellular accumulation of nanoparticles, cell membrane damage, H$_2$O$_2$ production, release of Zn^{2+} ions	Antibacterial creams, lotions and ointment, deodorant, self-cleaning glass and ceramics	Surface coating	[108,109]

4. Guidelines and Regulations on Thermal Spa Water Pools

The global scenario of the international regulations in the spa field is very heterogeneous and reflects the socio-economics and culture from the different countries (Table 4). In the USA, local and state regulations consider the routine inspection of aquatic environments for preventing risks and accidents [120]. Deaths due to pool entrapment have led to the enactment of the Virginia Graeme Baker Pool and Spa Safety Act [121,122]. The act outlines provisions to minimize the risk of entrapment, including mandatory requirements with respect to vacuum covers, pool barriers, and main drain requirements. For hygienic aspects, U.S. states have separate law or guidelines (e.g., Alabama and Kansas), although the point of reference remains the guidelines issued by the World Health Organization (WHO) [22,122]. In fact, since 1994, WHO had been promoting the development of guidelines for the use of recreational waters; these guidelines have now evolved to safety guidelines for recreational aquatic environments [22]. In Canada, British Columbia health authorities approve and inspect pools, hot tubs and other facilities to ensure safety in construction and operation, according to the Pool Regulation under the Public Health Act [123]. Hygienic-sanitary safety of thermal plants is addressed in the 2007 legislation, which has established the quality criteria for waters, including spas, and obligations for pool managers, following the Health Canada's Guidelines for Canadian Recreational Water Quality. These guidelines address potential health hazards, such as infections transmitted by disease-causing microorganisms, as well as aesthetics and nuisance conditions [124]. The Pool Standards have set specific technical thresholds pertaining to water quality and facility operations requirements under the Public Swimming Pools Regulation as well as other requirements, including: operator and user education, recirculation systems, water chemistry and microbiology indicators, water quality monitoring, anti-entrapment policies and other plans related to pool safety [125]. The standards also include a protocol for the management of contaminated public swimming pool water and the calculations for maximum bather load and flow rates through anti-entrapment suction outlets. These standards were developed in consultation with the pool industry, pool operators, and public health officials and recently revised in 2018 [125]. Australian swimming pool regulations was established in 1990 and revised in 1992, focusing also on spa pools, swimming pools and similar environments but does not include baths [126,127]. In the recent years, some regulations and technical standards have been introduced with regard to spas [128,129]. Europe is a rich continent in terms of natural hot springs, harbouring over 5000 springs and facilities, very popular since ancient times [8,56]. However, the European legislative situation in this matter seems very fragmented and inconsistent. A comprehensive community directive is still missing. The European reference 76/160/EEC concerning bathing water, as amended by 2006/7/EC, is not applicable to the spa and swimming pool waters or to the confined waters subjected to treatment or used for therapeutic purposes [130,131]. Austria had already issued regulations concerning swimming pools with the goal of preventing the spread of waterborne diseases [132]. Subsequent changes extended the scope of the legislation, but only in 2012 a new law has been passed regarding the technical and operational requirements for the water quality of traditional pools and bathing water, whirlpools, small natural pools, and ancillary facilities used for recreational or therapeutic activities [133–137]. The government of the Brussels-Capital region and the Walloon region in Belgium have issued specific ordinances on sectoral conditions related to swimming pools, saunas, and general artificial reservoirs designed for therapeutic, recreational, or sporting activities, but not domestic facilities [138–140]. In France, the current legislative framework related to swimming pools is based on the Public Health Code about the care and rehabilitation in thermal pools with an independent section concerning traditional pools [141,142]. Furthermore, in 2010, the Agency for Environmental Health and Safety (ANSES) published a document on health risks in swimming pools, indicating the thermal pools as "atypical" pools [143]. In 2013, ANSES published the part II of this document, focusing on hot tubs ("bains à remous") [144]. In England, Health and Safety Executive is the authority overlooking the pools of local authorities and schools. This institute together with the Health Protection Agency published the guidelines concerning the control of the risk of infections in thermal pools [145]. These protocols have been designed to improve the understanding about microbiological risks associated with the use of thermal baths and to provide advice on risk management [25,145]. Similarly, in Ireland, a country with a large number of geothermal pools, every swimming pool is a public spa that is managed in compliance with the Safety, Health and Welfare at Work Act of 2005 as well as a specific set of guidelines published to provide administrators with criteria and detailed information for management [146,147]. In Germany, the technical provisions for the management of swimming pools are summarized in the DIN 19643, which guarantees hygiene safety in swimming pools, saunas, whirlpools, and spas [148,149]. Periodically, the Federal Environment Agency publishes recommendations for health managers and authorities [150]. Recently, new developments in swimming pool hygiene required a revision of the standard series DIN 19643, with the introduction of new treatment processes based on ultrafiltration [151]. Czech Republic has a legislation concerning the spa sector, but it is not extended to the recreational applications of these waters or to the sanitary-hygiene related issues [152]. More specific standards concerning the management of water for therapeutic uses and thermal spas, are also available [153,154]. Iindependent standards are available in Portugal for specific regulations in spa facilities, focusing on licenses, organization, management, and control and attention is dedicated to the quality of public pools. However, Portugal uses a directive issued by the Council National Quality that does not apply to thermal pools for therapeutic use, indicating to other specific regulations [155,156]. In Slovakia, a country with a great spa tradition, water quality used for swimming is managed by the Public Health Authority and 36 regional health authorities, which overlook the pools supplied with thermal water [157]. In Spain, pool regulations are available since 1987 and the health authorities refer to the WHO guidelines [158–160]. The Ministry of Health, Social Services and Equality of Spain has developed the Real Decreto project to establish the water quality criteria for public pools, spas, private pools, and water parks but excludes natural pools and thermal waters used for medical therapeutic purposes [161]. An innovative appearance of this law is the consideration of water safety plans. Finland has included recommendations for public baths, spas, and swimming pools in the application law for the European directive n.2006/7/CE [162,163]. Other countries, namely Cyprus, Bulgaria, and Norway, have considered a different approach, not including this 2006 Directive along the specific rules for pools [164–166]. In Italy, the recreational use of spas has extensively increased in the last few years, but no specific guidelines have been established, yet. In fact, more recently, the Italian legislation started referring to the law of "the reorganization of the thermal system" established in 2000 for thermal waters [167]. This law reports the definition of thermal waters and the provisions concerning bottling and permitted uses but does not deal with the hygiene aspects related to the recreational use. The current legislation concerning swimming pools is the January 16th Agreement 2003 between the Minister of Health, the Regions, and the Autonomous Provinces of Trento and Bolzano [168]. This document is under revision and a public consultation was performed in 2016 [169]. The Agreement specifies that the swimming facilities can be supplied with different types of water, including thermal waters, but postponing the discipline of the latter to specific regional measures; moreover, additional guidelines for the spa hygiene are available for preventing Legionnaire's. This document has a chapter fully dedicated to swimming pool measures that underlines the need for adequate design of pool spa facilities because no specific treatment of these waters is allowed [170]. In summary, the complexity of the argument in the different countries does not seem to have fostered the development of unequivocal rules and shared strategies. Future joined projects and consensus documents would be welcome and useful on a local and international scale.

Table 4. International guidelines, regulation and recommendation regarding recreational water environments.

Country	Law	References
Australia	New South Wales Consolidated Acts. Swimming Pools Act 1990 n. 31.	[126–129]
	New South Wales Consolidated Acts. Swimming Pools Act 1992 n. 49.	
	Standard. Spa Pools Part 1: Public spas. 2007	
	Pool Water Quality and Operational Guidelines.	
Austria	Bundesgesetzblatt für die Republik Österreich 1978; 167:3053–63.	[132–136]
	Mitteilungen der Österreichischen Sanitätsverwaltung, 1992;93(11):358.	
	Bundesgesetzblatt für die Republik Österreich. 1996; 212:4617-24.	
	Mitteilungen der Österreichischen Sanitätsverwaltung. 1997;98(5):228–32.	
	Gesamte Rechtsvorschrift für Bäderhygienegesetz, Fassung vom 28.10.2012.	
Belgium	Belgio. Arrêté du Gouvernement wallon portant conditions sectorielles relatives aux bassins de natation.	[138–140]
	Belgio. Arrêté du Gouvernement de la Région de Bruxelles-Capitale fixant des conditions d'exploitation pour les bassins de natation.	
	Belgio. Arrete´ du Gouvernement de la Region de Bruxelles-Capitale fixant la liste des installations de classe IB, II et III en execution de l'article 4 de l'ordonnance du 5 juin 1997 relative aux permis d'environnement.	
Bulgaria	*D'rzaven vestnik* 1994; 65:1-14.	[160]
Canada	Réglement de sécurité, Fédération de natation du Québec (natation en bassin)	[122–125]
	Guidelines for Canadian Recreational Water Quality	
	Alberta Health Pool Standards	
Ciprium	*Ciprium Government Law N. 55(I)/92*	[164]
Czech Republic	Decree of Ministry of Health No.423/2001—On Spas and Sources	[152–154]
	Decree of Ministry of Health No.252/2004—Requirements on Cold and Hot Water in Health Care and Accommodation Facilities	
	Decree of Ministry of Health No.135/2004—Requirements on Swimming Pools, Saunas and Outdoor Playgrouds.	
Finland	Finlands Författningssamling 2008/70.	[162,163]
	Finlands Författningssamling 2014/47	
France	Code de la santé publique, 2010. Section V: Surveillance des établissements thermaux.	[141–144]
	Code de la santé publique, 2010. Section I: Normes d'hygiène et de sécurité applicables aux piscines et baignades aménagées	
	Afsset Evaluation des risques sanitaires liés aux piscines Partie I: piscines réglementées. Saisine Afsset «2006/11», Rapport final. 2010	
	Anses. Évaluation des risques sanitaires liés aux piscines Partie II: bains à remous. 10.13140/RG.2.1.2182.7043.	
England	Management of Spa Pools: Controlling the Risk of Infection. Health Protection Agency. March 2006.	[25,145]
	Health and Safety Executive (HSE). The control of Legionella and other infectious agents in spa-pool systems.	

Table 4. *Cont.*

Country	Law	References
Germany	DIN 19643. Aufbereitung von Schwimm- und Badebeckenwasser–Teil 1: Allgemeine Anforderungen.Beuth,Berlin	[148–151]
	Hygienische Anforderungen an Kleinbadeteiche. Empfehlung des Umweltbundesamtes. Bundesgesundhbl	
	Bundesgesundheitsbl-Gesundheitsforsch-Gesundheitsschutz	
	DIN 19643. Aufbereitung von Schwimm- und Badebeckenwasser–Teil 4: Verfahrenskombinationen mit Ultrafiltration	
Italy	Law of 24 October 2000, n. 323. Reorganization of the thermal sector. Official Gazette November 8, 2000, n. 261.	[167–170]
	Agreement between the Minister of Health, the Regions and the Autonomous Provinces of Trento and Bolzano G.U. March 3, 2003: 45, n. 51.	
	Guidelines with indications on legionellosis for managers of tourist accommodation and thermal facilities G.U. n 28 Febrary 5, 2005	
Ireland	Safety, Health and Welfare at Work Act", 2005. Health and Safety Authority	[146,147]
	Swimming Pool Safety Guidelines. Irish Water Safety, ILAM and Swim Ireland. 2010.	
Norway	*Norsk Lovtidend*, 1 sezione. 1996;11:767–73.	[166]
Portugal	Ministério da saúde Decreto-lei n. 142. 11 giugno 2004	[155,156]
	Directiva Conselho Nacional da Qualidade "A qualidade nas piscinas de uso público". n.° 23, 1993.	
Slovakia	*Zbierka zákonov Slovenskej Republiky* 1994;77:1350-1370.	[157]
Spain	Boletín Oficial del Ministerio de Sanidad y Consumo 1987;19:1147-52.	[158–161]
	Boletín Oficial del Ministerio de Sanidad y Consumo 1998, 80. por el que se regulan las condiciones higiénico-sanitarias de piscinas de uso colectivo.	
	Boletín Oficial orden 1319/2006	
	Real Decreto 742/2013	
USA	CDC's Model Aquatic Health Code	[120,122]
	Virginia Graeme baker Pool and Spa Safety Act	
	Dedicated law and guidelines for U.S. STATES	

5. Conclusions

Hot spring waters represent a unique natural fluid that humans have used since ancient times for health and recreational purposes. Spa facilities are present all over the world denoting a relevant resource for business that involves a large and growing number of users. The safeguard of the natural composition of spa waters clashes with the need of appropriate treatments in pools. Innovative strategies have been proposed, but further studies and validations are required. In addition to traditional chemical-physical parameters, the possibility to characterize the biological component is opening new perspectives for the classification and fingerprinting of spa waters through mfDNA (microflora DNA) analysis and the definition of spa microbiota patterns. Recent advancements in massive sequencing and bioinformatics are supporting this process, providing new tools for hygiene and knowledge on properties of spa water. The heterogeneity of spa waters and their uses may suggest an individualized approach to design and carry on a sustainable management through dedicated technical solutions and water safety plans. Public health regulations for the use of spa waters in pools are mainly lacking and a consensus at international level would be needed and welcome for providing agreements and shared guidelines.

Author Contributions: V.R.S.: conception, design and supervision of the study; F.V., L.M.M.: selection and analysis of the articles, collection of data of interest in a structured form; F.V., V.R.S.: Writing-Original Draft Preparation. All authors approved the final version of the manuscript.

Funding: This research was supported by Fondazione per la Ricerca Scientifica Termale (FORST) grants, grant number 1121.

Conflicts of Interest: The authors declare no conflict of interest.

References

1. Giampaoli, S.; Romano Spica, V. Health and safety in recreational waters. *Bull World Health Organ.* **2014**, *92*, 79. [CrossRef] [PubMed]
2. Van Tubergen, A.; van der Linden, S. A Brief History of Spa Therapy. *Ann. Rheum. Dis.* **2002**, *61*, 273–275. [CrossRef] [PubMed]
3. Routh, H.B.; Bhowmik, K.R.; Parish, L.C.; Witkowski, J.A. Balneology, mineral water, and spas in historical perspective. *Clin. Dermatol.* **1996**, *14*, 551–554. [CrossRef]
4. Frosh, W.A. "Taking the waters"—Springs, wells and spas. *FASEB J.* **2007**, *21*, 1948–1950. [CrossRef] [PubMed]
5. Frost, G.J. The spa as a model of an optimal healing environment. *J. Altern. Complement. Med.* **2004**, *10*, 85–92. [CrossRef]
6. Croutier, A.L. *Taking the Waters: Spirit, Art, Sensuality*, 1st ed.; Abbeville Press: New York, NY, USA, 1992.
7. Jackson, R. Waters and spas in the classical world. *Med. History* **1990**, *34*, 1–13. [CrossRef]
8. Global Wellness Institute. Global Spa & Wellness Economy Monitor Global Wellness Institute. 2014. Available online: www.gsws.org (accessed on 29 May 2018).
9. Mavridou, A.; Pappa, O.; Papatzitze, O.; Blougoura, A.; Drossos, P. An overview of pool and spa regulations in Mediterranean countries with a focus on the tourist industry. *J. Water Health* **2014**, *12*, 359–371. [CrossRef] [PubMed]
10. Giampaoli, S.; Valeriani, F.; Romano Spica, V. Thermal water for recreational use: Overview of international standards. *Igiene e Sanita Pubblica* **2012**, *68*, 863–873. [PubMed]
11. Özkuk, K.; Uysal, B.; Ateş, Z.; Ökmen, B.M.; Sezer, R.; Dilek, G. The effects of inpatient versus outpatient spa therapy on pain, anxiety, and quality of life in elderly patients with generalized osteoarthritis: A pilot study. *Int. J. Biometeorol.* **2018**, *62*, 1823–1832. [CrossRef] [PubMed]
12. Morer, C.; Roques, C.F.; Françon, A.; Forestier, R.; Maraver, F. The role of mineral elements and other chemical compounds used in balneology: Data from double-blind randomized clinical trials. *Int. J. Biometeorol.* **2017**, *61*, 2159–2173. [CrossRef] [PubMed]
13. Harzy, C.; Ghani, N.; Akasbi, N.; Bono, W.; Nejjari, C. Short- and long-term therapeutic effects of thermal mineral waters in knee osteoarthritis: A systematic review of randomized controlled trials. *Clin. Rheumatol.* **2008**, *28*, 501–507. [CrossRef] [PubMed]

14. Güleç, A.T. Natural Thermal Spa Water Versus Hyperthermic Tap Water for Treatment of Recalcitrant Hand Warts in Organ Transplant Recipients: A Patient-Blinded, Comparative Preliminary Study. *Exp. Clin. Transp.* **2018**, *16*, 189–193.

15. Matsumoto, S. Evaluation of the Role of Balneotherapy in Rehabilitation Medicine. *J. Nippon Med. Sch.* **2018**, *85*, 196–203. [CrossRef] [PubMed]

16. Baron, P.A.; Willeke, K. Respirable droplets from whirlpools: Measurements of size distribution and estimation of disease potential. *Environ. Res.* **1986**, *39*, 8–18. [CrossRef]

17. Insler, M.S.; Gore, H. Pseudomonas Keratitis and Folliculitis from Whirlpool Exposure. *Am. J. Ophthalmol.* **1986**, *101*, 41–43. [CrossRef]

18. Briancesco, R.; Meloni, P.; Semproni, M.; Bonadonna, L. Non-tuberculous mycobacteria, amoebae and bacterial indicators in swimming pool and spa. *Microchem. J.* **2014**, *113*, 48–52. [CrossRef]

19. Jernigan, D.B.; Hofmann, J.; Cetron, M.S.; Nuorti, J.P.; Fields, B.S.; Benson, R.F.; Breiman, R.F.; Lipman, H.B.; Carter, R.J.; Genese, C.A.; et al. Outbreak of Legionnaires' disease among cruise ship passengers exposed to a contaminated whirlpool spa. *Lancet* **1996**, *347*, 494–499. [CrossRef]

20. Silverman, A.R.; Nieland, M.L. Hot tub dermatitis: A familial outbreak of Pseudomonas folliculitis. *J. Am. Acad. Dermatol.* **1983**, *8*, 153–156. [CrossRef]

21. Leoni, E.; Catalani, F.; Marini, S.; Dallolio, L. Legionellosis Associated with Recreational Waters: A Systematic Review of Cases and Outbreaks in Swimming Pools, Spa Pools, and Similar Environments. *Int. J. Environ. Res. Public Health* **2018**, *15*, 1612. [CrossRef] [PubMed]

22. World Health Organization (WHO). *Guidelines for Safe Recreational Water Environments*; WHO Press: Geneva, Switzerland, 2006; Volume 2, Available online: http://apps.who.int/iris/bitstream/10665/43336/1/9241546808_eng.pdf (accessed on 29 May 2018).

23. Andreassi, L.; Flori, L. Mineral water and spas in Italy. *Clin. Dermatol.* **1996**, *14*, 627–632. [CrossRef]

24. Giampaoli, S.; Valeriani, F.; Gianfranceschi, G.; Vitali, M.; Delfini, M.; Festa, M.R.; Bottari, E.; Romano Spica, V. Hydrogen sulfide in thermal spring waters and its action on bacteria of human origin. *Microchem. J.* **2013**, *108*, 210–214. [CrossRef]

25. Health and Safety Executive (HSE). The Control of Legionella and Other Infectious Agents in Spa-Pool Systems. 2014. Available online: www.hse.gov.uk/pubns/books/hsg282.htm (accessed on 29 May 2018).

26. Signorelli, C.; Pasquarella, C.; Saccani, E.; Sansebastiano, G. Treatment of thermal pool waters. *Ig Sanita Pubbl.* **2006**, *62*, 539–552. [PubMed]

27. Fazlzadeh, M.; Sadeghi, H.; Bagheri, P.; Poureshg, Y.; Rostami, R. Microbial quality and physical-chemical characteristics of thermal Springs. *Environ. Geochem. Health* **2016**, *38*, 413–422. [CrossRef] [PubMed]

28. Barna, Z.; Kádár, M. The risk of contracting infectious diseases in public swimming pools. A review. *Annali Dell'istituto Superiore di Sanita* **2012**, *48*, 374–386. [CrossRef] [PubMed]

29. Ferretti, E.; Fantuzzi, G.; Romano Spica, V.; Caroli, S.; Bonadonna, L. Fifth International Conference Swimming Pool & Spa. ISTISAN Congressi 13/C1 ISSN 0393-5620. Rome. 2013. Available online: https://www.researchgate.net/publication/236157805_Free-living_amoebae_and_enteric_protozoa_isolated_in_swimming_pool (accessed on 19 November 2018).

30. Chong, M.N.; Jin, B.; Chow, C.W.; Saint, C. Recent developments in photocatalytic water treatment technology: A review. *Water Res.* **2010**, *44*, 2997–3027. [CrossRef] [PubMed]

31. Csirmaz, É.; Pető, K. International Trends in Recreational and Wellness Tourism. *Procedia Econ. Finance* **2015**, *32*, 755–762. [CrossRef]

32. Atanga Adongo, C.; Amuquandoh, F.E.; Amenumey, E.K. Modelling spa-goers' choices of therapeutic activities. *J. Hosp. Tour. Manag.* **2017**, *31*, 105–113. [CrossRef]

33. Loureiro, S.M.C.; Almeida, M.; Rita, P. The effect of atmospheric cues and involvement on pleasure and relaxation: The spa hotel context. *Int. J. Hosp. Manag.* **2013**, *35*, 35–43. [CrossRef]

34. McCarthy, J. Global spa & wellness trends Psychology of Spas and Wellbeing. 2017. Available online: http://psychologyofwellbeing.com/201701/2017-global-spa-wellness-trends.html (accessed on 29 May 2018).

35. Dryglas, D.; Salamaga, M. Segmentation by push motives in health tourism destinations: A case study of Polish spa resorts. *J. Destin. Market. Manag.* **2018**, *9*, 234–246. [CrossRef]

36. Han, H.; Kiatkawsin, K.; Kim, W.; Lee, S. Investigating customer loyalty formation for wellness spa: Individualism vs. Collectivism. *Int. J. Hosp. Manag.* **2017**, *67*, 11–23. [CrossRef]

37. Tunstall, J. Clinical remarks upon the effects of the bath thermal waters in the treatment of chronic rheumatism. *Assoc. Med. J.* **1853**, *1*, 8–10. [CrossRef] [PubMed]
38. Brues, C.T. Observations on the Fauna of Thermal Waters. *Proc. Natl. Acad. Sci. USA* **1924**, *10*, 484–486. [CrossRef] [PubMed]
39. Oliveira, D. Indications & contraindications of thermal waters. *Rev. Bras. Med.* **1957**, *14*, 635–638. [PubMed]
40. Alberti, S.; Tonolo, A.; De Felip, G. Preliminary observations on the microbial flora of thermal waters of Viterbo in the nature of sulfobacteria. *Rendiconti-Istituto Superiore di Sanita* **1959**, *22*, 1018–1024. [PubMed]
41. Araujo, A.R.T.S.; Sarraguça, M.C.; Ribeiro, M.P.; Coutinho, P. Physicochemical fingerprinting of thermal waters of Beira Interior region of Portugal. *Environ. Geochem. Health.* **2017**, *39*, 483–496. [CrossRef] [PubMed]
42. Directive 2009/54/EC of the European Parlament and the Concil of 18 June 2009 on the Exploitation and Marketing of Natural Mineral Water. Available online: https://eur-lex.europa.eu/legal-content/en/ALL/?uri=CELEX%3A32009L0054 (accessed on 19 November 2018).
43. Karakaya, M.Ç.; Doğru, M.; Karakaya, N.; Kuluöztürk, F.; Nalbantçılar, M.T. Radioactivity and hydrochemical properties of certain thermal Turkish spa waters. *J. Water Health* **2017**, *15*, 591–601. [CrossRef] [PubMed]
44. Gomes, C.; Carretero, M.I.; Pozo, M.; Maraver, F.; Cantista, P.; Armijo, F.; Legido, J.L.; Teixeira, F.; Rautureau, M.; Delgado, F. Peloids and pelotherapy: Historical evolution, classification and glossary. *Appl. Clay Sci.* **2013**, *75*, 28–38. [CrossRef]
45. Valeriani, F.; Biagini, T.; Giampaoli, S.; Crognale, S.; Santoni, D.; Romano Spica, V. Draft Genome Sequence of Tepidimonas taiwanensis Strain VT154-175. *Genome Announc.* **2016**, *4*, e00942-16. [CrossRef] [PubMed]
46. Yang, L.; Muhadesi, J.B.; Wang, M.M.; Wang, B.J.; Liu, S.J.; Jiang, C.Y. Thauera hydrothermalis sp. nov.; a thermophilic bacterium isolated from hot spring. *Int. J. Syst. Evol. Microbiol.* **2018**, *68*, 3163–3168. [CrossRef] [PubMed]
47. Jiang, X.; Takacs-Vesbach, C.D. Microbial community analysis of pH 4 thermal springs in Yellowstone National Park. *Extremophiles* **2017**, *21*, 135–152. [CrossRef] [PubMed]
48. Borella, P.; Montagna, M.T.; Romano-Spica, V.; Stampi, S.; Stancanelli, G.; Triassi, M.; Marchesi, I.; Bargellini, A.; Neglia, R.; Paglionico, N.; et al. Relationship between mineral content of domestic hot water and microbial contamination. *J. Trace Elem. Med. Biol.* **2003**, *17*, 37–43. [PubMed]
49. Romano Spica, V. Advances in Microbiota Knowledge and NGS Technologies: Perspectives for Surveillance in Recreational Waters. ICSPS 2019. Available online: https://8thswimpoolspa.sciencesconf.org/resource/page/id/20 (accessed on 19 November 2018).
50. Valeriani, F.; Protano, C.; Gianfranceschi, G.; Leoni, E.; Galasso, V.; Mucci, N.; Vitali, M.; Romano Spica, V. Microflora Thermarum Atlas project: Biodiversity in thermal spring waters and natural SPA pools. *Water Sci. Technol. Water Supply* **2018**, *18*, 1472–1483. [CrossRef]
51. Valeriani, F.; Agodi, A.; Casini, B.; Cristina, M.L.; D'Errico, M.M.; Gianfranceschi, G.; Liguori, G.; Liguori, R.; Mucci, N.; Mura, I.; et al. Potential testing of reprocessing procedures by real-time polymerase chain reaction: A multicenter study of colonoscopy devices. *Am. J. Infect. Control* **2018**, *46*, 159–164. [CrossRef] [PubMed]
52. Giampaoli, S.; Berti, A.; Valeriani, F.; Gianfranceschi, G.; Piccolella, A.; Buggiotti, L.; Rapone, C.; Valentini, A.; Ripani, L.; Romano Spica, V. Molecular identification of vaginal fluid by microbial signature. *Forensic Sci. Int. Genet.* **2012**, *6*, 559–564. [CrossRef] [PubMed]
53. Fortney, N.W.; He, S.; Converse, B.J.; Boyd, E.S.; Roden, E.E. Investigating the Composition and Metabolic Potential of Microbial Communities in Chocolate Pots Hot Springs. *Front. Microbiol.* **2018**, *9*, 2075. [CrossRef] [PubMed]
54. Amin, A.; Ahmed, I.; Salam, N.; Kim, B.Y.; Singh, D.; Zhi, X.Y.; Xiao, M.; Li, W.J. Diversity and Distribution of Thermophilic Bacteria in Hot Springs of Pakistan. *Microb. Ecol.* **2017**, *74*, 116–127. [CrossRef] [PubMed]
55. The Earth Microbiome Project. Available online: www.earthmicrobiome.org (accessed on 19 November 2018).
56. Valeriani, F.; Crognale, S.; Protano, C.; Gianfranceschi, G.; Orsini, M.; Vitali, M.; Romano Spica, V. Metagenomic analysis of bacterial community in a travertine depositing hot spring. *New Microbiol.* **2018**, *41*, 126–135. [PubMed]
57. Paduano, S.; Valeriani, F.; Romano Spica, V.; Bargellini, A.; Borella, P.; Marchesi, I. Microbial biodiversity of thermal water and mud in an Italian spa by metagenomics: A pilot study. *Water Sci. Technol. Water Supply* **2018**, *18*, 1456–1465. [CrossRef]

58. Baron, J.L.; Vikram, A.; Duda, S.; Stout, J.E.; Bibby, K. Shift in the microbial ecology of a hospital hot water system following the introduction of an on-site monochloramine disinfection system. *PLoS ONE* **2014**, *9*, 102679. [CrossRef] [PubMed]

59. Ma, X.; Baron, J.L.; Vikram, A.; Stout, J.E.; Bibby, K. Fungal diversity and presence of potentially pathogenic fungi in a hospital hot water system treated with on-site monochloramine. *Water Res.* **2015**, *71*, 197–206. [CrossRef] [PubMed]

60. Valeriani, F.; Giampaoli, S.; Buggiotti, L.; Gianfranceschi, G.; Romano Spica, V. Molecular enrichment for detection of *S. aureus* in recreational waters. *Water Sci. Technol.* **2012**, *66*, 2305–2310. [CrossRef] [PubMed]

61. Tartanson, M.A.; Soussan, L.; Rivallin, M.; Chis, C.; Penaranda, D.; Lapergue, R.; Calmels, P.; Faur, C. A new silver based composite material for SPA water disinfection. *Water Res.* **2014**, *63*, 135–146. [CrossRef] [PubMed]

62. Guida, M.; Di Onofrio, V.; Gallè, F.; Gesuele, R.; Valeriani, F.; Liguori, R.; Romano Spica, V.; Liguori, G. Pseudomonas aeruginosa in Swimming Pool Water: Evidences and Perspectives for a New Control Strategy. *Int. J. Environ. Res. Public Health* **2016**, *13*, 919. [CrossRef] [PubMed]

63. Varga, C.; László, M.; Gerencsér, G.; Gyöngyi, Z.; Szendi, K. Natural UV-protective organic matter in thermal water. *J Photochem Photobiol B.* **2015**, *144*, 8–10. [CrossRef] [PubMed]

64. Valeriani, F.; Protano, C.; Vitali, M.; Romano Spica, V. Swimming attendance during childhood and development of asthma: Meta-analysis. *Pediatr. Int.* **2017**, *59*, 614–621. [CrossRef] [PubMed]

65. Carter, R.A.A.; Joll, C.A. Occurrence and formation of disinfection by-products in the swimming pool environment: A critical review. *J. Environ. Sci.* **2017**, *58*, 19–50. [CrossRef] [PubMed]

66. Cortés, C.; Marcos, R. Genotoxicity of disinfection byproducts and disinfected waters: A review of recent literature. *Mutat. Res.* **2018**, *831*, 1–12. [CrossRef] [PubMed]

67. WHO. Water Safety in Buildings. Available online: http://www.who.int/water_sanitation_health/publications/2011/9789241548106/en/ (accessed on 29 May 2018).

68. Napoli, C.; Giampaoli, S.; Gallè, F.; Frangella, C.; Di Onofrio, V.; Bonadonna, L.; Romano Spica, V.; Liguori, G. World Health Organization document "water safety in buildings": Italian translation. *Igiene e Sanita Pubblica* **2012**, *68*, 613–624. [PubMed]

69. Lee, J.; Jun, M.-J.; Lee, M.-H.; Lee, M.-H.; Eom, S.-W.; Zoh, K.-D. Production of various disinfection byproducts in indoor swimming pool waters treated with different disinfection methods. *Int. J. Hyg. Environ. Health* **2010**, *213*, 465–474. [CrossRef] [PubMed]

70. Valeriani, F.; Gianfranceschi, G.; Vitali, M.; Protano, C.; Romano Spica, V. Development of the laboratory prototype "CavyPool" for assessing treatments and materials for swimming pools. *Annali di Igiene Medicina Preventiva e di Comunita* **2017**, *29*, 548–560. [PubMed]

71. Fantuzzi, G.; Aggazzotti, G.; Righi, E.; Predieri, G.; Castiglioni, S.; Riva, F.; Zuccato, E. Illicit drugs and pharmaceuticals in swimming pool waters. *Sci. Total Environ.* **2018**, *635*, 956–963. [CrossRef] [PubMed]

72. Tang, H.L.; Xie, Y.F. Biologically active carbon filtration for haloacetic acid removal from swimming pool water. *Sci. Total Environ.* **2016**, *541*, 58–64. [CrossRef] [PubMed]

73. Zwiener, C.; Richardson, S.D.; De Marini, D.M.; Grummt, T.; Glauner, T.; Frimmel, F.H. Drowning in disinfection byproducts? Assessing swimming pool water. *Environ. Sci. Technol.* **2007**, *41*, 363–372. [CrossRef] [PubMed]

74. Manasfi, T.; Méo, M.D.; Coulomb, B.; Giorgio, C.D.; Boudenne, J.-L. Identification of disinfection by-products in freshwater and seawater swimming pools and evaluation of genotoxicity. *Environ. Int.* **2016**, *88*, 94–102. [CrossRef] [PubMed]

75. Kim, H.; Shim, J.; Lee, S. Formation of disinfection by-products in chlorinated swimming pool water. *Chemosphere* **2002**, *46*, 123–130. [CrossRef]

76. Liu, R.; Tian, C.; Hu, C.; Qi, Z.; Liu, H.; Qu, J. Effects of bromide on the formation and transformation of disinfection by-products during chlorination and chloramination. *Sci. Total Environ.* **2018**, *625*, 252–261. [CrossRef] [PubMed]

77. Glauner, T.; Kunz, F.; Zwiener, C.; Frimmel, F.H. Elimination of swimming pool water disinfection byproducts with advanced oxidation processes (AOPs). *Acta Hydrochim. Hydrobiol.* **2005**, *33*, 585–594. [CrossRef]

78. Lee, J.; Ha, K.-T.; Zoh, K.-D. Characteristics of trihalomethane (THM) production and associated health risk assessment in swimming pool waters treated with different disinfection methods. *Sci. Total Environ.* **2009**, *407*, 1990–1997. [CrossRef] [PubMed]

79. Hang, C.; Zhang, B.; Gong, T.; Xian, Q. Occurrence and health risk assessment of halogenated disinfection byproducts in indoor swimming pool water. *Sci. Total Environ.* **2016**, *543*, 425–431. [CrossRef] [PubMed]

80. Daiber, E.J.; DeMarini, D.M.; Ravuri, S.A.; Liberatore, H.K.; Cuthbertson, A.A.; Thompson-Klemish, A.; Byer, J.D.; Schmid, J.E.; Afifi, M.Z.; et al. Progressive increase in disinfection byproducts and mutagenicity from source to tap to swimming pool and spa water: Impact of human inputs. *Environ. Sci. Technol.* **2016**, *50*, 6652–6662. [CrossRef] [PubMed]

81. Hansen, K.M.S.; Spiliotopoulou, A.; Cheema, W.A.; Andersen, H.R. Effect of ozonation of swimming pool water on formation of volatile disinfection by-products—A laboratory study. *Chem. Eng. J.* **2016**, *289*, 277–285. [CrossRef]

82. Spiliotopoulou, A.; Hansen, K.M.S.; Andersen, H.R. Secondary formation of disinfection by-products by UV treatment of swimming pool water. *Sci. Total Environ.* **2015**, *520*, 96–105. [CrossRef] [PubMed]

83. Hijnen, W.A.M.; Beerendonk, E.F.; Medema, G.J. Inactivation credit of UV radiation for viruses, bacteria and protozoan (oo)cysts in water: A review. *Water Res.* **2006**, *40*, 3–22. [CrossRef] [PubMed]

84. Craik, S.A.; Weldon, D.; Finch, G.R.; Bolton, J.R.; Belosevic, M. Inactivation of Cryptosporidium parvum oocysts using medium- and low-pressure ultraviolet radiation. *Water Res.* **2001**, *35*, 1387–1398. [CrossRef]

85. Chang, J.C.H.; Ossoff, S.F.; Lobe, D.C.; Dorfman, M.H.; Dumais, C.M.; Qualls, R.G.; Johnson, J.D. UV inactivation of pathogenic and indicator microorganisms. *Appl. Environ. Microbiol.* **1985**, *49*, 1361–1365. [PubMed]

86. Cheema, W.A.; Manasfi, T.; Kaarsholm, K.M.S.; Andersen, H.R.; Boudenne, J.-L. Effect of medium-pressure UV-lamp treatment on disinfection by-products in chlorinated seawater swimming pool. *Sci. Total Environ.* **2017**, *599–600*, 910–917. [CrossRef] [PubMed]

87. Li, J.; Blatchley, E.R., III. UV photodegradation of inorganic chloramines. *Environ. Sci. Technol.* **2009**, *43*, 60–65. [CrossRef] [PubMed]

88. Cimetiere, N.; De Laat, J. Effects of UV-dechloramination of swimming pool water on the formation of disinfection by-products: A lab-scale study. *Microchem. J.* **2014**, *112*, 34–41. [CrossRef]

89. Afifi, M.Z.; Blatchley, E.R., III. Effects of UV-based treatment on volatile disinfection byproducts in a chlorinated, indoor swimming pool. *Water Res.* **2016**, *105*, 167–177. [CrossRef] [PubMed]

90. Sisti, M.; Pieretti, B.; De Santi, M.; Brandi, G. Inactivation of pathogenic dermatophytes by ultraviolet irradiation in swimming pool thermal water. *Int. J. Environ. Health Res.* **2014**, *24*, 412–417. [CrossRef] [PubMed]

91. Florentin, A.; Hautemanière, A.; Hartemann, P. Health effects of disinfection by-products in chlorinated swimming pools. *Int. J. Hyg. Environ. Health* **2011**, *214*, 461–469. [CrossRef] [PubMed]

92. World Health Organization. Alternative Drinking-Water Disinfectants: Bromine, Iodine and Silver. Available online: http://www.who.int/water_sanitation_health/publications/alternative-disinfectants/en/ (accessed on 19 November 2018).

93. Schwake, A.; Ross, B.; Cammann, K. Chrono amperometric determination of hydrogen peroxide in swimming pool water using an ultramicroelectrode array. *Sens. Actuators B Chem.* **1998**, *46*, 242–248. [CrossRef]

94. World Water Development Report 19 March, 2018. Available online: http://www.unwater.org/publications/world-water-development-report-2018/ (accessed on 19 November 2018).

95. Inoue, T.; Inoue, S.; Kubota, K. Bactericidal activity of manganese and iodide ions against Staphylococcus aureus: A possible treatment for acute atopic dermatitis. *Acta Derm. Venereol.* **1999**, *79*, 360–362. [PubMed]

96. Akiyama, H.; Yamasaki, O.; Tada, J.; Kubota, K.; Arata, J. Antimicrobial effects of acidic hot-spring water on Staphylococcus aureus strains isolated from atopic dermatitis patients. *J. Dermatol. Sci.* **2000**, *24*, 112–118. [CrossRef]

97. Barbot, E.; Moulin, P. Swimming pool water treatment by ultrafiltration–adsorption process. *J. Membr. Sci.* **2008**, *314*, 50–57. [CrossRef]

98. Gitis, V.; Hankins, N. Water treatment chemicals: Trends and challenges. *J. Water Process Eng.* **2018**, *25*, 34–38. [CrossRef]

99. Yao, K.M.; Habibian, M.T.; O'Melia, C.R. Water and waste water filtration. Concepts and applications. *Environ. Sci. Technol.* **1971**, *5*, 1105–1112. [CrossRef]

100. Wang, X.; Ma, B.; Bai, Y.; Lan, H.; Liu, H.; Qu, J. The effects of hydrogen peroxide pre-oxidation on ultrafiltration membrane biofouling alleviation in drinking water treatment. *J. Environ. Sci.* **2018**, *73*, 117–126. [CrossRef] [PubMed]

101. Li, Q.; Mahendra, S.; Lyon, D.Y.; Brunet, L.; Liga, M.V.; Li, D.; Alvarez, P.J. Antimicrobial nanomaterials for water disinfection and microbial control: Potential applications and implications. *Water Res.* **2008**, *42*, 4591–4602. [CrossRef] [PubMed]

102. Gazit, E. Self-assembled peptide nanostructures: The design of molecular building blocks and their technological utilization. *Chem. Soc. Rev.* **2007**, *36*, 1263–1269. [CrossRef] [PubMed]

103. Badawy, M.E.I.; Rabea, E.I.; Rogge, T.M.; Stevens, C.V.; Steurbaut, W.; Hofte, M.; Smagghe, G. Fungicidal and insecticidal activity of O-acyl chitosan derivatives. *Polym. Bull.* **2005**, *54*, 279–289. [CrossRef]

104. Rabea, E.I.; Badawy, M.E.; Stevens, C.V.; Smagghe, G.; Steurbaut, W. Chitosan as antimicrobial agent: Applications and mode of action. *Biomacromolecules* **2003**, *4*, 1457–1465. [CrossRef] [PubMed]

105. Chirkov, S.N. The antiviral activity of chitosan (review). *Appl. Biochem. Microbiol.* **2002**, *38*, 1–8. [CrossRef]

106. Don, T.M.; Chen, C.C.; Lee, C.K.; Cheng, W.Y.; Cheng, L.P. Preparation and antibacterial test of chitosan/PAA/PEGDA bilayer composite membranes. *J. Biomater. Sci. Polym. Ed.* **2005**, *16*, 1503–1519. [CrossRef] [PubMed]

107. Rani, D.; Singla, P.; Agarwal, J. 'Chitosan in water' as an eco-friendly and efficient catalytic system for Knoevenagel condensation reaction. *Carbohydr. Polym.* **2018**, *202*, 355–364. [CrossRef] [PubMed]

108. Ibrahim, M.M.; Asal, S. Physicochemical and photocatalytic studies of Ln^{3+}-ZnO for water disinfection and wastewater treatment applications. *J. Mol. Struct.* **2017**, *1149*, 404–413. [CrossRef]

109. Jeon, S.K.; Kim, E.J.; Lee, J.; Lee, S. Potential risks of TiO_2 and ZnO nanoparticles released from sunscreens into outdoor swimming pools. *J. Hazard. Mater.* **2016**, *317*, 312–318. [CrossRef] [PubMed]

110. World Health Organization (WHO) and International agency for Research on Cancer (IARC). Monographs on the Evaluation of Carcinogenic Risks to Humans. Carbon Black, Titanium Dioxide and Talc. Vol, 93, Lyon France. Available online: https://monographs.iarc.fr/wp-content/uploads/2018/06/mono93.pdf (accessed on 29 May 2018).

111. Seltenrich, N. Nanosilver: Weighing the risks and benefits. *Environ. Health Perspect.* **2013**, *121*, 220–225. [CrossRef] [PubMed]

112. Nowack, B.; Krug, H.F.; Height, M. 120 years of nanosilver history: Implications for policy makers. *Environ. Sci. Technol.* **2011**, *45*, 1177–1183. [CrossRef] [PubMed]

113. Gehrke, I.; Geiser, A.; Somborn-Schulz, A. Innovations in nanotechnology for water treatment. *Nanotechnol. Sci. Appl.* **2015**, *8*, 1–17. [CrossRef] [PubMed]

114. Shrestha, B.; Acosta-Martinez, V.; Cox, S.B.; Green, M.J.; Li, S.; Canas-Carrell, J.E. An evaluation of the impact of multiwalled carbon nanotubes on soil microbial community structure and functioning. *J. Hazard. Mater.* **2013**, *261*, 188–197. [CrossRef] [PubMed]

115. Shvedova, A.A.; Pietroiusti, A.; Fadeel, B.; Kagan, V.E. Mechanisms of carbon nanotube-induced toxicity: Focus on oxidative stress. *Toxicol. Appl. Pharmacol.* **2012**, *261*, 121–133. [CrossRef] [PubMed]

116. Van Aken, B. Gene expression changes in plants and microorganisms exposed to nanomaterials. *Curr. Opin. Biotechnol.* **2015**, *33*, 206–219. [CrossRef] [PubMed]

117. Zhu, B.; Xia, X.; Zhang, S.; Tang, Y. Attenuation of bacterial cytotoxicity of carbon nanotubes by riverine suspended solids in water. *Environ. Pollut.* **2018**, *234*, 581–589. [CrossRef] [PubMed]

118. Ko, K.; Kim, M.J.; Lee, J.Y.; Kim, W.; Chung, H. Effects of graphene oxides and silver-graphene oxides on aquatic microbial activity. *Sci. Total Environ.* **2019**, *651*, 1087–1095. [CrossRef] [PubMed]

119. Shen, L.; Jin, Z.; Wang, D.; Wang, Y.; Lu, Y. Enhance wastewater biological treatment through the bacteria induced graphene oxide hydrogel. *Chemosphere* **2018**, *190*, 201–210. [CrossRef] [PubMed]

120. Centers for Disease Control and Prevention (CDC). The Model Aquatic Health Code (MAHC): An All-inclusive Model Public Swimming Pool and Spa Code. Available online: https://www.cdc.gov/mahc/index.html (accessed on 29 May 2018).

121. *Virginia Graeme baker Pool and Spa Safety Act Guidelines for Entrapment Hazards: Making Pools and Spas Safer; Virginia Graeme Baker Pool and Spa Safety Act, Title 14 of the U.S. Energy Independence and Security Act*; U.S. Consumer Product Safety Commission: Washington, DC, USA, 2007. Available online: https://www.govtrack.us/congress/bills/110/hr6/text (accessed on 29 May 2018).

122. Centers for Disease Control and Prevention (CDC). Available online: http://www.cdc.gov/healthywater/swimming/pools/regulation/index.html (accessed on 29 May 2018).

123. Règlement de Sécurité, Fédération de Natation du Québec (Natation En Bassin) Janvier 2009. Available online: http://www.fnq.qc.ca/doc/doc/00000519_safety.pdf (accessed on 29 May 2018).

124. Guidelines for Canadian Recreational Water Quality—Third Edition, Published by Authority of the Minister of Health. Available online: http://www.healthcanada.gc.ca/ (accessed on 29 May 2018).

125. Alberta. Health Pool Standards July 2014 (Amended January 2018). Available online: https://open.alberta.ca/publications/9781460137215 (accessed on 29 May 2018).

126. Australia. New South Wales Consolidated Acts. Swimming Pools Act 1990 n. 31. Available online: http://www.austlii.edu.au/au/legis/nsw/num_act/spa1990n31219.pdf (accessed on 29 May 2018).

127. Australia. New South Wales Consolidated Acts. Swimming Pools Act 1992 n. 49. Available online: http://classic.austlii.edu.au/au/legis/nsw/consol_act/spa1992192/ (accessed on 29 May 2018).

128. Standards Australia. Swimming and Spa Pools Part 1: Public spas2007 (Reconfirmed 2016), Standards Australia. Available online: https://www.standards.org.au/standards-catalogue/sa-snz/building/cs-034/as--2610-dot-1-2007 (accessed on 29 May 2018).

129. Queensland Department of Health. *Swimming and Spa Pool Water Quality and Operational Guidelines*; Queensland Department of Health, Australian Capital Territory, 2004. Available online: https://www.health.qld.gov.au/__data/assets/pdf_file/0021/444612/guidelines-pool-spa.pdf (accessed on 29 May 2018).

130. Council Directive 76/160/EEC of 8 December 1975 Concerning the Quality of Bathing Water. GUCE 8 December 1975 n. L 76. Available online: https://eur-lex.europa.eu/legal-content/EN/TXT/?uri=CELEX:31976L0160 (accessed on 29 May 2018).

131. Directive 2006/7/EC of the European Parliament and of the Council of 15 February 2006 Concerning the Management of Bathing Water Quality and Repealing Directive 76/160/EEC. Available online: https://eur-lex.europa.eu/legal-content/EN/TXT/?uri=CELEX:32006L0007 (accessed on 29 May 2018).

132. Verordnung des Bundesministers für Gesundheit und Umweltschutz vom 26 Juli 1978 über Hygiene in Bädern. *Bundesgesetzblatt für die Republik Österreich* **1978**, *167*, 3053–3063.

133. Volksgesundheitsamt, Oberster Sanitätsrat. *Mitteilungen der Österreichischen Sanitätsverwaltung* **1992**, *93*, 358.

134. Austria. Bundesgesetzblatt für die Republik Österreich. **1996**, *212*, 4617–4624. Available online: https://ris.bka.gv.at/Dokumente/BgblPdf/1996_658_0/1996_658_0.pdf (accessed on 29 May 2018).

135. Volksgesundheitsamt, Oberster Sanitätsrat. *Mitteilungen der Österreichischen Sanitätsverwaltung* **1997**, *98*, 228–232.

136. Austria. Gesamte Rechtsvorschrift für Bäderhygienegesetz, Fassung vom 28.10.2012. Available online: https://hygiene.medunigraz.at/fileadmin/institute-oes/hygiene/pdf/wasseruntersuchungen/downloads/Bäderhygienegesetz.pdf (accessed on 29 May 2018).

137. Giampaoli, S.; Garrec, N.; Donzé, G.; Valeriani, F.; Erdinger, L.; Romano Spica, V. Regulations concerning natural swimming ponds in Europe: Considerations on public health issues. *J. Water Health.* **2014**, *12*, 564–572. [CrossRef] [PubMed]

138. Belgium. Arrêté du Gouvernement Wallon Portant Conditions Sectorielles Relatives Aux Bassins De Natation. March 13, 2003 (Repealing 26.05.2004 e M.B. 30.01.2007). Available online: http://formpe.environnement.wallonie.be/html/CS%20Piscines%20(cl_2).pdf (accessed on 29 May 2018).

139. Belgium. Arrêté du Gouvernement de la Région de Bruxelles-Capitale Fixant des Conditions d'exploitation Pour les Bassins de Natation. October 10 Ottobre 2002. Available online: https://vlex.be/vid/arr-conditions-exploitation-bassins-natation-29702709 (accessed on 29 May 2018).

140. Belgium. Arrete´ du Gouvernement de la Region de Bruxelles-Capitale Fixant la Liste des Installations de Classe IB, II et III en Execution de l'article 4 de L'ordonnance du 5 juin 1997 Relative aux Permis D'environnement. 4 March 1999. Available online: http://www.etaamb.be/fr/arrete-du-gouvernement-de-la-region-de-bruxellescapit_n1999031224.html (accessed on 29 May 2018).

141. Francia. Code de la Santé Publique. 2010. Section 5: Surveillance des Etablissements Thermaux. Article R1322-45 a R1322-51 (Dernière Modification: 6 octobre 2018). Available online: http://www.codes-et-lois.fr/code-de-la-sante-publique/article-r1322-47 (accessed on 29 May 2018).

142. Francia. Code de la Santé Publique, 2010. Section I: Normes d'hygiène et de Sécurité Applicables aux Piscines et Baignades Aménagées—Articles D1332-1 a D1332-13 (Dernière Modification: 6 octobre 2018). Available online: https://www.legifrance.gouv.fr/affichCode.do?idSectionTA=LEGISCTA000006190970&cidTexte=LEGITEXT000006072665&dateTexte=20080921 (accessed on 29 May 2018).

143. Francia. Afsset Evaluation des Risques Sanitaires liés Aux Piscines Partie I: Piscines Réglementées. Saisine Afsset «2006/11». Rapport Final. 2010. Available online: https://www.anses.fr/fr/system/files/EAUX2007sa0409Ra.pdf (accessed on 29 May 2018).

144. Boudenne, J.-L. Évaluation des Risques Sanitaires liés aux Piscines Partie II: Bains à Remous. 10.13140/RG.2.1.2182.7043. 2015. Available online: https://www.researchgate.net/publication/282245336_ Evaluation_des_risques_sanitaires_lies_aux_piscines_Partie_II_bains_a_remous (accessed on 29 May 2018).

145. Health Protection Agency. *Management of Spa Pools: Controlling the Risk of Infection*; Health Protection Agency: London, UK, March 2006.

146. Ireland. Safety, Health and Welfare at Work Act. 2005. Health and Safety Authority. Available online: http://www.irishstatutebook.ie/eli/2005/act/10/enacted/en/print (accessed on 29 May 2018).

147. Ireland. Swimming Pool Safety Guidelines. Irish Water Safety, ILAM and Swim Ireland. 2010. Available online: http://www.irelandactive.ie/contentfiles/Swimming-Pool-Safety-Guidelines1.pdf (accessed on 29 May 2018).

148. Germany. DIN 19643. Aufbereitung von Schwimm-und Badebeckenwasser–Teil 1: Allgemeine Anforderungen.Beuth ; Englischer Titel: Treatment of the water of swimming-pools and baths—Part 1: General requirements Ausgabedatum 1997-04 1997, Ausgabe:1997-04. Available online: https://www.beuth. de/de/norm/din-19643-1/2936483 (accessed on 29 May 2018).

149. Germany. Hygienische Anforderungen an Kleinbadeteiche. Empfehlung des Umweltbundesamtes. *Bundesgesundhbl Gesundheitsschutz* **2003**, *46*, 527–529. Available online: https://link.springer.com/article/10. 1007/s00103-003-0627-0 (accessed on 29 May 2018). [CrossRef]

150. Germany. Empfehlung des Umweltbundesamtes. *Bundesgesundheitsbl-Gesundheitsforsch-Gesundheitsschutz* **2006**, *49*, 926–937. Available online: https://doi.org/10.1007/s00103-006-0030-8 (accessed on 29 May 2018).

151. Germany. DIN 19643. Aufbereitung von Schwimm-und Badebeckenwasser—Teil 4: Verfahrenskombinationen Mit Ultrafiltration. Englischer Titel: Treatment of water of swimming pools and baths—Part 4: Combinations of process with ultrafiltration. 2018. Available online: https://www.beuth.de/de/norm/din-19643-4/164174207 (accessed on 29 May 2018).

152. Czech Republic. Decree of the Ministry of Health 423/2001—On Spas and Sources. Available online: http://www.mzcr.cz/obsah/souvisejici-legislativa_1757_3.html (accessed on 29 May 2018).

153. Czech Republic. Decree of Ministry of Health 252/2004 (update 70/2018)—Requirements on Cold and Hot Water in Health Care and Accommodation Facilities. Available online: http://www.mzcr.cz/obsah/ souvisejici-legislativa_1757_3.html (accessed on 29 May 2018).

154. Czech Republic. Decree of Ministry of Health 135/2004—Requirements on Swimming Pools, Saunas and Outdoor Playgrouds. Available online: https://publications.europa.eu/en/publication-detail/-/ publication/b52fa07c-8be9-454f-a2f0-417ae2d9f798 (accessed on 19 November 2018).

155. Portugal. Ministério da saúde Decreto-lei n. 142. 11 giugno 2004. Diário da República n. 136/2004, Série I-A de 2004-06-11. Available online: https://dre.pt/web/guest/pesquisa/-/search/286109/details/normal?q= 142%2F2004 (accessed on 29 May 2018).

156. Conselho Nacional da Qualidade. Directiva CNQ n.º 23/93 de 24 de Maio—A qualidade das piscinas de uso público. Lisboa, 1993.

157. Matisova, E. *Report on Monitoring of Hygienic Situation on Natural and Artificial Pools in Year 2004*; Authority of Public Health of the Slovak Republic: Batislava, 2004; Available online: http://www.dinax.hu/dok/spa_ conference_2005_HUN/02/03.pdf (accessed on 29 May 2018).

158. Spain. Boletin Oficial del Ministerio de Sanidad y Consumo. 1987, 19, pp. 1147–1152. Available online: https://www.boe.es (accessed on 19 November 2018).

159. Spain. Boletin Oficial del Ministerio de Sanidad y Consumo 1998, 80, por el que se regulan las condiciones higiénico–sanitarias de piscinas de uso colectivo. Available online: http://www.bocm.es/boletin/CM_ Boletin_BOCM/19980527_B/12400.pdf (accessed on 19 November 2018).

160. Spain. La Orden 1319/2006 de 27 de junio de la Consejería de Sanidad y Consumo de la Comunidad de Madrid, por la que se establecen los criterios que permitan establecer los niveles de formación del personal que preste sus servicios como socorrista en piscinas, instalaciones acuáticas y medio natura. Available online: http://www.bocm.es/boletin/CM_Boletin_BOCM/20060714_B/16600.pdf (accessed on 19 November 2018).

161. Spain. Real Decreto 742/13 de 27 de Septiembre, Por el que se Establecen los Criterios Técnico-Srios de las Piscinas. Available online: https://www.boe.es/boe/dias/2013/10/11/pdfs/BOE-A-2013-10580.pdf (accessed on 19 November 2018).

162. *Finlands Författningssamling: Ålands landskapsregerings beslut om kvalitetskrav på och kontroll av vattnet vid allmänna ytvattenbadplatser*; Official publication: Ålands Författningssamling (ÅFS), Number: 2008/70; Available online: https://eur-lex.europa.eu/legal-content/EN/NIM/?uri=CELEX:32006L0007 (accessed on 19 November 2018).

163. *Finlands Författningssamling: Ålands landskapsregerings beslut om kvalitetskrav på och kontroll av vattnet vid allmänna ytvattenbadplatser (2014/47) 16/10/2014*; Official publication: Ålands Författningssamling (ÅFS), Number: 2014/47; Available online: https://eur-lex.europa.eu/legal-content/EN/NIM/?uri=CELEX: 32006L0007 (accessed on 19 November 2018).

164. Ciprium Government. Law N. 55(I)/92 (2). 1992, Ciprium. Available online: www.cyprus.gov.cy (accessed on 19 November 2018).

165. Bulgar. D'rzaven Vestnik. 1994, 6, pp. 1–14. Available online: http://lexbg/laws (accessed on 29 May 2018).

166. Norway. Norsk Lovtidend, section 1. 1996, 11, pp. 767–773. Available online: https://lovdata.no/register/lovtidend (accessed on 19 November 2018).

167. Italy. Law of 24 October 2000, n. 323. Reorganization of the Thermal Sector. Official Gazette November 8, 2000, n. 261. (GU Serie Generale n.261 del 08-11-2000). Available online: http://www.gazzettaufficiale.it/eli/id/2000/11/08/000G0377/sg (accessed on 19 November 2018).

168. Italy. Agreement between the Minister of Health, the Regions and the Autonomous Provinces of Trento and Bolzano Concerning the Sanitary-Hygiene Aspects for the Construction, Maintenance and Supervision of Swimming Pools for Swimming (16.01.2003). G.U. March 3, 2003: 45, n. 51. Available online: http://www.salute.gov.it/imgs/C_17_normativa_1911_allegato.pdf (accessed on 19 November 2018).

169. Valeriani, F.; Briancesco, R.; Sanzari, S.; Gianfranceschi, G.; Ferretti, E.; Bonadonna, L.; Romano Spica, V. Some considerations on revision of legislation Hygiene-sanitary for the management of swimming pools for swimming-pool use and the National Consultation of the Ministry of Health. *Igiene e Sanita Pubblica* **2017**, *73*, 247–266. [PubMed]

170. Italy. Guidelines with Indications on Legionellosis for Managers of Tourist Accommodation and Thermal Facilities (13/01/2005). Official Gazette February 4, 2005, n. 28. Available online: http://www.salute.gov.it/portale/documentazione/p6_2_2_1.jsp?id=2362 (accessed on 19 November 2018).

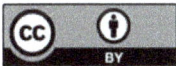

MDPI

St. Alban-Anlage 66

4052 Basel

Switzerland

Tel. +41 61 683 77 34

Fax +41 61 302 89 18

www.mdpi.com

International Journal of Environmental Research and Public Health Editorial Office

E-mail: ijerph@mdpi.com

www.mdpi.com/journal/ijerph